Veterans and Agent Orange

Update 1996

Committee to Review the Health Effects in
Vietnam Veterans of Exposure to Herbicides

Division of Health Promotion and
Disease Prevention

INSTITUTE OF MEDICINE

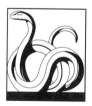

NATIONAL ACADEMY PRESS
Washington, D.C. 1996

National Academy Press • 2101 Constitution Avenue, N.W. • Washington, D.C. 20418

NOTICE: The project that is the subject of this report was approved by the Governing Board of the National Research Council, whose members are drawn from the councils of the National Academy of Sciences, the National Academy of Engineering, and the Institute of Medicine. The members of the committee responsible for the report were chosen for their special competences and with regard for appropriate balance.

This report has been reviewed by a group other than the authors according to procedures approved by a Report Review Committee consisting of members of the National Academy of Sciences, the National Academy of Engineering, and the Institute of Medicine.

The Institute of Medicine was chartered in 1970 by the National Academy of Sciences to enlist distinguished members of the appropriate professions in the examination of policy matters pertaining to the health of the public. In this, the Institute acts under the Academy's 1863 congressional charter responsibility to be an adviser to the federal government and its own initiative in identifying issues of medical care, research, and education. Dr. Kenneth I. Shine is president of the Institute of Medicine.

Support for this study was provided by the Department of Veterans Affairs (contract no. V101(93)P-1331).

Veterans and Agent Orange: Update 1996 is available for sale from the National Academy Press, 2101 Constitution Avenue, N.W., Lock Box 285, Washington, DC, 20055. Call 800-624-6242 or 202-334-3938 (in the Washington Metropolitan Area).

The Executive Summary of *Veterans and Agent Orange: Update 1996* is available on-line at **http://www.nap.edu/nap/online/veterans/**.

The serpent has been a symbol of long life, healing, and knowledge among almost all cultures and religions since the beginning of recorded history. The image adopted as a logo-type by the Institute of Medicine is based on a relief carving from ancient Greece, now held by the Staatlichemusseen in Berlin.

KEN RAMOS, Associate Professor, Department of Physiology and Pharmacology, College of Veterinary Medicine, Texas A&M University, College Station, Texas

NOEL ROSE, Professor, Department of Molecular Microbiology and Immunology, Johns Hopkins University School of Hygiene and Public Health, Baltimore, Maryland

Project Staff

MICHAEL A. STOTO, Director, Division of Health Promotion and Disease Prevention

DAVID A. BUTLER, Study Director (as of January 1996)

KELLEY BRIX, Study Director (through November 1995)

CYNTHIA ABEL, Program Officer

DEBORAH KATZ, Research Assistant

AMY NOEL O'HARA, Project Assistant

DONNA D. THOMPSON, Division Assistant

MONA BRINEGAR, Financial Associate

Staff Consultants

CAROL MACZKA, Director of Toxicology and Risk Assessment, Institute of Medicine

DIANE J. MUNDT, Senior Program Officer, Institute of Medicine

CATHARYN LIVERMAN, Program Office, Institute of Medicine

TOM BURROWS, Contract Editor

Preface

In response to the concerns voiced by Vietnam veterans and their families, Congress called upon the National Academy of Sciences (NAS) to review the scientific evidence on the possible health effects of exposure to Agent Orange and other herbicides (Public Law 102-4, signed on February 6, 1991). The creation of the first NAS Institute of Medicine committee, in 1992, underscored the critical importance of approaching these questions from a scientific standpoint. The original Committee to Review the Health Effects in Vietnam Veterans of Exposure to Herbicides realized from the beginning that it could not conduct a credible scientific review without a full understanding of the experiences and perspectives of veterans. Thus, to supplement its standard scientific process, the original committee opened several of its meetings to the public in order to allow veterans and other interested individuals to voice their concerns and opinions, to provide personal information about individual exposure to herbicides and associated health effects, and to educate the original committee on recent research results and studies still under way. This information provided a meaningful backdrop for the numerous scientific articles that the original committee reviewed and evaluated.

In its 1994 report *Veterans and Agent Orange: Health Effects of Herbicides Used in Vietnam*, the committee reviewed and evaluated the available scientific evidence regarding the association between exposure to dioxin or other chemical compounds contained in herbicides used in Vietnam and a wide range of health effects and provided the committee's findings to the Secretary of Veterans Affairs to consider as the Department of Veterans Affairs carried out its responsibilities to Vietnam veterans. The report also described areas in which the available scientific data were insufficient to determine whether an association exists and provided the committee's recommendations for future research.

Public Law 102-4 also asked the IOM to conduct biennial updates that would review newly published scientific literature regarding statistical associations between health outcomes and exposure to dioxin and other chemical compounds in these herbicides. The focus of this first updated review is on new scientific studies published since the release of *Veterans and Agent Orange (VAO)* and on updates of scientific studies previously reviewed in *VAO*. To conduct this review, the IOM established a new committee of 16 members representing a wide range of expertise to take a fresh look at the studies reviewed in *VAO* and new scientific studies to determine whether an association exists between herbicide exposure and specific health outcomes. In order to provide a link to *VAO*, half of the committee members had also served on the original committee. All committee members were selected because they are leading experts in their fields, have no conflicts of interest with regard to the matter under study, and have taken no public positions concerning the potential health effects of herbicides in Vietnam veterans or related aspects of herbicide or dioxin exposure. Biographical sketches of committee members and staff appear in Appendix C.

The committee worked on several fronts in conducting this updated review, always with the goal of seeking the most accurate information and advice from the widest possible range of knowledgeable sources. Consistent with procedures of the IOM, the committee met in a series of closed sessions and working group meetings in which members could freely examine, characterize, and weigh the strengths and limitations of the evidence. Given the nature of the controversy surrounding this issue, the committee deemed it vital to convene an open meeting as well. The public meeting was held in conjunction with the committee's first meeting, in April 1995, and provided the opportunity for veterans and veterans service organizations, researchers, policymakers, and other interested parties to present their concerns, review their research, and exchange information directly with committee members. To solicit broad participation, the committee sent announcements to nearly 1,300 individuals and organizations known to have an interest in this issue. The oral presentations and written statements submitted to the committee are described in detail in Appendix A.

In addition to its formal meetings, the committee actively and continuously sought information from, and explained its mission to, a broad array of individuals and organizations with interest or expertise in assessing the effects of exposure to herbicides. These interactions included meetings with representatives of veterans service organizations, congressional committees, federal agencies, and scientific organizations. The committee also heard from the public through telephone calls and letters, each of which received a response from the IOM staff.

Most of the committee's work involved reviewing the scientific literature bearing on the association between herbicides or dioxin and various health outcomes. The literature included studies of people exposed in occupational and environmental settings to the types of herbicides used in Vietnam, as well as studies of Vietnam veterans. The committee reviewed the original publications themselves rather than summaries or commentaries. Such secondary sources were used to check the completeness of the review. The committee also reviewed the primary and secondary literature on basic toxicological and animal studies related to dioxin and other herbicides in question.

As explained in the Executive Summary on page 14, the committee found that, in general, it is not possible to quantify the degree of risk likely to be experienced by Vietnam veterans because of their exposure to herbicides in Vietnam. Two members of the committee believe that there are certain circumstances under which the risk to veterans can be quantified. Appendix B presents their analysis and estimates; it represents their opinion alone.

Kelley Brix served as the original study director for this project and deserves credit for drafting sections of the report. The committee would also like to acknowledge the excellent work of the staff members, David Butler, Deborah Katz, and Amy Noel O'Hara. The committee would also like to thank Michael Stoto, Cynthia Abel, Diane Mundt, and Catharyn Liverman, who also served as staff members for the original committee; their knowledge of the subject was helpful in completing the report. Thanks are also extended to Mona Brinegar, who handled the finances for the project; Thomas Burroughs, who provided excellent editorial skills; Michael Edington, who supervised the report through the editorial and publication phases; and Donna Thompson, who provided assistance with editorial changes to the manuscript.

David Tollerud, *Chairman*

Contents

Veterans
and Agent
Orange

Update 1996

1

Executive Summary

Because of continuing uncertainty about the long-term health effects of exposure to herbicides used in Vietnam, Congress passed Public Law 102-4, the "Agent Orange Act of 1991." This legislation directed the Secretary of Veterans Affairs to request the National Academy of Sciences (NAS) to conduct a comprehensive review and evaluation of scientific and medical information regarding the health effects of exposure to Agent Orange, other herbicides used in Vietnam, and the various chemical components of these herbicides, including dioxin. The Institute of Medicine (IOM) of the NAS conducted this review and in 1994 published a comprehensive report, entitled *Veterans and Agent Orange: Health Effects of Herbicides Used in Vietnam* (IOM, 1994).

Public Law 102-4 also called for the NAS to conduct subsequent reviews at least every two years for a period of ten years from the date of the first report. The NAS was instructed to conduct a comprehensive review of the evidence that has become available since the previous IOM committee report; and reassess its determinations and estimates of statistical association, risk, and biological plausibility.

This IOM report presents the first updated review and evaluation of the newly published scientific evidence regarding associations between diseases and exposure to dioxin and other chemical compounds in herbicides used in Vietnam. For each disease, the IOM was asked to determine, to the extent that available data permitted meaningful determinations: 1) whether a statistical association with herbicide exposure exists, taking into account the strength of the scientific evidence and the appropriateness of the statistical and epidemiological methods used to detect the association; 2) the increased risk of the disease among those exposed to herbicides during Vietnam service; and 3) whether there is a plausible biological mechanism or other evidence of a causal relationship between herbicide exposure and the disease.

In addition to bringing the earlier scientific evidence up to date, the committee has addressed several specific areas of concern, as requested by the Department of Veterans Affairs (DVA). These are: 1) the relationship between exposure to herbicides and the development of acute and subacute peripheral neuropathy; 2) the relationship between exposure to herbicides and the development of prostate cancer, hepatobiliary cancer, and nasopharyngeal cancer; and 3) the relationship between the length of time since first exposure and the possible risk of cancer development.

In conducting its study, the IOM committee operated independently of the DVA and other government agencies. The committee was not asked to and did not make judgments regarding specific cases in which individual Vietnam veterans have claimed injury from herbicide exposure. Rather, the study provides scientific information for the Secretary of Veterans Affairs to consider as the DVA exercises its responsibilities to Vietnam veterans.

ORGANIZATION AND FRAMEWORK

The conclusions in this updated report are based on cumulative evidence from the scientific literature reviewed in *Veterans and Agent Orange: Health Effects of Herbicides Used in Vietnam*, which will be abbreviated here as *VAO*. This update is intended to supplement rather than replace *VAO*; therefore, most of the background information has not been repeated. Most chapter sections begin with brief summaries of the scientific data in *VAO*, followed by a more thorough discussion of the newly published data and their interpretation. The reader is referred to relevant sections of *VAO* for additional detail and explanation.

Chapter 2 provides an overview of the methods and conclusions of *VAO*. In addition, it provides a summary of the recent activities of several federal government agencies that are relevant to the health effects of Agent Orange and other herbicides used in Vietnam. Chapter 3 provides an update of the recent experimental toxicology data on the effects of the herbicides and of TCDD, a compound found as a contaminant in the herbicide 2,4,5-trichlorophenoxyacetic acid (2,4,5-T). These data serve as the basis for the biological plausibility of potential health effects in human populations. Chapter 4 describes the methodological considerations that guided the committee's review and its evaluation. Chapter 5 updates the exposure assessment issues in *VAO*. Chapter 8 reviews the methods used to study latency, or time-related effects—a topic of special interest to the DVA—and evaluates the evidence on latency for the cancers under study.

The committee focused most of its efforts on reviewing and interpreting epidemiologic studies, in order to judge whether each of the human health effects is associated with exposure to herbicides or dioxin. The committee weighed the strengths and limitations of the scientific data in *VAO* as well as the newly published scientific data, and reached its conclusions by interpreting the new evidence in the context of the original report. In particular, each disease has been placed into one of four categories, depending on the strength of evidence for an association (see Conclusions about Health Outcomes, below). The committee used the same criteria to categorize diseases as were used in *VAO*.

In the chapters on the various health outcomes (7, 9, 10, and 11), the committee relied on many of the same epidemiologic studies when assessing the potential associations with herbicides. Therefore, Chapter 6 provides a framework for the methods used in the epidemiologic studies. The chapter is organized to reflect similarities and differences in the nature of exposure among three types of study populations: occupationally exposed, environmentally exposed, and Vietnam veterans.

TOXICOLOGY SUMMARY

Chapter 3 reviews the results of animal studies published during the past three years that investigated the toxicokinetics, mechanism of action, and disease outcomes of TCDD, plus the herbicides themselves.

TCDD elicits a diverse spectrum of biological sex-, strain-, age-, and species-specific effects, including carcinogenicity, immunotoxicity, reproductive/ developmental toxicity, hepatotoxicity, neurotoxicity, chloracne, and loss of body weight. These effects vary according to the age, sex, species, and strain of the animals involved. To date, the scientific consensus is that TCDD is not genotoxic and that its ability to influence the carcinogenic process is mediated via epigenetic events such as enzyme induction, cell proliferation, apoptosis, and intracellular communication.

Recent studies on the effects of TCDD and related substances on the immune system amplify earlier findings and suggest that these compounds affect primarily the T-cell arm of the immune response. Direct effects of TCDD on T cells in vitro, however, have not been demonstrated suggesting that the action of TCDD may be indirect. In contrast, a number of animal studies of the reproductive and developmental toxicity of TCDD suggests that developing animals may be particularly sensitive to the effects of TCDD. Specifically, male reproductive function has been reported to be altered following perinatal exposure to TCDD. In addition, experimental studies of the effects of TCDD in the peripheral nervous system suggest that TCDD can cause a toxic polyneuropathy in rats after a single, low dose. Other recent studies provide evidence that hepatotoxicity of TCDD involves AhR-dependent mechanisms.

The most recent studies have focused on the elucidation of the molecular mechanism of TCDD toxicity. The evidence further supports the concept that the toxic effects of TCDD involve AhR-dependent mechanisms. A better appreciation of the complexity of TCDD effects in target cells has led to the development of refined, physiologically based pharmacokinetic models. These models take into account intracellular diffusion, receptor and protein binding, and liver induction to establish the fractional distribution of the total body burden as a function of the overall body concentration. The association of TCDD with the cytosolic AhR has been shown to require a second protein, known as ARNT, for DNA binding capability and transcriptional activation of target genes. There is also increasing evidence suggesting that events other than receptor binding influence biological response to TCDD. It is now clear that AhR-related signaling influences, and is itself influenced by, other signal transduction mechanisms at low concentrations. Signaling interactions explaining the toxic effects of TCDD may involve growth factors, free radicals, the interaction of TCDD with the estrogen transduction pathway, and protein kinases.

The toxicity of the herbicides used in Vietnam remains poorly studied. In general, the herbicides 2,4-D, 2,4,5-T, cacodylic acid, and picloram have not been identified as particularly toxic substances since high concentrations are often required to modulate cellular and biochemical processes. Impairment of motor function has been reported in rats administered high single oral doses of 2,4-D. The ability of 2,4,5-T to interfere with calcium homeostasis in vitro has been documented and linked to the teratogenic effects of 2,4,5-T on the early development of sea urchin eggs. There is evidence suggesting that both 2,4-D and 2,4,5-T are capable of inducing renal lesions in rats. A series of studies indicates that high concentrations of cacodylic acid results in the formation of a toxic intermediate, the dimethylarsenic radical. No recent studies pertaining to the toxicity of picloram have been published. The half-life in the body of 2,4-D and 2,4,5-T is relatively short and does not appear to extend beyond two weeks. 2,4-D binds covalently to hepatic proteins and lipids, but the molecular basis of this interaction and its biologic consequences are unknown.

EXPOSURE ASSESSMENT

Assessment of individual exposure to herbicides and dioxin is a key element in determining whether specific health outcomes are linked to these compounds. The committee has found, however, that the definition and quantification of exposure are the weakest methodologic aspects of the epidemiologic studies. Although different approaches have been used to estimate exposure among Vietnam veterans and among various occupationally and environmentally exposed groups, each approach is limited in its ability to determine precisely the intensity and duration of individual exposure.

Since the publication of *VAO*, there has been considerable progress in the use of serum TCDD levels and/or quantitative exposure indices, as summarized in Chapter 5. There also has been progress in characterizing the TCDD body burdens in several groups, including the Ranch Hand cohort, Seveso residents, German herbicide production employees, and Vietnamese civilians (Michalek et al., 1996; Needham et al., 1994; Flesch-Janys et al., 1994; Ott et al., 1993; and Verger et al., 1994). The mean half-life of TCDD in humans has been calculated to be about 8.7 years in the Ranch Hand cohort (Michalek et al., 1996). Serum TCDD measurements may provide valuable information about past herbicide exposure under some conditions, and they are best used to detect differences in exposure levels among large groups in epidemiologic studies. This additional information on TCDD body burdens in specific groups and information on half-lives allow more accurate comparisons of relative levels of exposure to TCDD among cohorts.

Although definitive data are lacking, the available evidence suggests that Vietnam veterans as a group had substantially lower exposure to herbicides and dioxin than did the subjects in many occupational studies. The participants in Operation Ranch Hand and the Army Chemical Corps are exceptions to this pattern, and it is likely that there are others who served in Vietnam who had exposures comparable in intensity to members of the occupationally exposed cohorts. It is currently not possible to identify this heavily exposed fraction of Vietnam veterans, although exposure reconstruction methods with this capability could perhaps be developed and validated.

CONCLUSIONS ABOUT HEALTH OUTCOMES

Chapters 7, 9, 10, and 11 provide a detailed evaluation of the epidemiologic studies reviewed by the committee and their implications for cancer, reproductive effects, neurobehavioral effects, and other health effects. As is detailed in Chapter 4, the committee used the epidemiologic evidence it reviewed to assign each of the health outcomes being studied into one of the four categories listed in Table 1-1. The definitions of the categories and the criteria for assigning a particular health outcome to them are described in the table, and the specific rationale for each of the findings is detailed in Chapters 7, 9, 10 and 11.

Consistent with the mandate of Public Law 102-4, the distinctions between categories are based on "statistical association," not on causality, as is common in scientific reviews. Thus, standard criteria used in epidemiology for assessing causality (Hill, 1971) do not strictly apply. The committee was charged with reviewing the scientific evidence rather than making recommendations regarding DVA policy, and Table 1-1 is not intended to imply or suggest any policy decisions; these must rest with the Secretary of Veterans Affairs.

Health Outcomes with Sufficient Evidence of an Association

In *VAO*, the committee found sufficient evidence of an association with herbicides and/or TCDD for five diseases: soft-tissue sarcoma, non-Hodgkin's lymphoma, Hodgkin's disease, chloracne, and porphyria cutanea tarda (in genetically susceptible individuals). The recent scientific literature continues to sup-

TABLE 1-1   Updated Summary of Findings in Occupational, Environmental, and Veterans Studies Regarding the Association Between Specific Health Problems and Exposure to Herbicides

---

Sufficient Evidence of an Association

Evidence is sufficient to conclude that there is a positive association. That is, a positive association has been observed between herbicides and the outcome in studies in which chance, bias, and confounding could be ruled out with reasonable confidence. For example, if several small studies that are free from bias and confounding show an association that is consistent in magnitude and direction, there may be sufficient evidence for an association. There is sufficient evidence of an association between exposure to herbicides and the following health outcomes:

> Soft-tissue sarcoma
> Non-Hodgkin's lymphoma
> Hodgkin's disease
> Chloracne

Limited/Suggestive Evidence of an Association

Evidence is suggestive of an association between herbicides and the outcome but is limited because chance, bias, and confounding could not be ruled out with confidence. For example, at least one high-quality study shows a positive association, but the results of other studies are inconsistent. There is limited/suggestive evidence of an association between exposure to herbicides and the following health outcomes:

> Respiratory cancers (lung, larynx, trachea)
> Prostate cancer
> Multiple myeloma
> *Acute and subacute peripheral neuropathy (new disease category)*
> *Spina bifida (new disease category)*
> *Porphyria cutanea tarda (category change in 1996)*

Inadequate/Insufficient Evidence to Determine Whether an Association Exists

The available studies are of insufficient quality, consistency, or statistical power to permit a conclusion regarding the presence or absence of an association. For example, studies fail to control for confounding, have inadequate exposure assessment, or fail to address latency. There is inadequate or insufficient evidence to determine whether an association exists between exposure to herbicides and the following health outcomes:

> Hepatobiliary cancers
> Nasal/nasopharyngeal cancer
> Bone cancer
> Female reproductive cancers (cervical, uterine, ovarian)
> Breast cancer

TABLE 1-1 Continued

Inadequate/Insufficient Evidence to Determine Whether an Association Exists
(continued)

> Renal cancer
> Testicular cancer
> Leukemia
> Spontaneous abortion
> Birth defects (other than spina bifida)
> Neonatal/infant death and stillbirths
> Low birthweight
> Childhood cancer in offspring
> Abnormal sperm parameters and infertility
> Cognitive and neuropsychiatric disorders
> Motor/coordination dysfunction
> Chronic peripheral nervous system disorders
> Metabolic and digestive disorders (diabetes, changes in liver enzymes,
>   lipid abnormalities, ulcers)
> Immune system disorders (immune suppression and autoimmunity)
> Circulatory disorders
> Respiratory disorders
> *Skin cancer (category change in 1996)*

Limited/Suggestive Evidence of *No* Association
Several adequate studies, covering the full range of levels of exposure that human beings are known to encounter, are mutually consistent in not showing a positive association between exposure to herbicides and the outcome at any level of exposure. A conclusion of "no association" is inevitably limited to the conditions, level of exposure, and length of observation covered by the available studies. *In addition, the possibility of a very small elevation in risk at the levels of exposure studied can never be excluded.* There is limited/suggestive evidence of *no* association between exposure to herbicides and the following health outcomes:

> Gastrointestinal tumors (stomach cancer, pancreatic
>   cancer, colon cancer, rectal cancer)
> Bladder cancer
> Brain tumors

NOTE: "Herbicides" refers to the major herbicides used in Vietnam: 2,4-D (2,4-dichlorophenoxyacetic acid); 2,4,5-T (2,4,5-trichlorophenoxyacetic acid) and its contaminant TCDD (2,3,7,8-tetrachlorodibenzo-*p*-dioxin); cacodylic acid; and picloram. The evidence regarding association is drawn from occupational and other studies in which subjects were exposed to a variety of herbicides and herbicide components.

port the classification of the first four of these diseases in the category of sufficient evidence. Based on the recent literature, the committee has reclassified porphyria cutanea tarda into the category of limited/suggestive evidence, as described below. Based on the recent literature, there are no additional diseases that satisfy this category's criteria—that a positive association between herbicides and the outcome must be observed in studies in which chance, bias, and confounding can be ruled out with reasonable confidence. The committee regards evidence from several small studies that are free from bias and confounding, and that show an association that is consistent in magnitude and direction, as sufficient evidence for an association. The evidence that supports the committee's conclusions for the three cancers is detailed in Chapter 7; for chloracne in Chapter 11.

Health Outcomes with Limited/Suggestive Evidence of Association

In *VAO*, the committee found limited/suggestive evidence of an association for three cancers: respiratory cancer, prostate cancer, and multiple myeloma. The recent scientific literature continues to support the classification of these diseases in the category of limited/suggestive evidence. The literature also indicates that three additional conditions satisfy the criteria necessary for this category: spina bifida, acute and subacute (transient) peripheral neuropathy, and porphyria cutanea tarda (PCT). For outcomes in this category, the evidence must be suggestive of an association with herbicides, but the association may be limited because chance, bias, or confounding could not be ruled out with confidence. Typically, at least one high-quality study indicates a positive association, but the results of other studies may be inconsistent.

The evidence that supports the committee's conclusions for respiratory cancer and multiple myeloma is detailed in Chapter 7 and is not substantially changed from *VAO*. Because prostate cancer is one of the three cancer types of special interest to the DVA, a brief summary of the relevant scientific evidence is provided here. Because spina bifida, acute and subacute (transient) peripheral neuropathy, and porphyria cutanea tarda have been classified in the category of limited/suggestive since *VAO*, evidence for these associations is also provided.

Several studies have shown an elevated risk for prostate cancer in agricultural or forestry workers. In a large cohort study of Canadian farmers (Morrison et al., 1993), an elevated risk of prostate cancer was associated with herbicide spraying, and the risk increased with increasing number of acres sprayed. The proportionate mortality from prostate cancer was elevated in a study of USDA forest conservationists (PMR = 1.6, CI 0.9-3.0) (Alavanja et al., 1989), and a case-control study of white male Iowans who died of prostate cancer (Burmeister et al., 1983) found a significant association with farming (OR = 1.2) that was not associated with any particular agricultural practice. These results are strengthened by a consistent pattern of nonsignificant elevated risks in studies of chemical production workers, agricultural workers, pesticide applicators, paper and pulp workers, and the population of Seveso, Italy. The largest recent study demonstrated a significantly increased risk of death from prostate cancer in both white and nonwhite farmers in 22 of the 23 states that were studied (Blair et al., 1993). Studies of prostate cancer among Vietnam veterans or among people who have been exposed environmentally, have not consistently shown an association. However, prostate cancer is generally a disease of older men, and the risk among Vietnam veterans would not be detectable in today's epidemiologic studies. Because there was a strong indication of a dose-response relationship in one study (Morrison et al., 1993) and a consistent positive association in a number of others, the committee felt that the evidence for association with herbicide exposure was limited/suggestive for prostate cancer.

There have been three epidemiologic studies that suggest an association between paternal herbicide exposure and an increased risk of spina bifida. In the Ranch Hand study (Wolfe et al., 1995), neural tube defects (spina bifida, anencephaly) were increased among offspring of Ranch Hands with four total (rate of 5 per 1,000), in contrast to none among the comparison infants (exact p = .04). The Centers for Disease Control and Prevention (CDC) VES cohort study (Centers for Disease Control, 1989) found that more Vietnam veterans reported that their children had a central nervous system anomaly (OR = 2.3; 95% CI 1.2-4.5) than did non-Vietnam veterans. The odds ratio for spina bifida was 1.7 (CI 0.6-5.0). In a substudy, hospital records were examined in an attempt to validate the reported cerebrospinal defects (spina bifida, anencephaly, hydrocephalus). While a difference was detected, its interpretation is limited by differential participation between the veteran groups and failure to validate negatives reported; that is, the veterans not reporting their children having a birth defect. Thus, the issue of a recall bias is of major concern with this study. In the CDC Birth Defects Study which utilized the population-based birth defects registry system in the metropolitan Atlanta area (Erickson et al., 1984), there was no association between Vietnam veteran status and the risk of spina bifida (OR = 1.1, CI 0.6-1.7) or anencephaly (OR = 0.9, CI 0.5-1.7). However, the exposure opportunity index (EOI) based upon interview data was associated with an increased risk of spina bifida; for the highest estimated level of exposure (EOI-5) the OR was 2.7 (CI 1.2-6.2). There was no similar pattern of association for anencephaly. Thus, all three epidemiologic studies (Ranch Hand, VES, CDC Birth Defects Study) suggest an association between herbicide exposure and an increased risk of spina bifida in offspring.

In contrast to most other diseases, for which the strongest data have been from occupationally exposed workers, these studies focused on Vietnam veterans. Although the studies were judged to be of relatively high quality, they suffer from methodologic limitations, including possible recall bias, nonresponse bias, small sample size, and misclassification of exposure. For these reasons, the committee concludes that there is limited/suggestive evidence for an association between exposure to herbicides used in Vietnam and spina bifida in offspring.

There is also limited/suggestive evidence of an association between exposure to herbicides and acute and subacute (transient) peripheral neuropathy. There are several published studies relevant to this health outcome, but they are primarily case histories from occupational studies and chemical reports following the Seveso accident, which describe transient symptoms of peripheral neuropathies in highly exposed intervals (Todd, 1962; Berkley and Magee, 1963; Goldstein et al., 1959; Boeri et al., 1978; Pocchiari et al., 1979; Filippini et al., 1981). Todd (1962) reported a sprayer of 2,4-D weedkiller who developed a gastrointestinal disturbance and, within days, after contact with the chemical, a severe sensory/motor polyneuropathy. Recovery occurred over a period of months. Berkley and Magee (1963) reported another patient who developed a polyneuropathy four days after exposure to a liquid solution of 2,4-D, which was being sprayed in a cornfield. The neuropathy was purely sensory in type. The patient's symptoms gradually resolved over months. Goldstein et al. described three patients with sensory/motor polyneuropathies that developed over several days and progressed over several weeks after exposure to 2,4-D. All had incomplete recovery after several years. Although these patients were not examined neurologically before their exposure, the temporal relationship between the development of their clinical deficit and the herbicide exposure was clearly documented in the study (1959). Nonetheless, the possibility that their occurrence was unrelated to the herbicide exposure and was due to other disorders such as idiopathic Guillain-Barre syndrome cannot be entirely excluded. The trend to recovery in the individual cases reported and the negative findings of many long-term follow-up studies of peripheral neuropathy suggest that if a peripheral neuropathy indeed develops, it resolves with time.

Case reports and animal studies led to the conclusion in *VAO* that porphyria cutanea tarda (PCT) was associated with TCDD or herbicide exposure in genetically predisposed individuals. However, three recent reports (Jung et al., 1994; Calvert et al., 1994; and Von Benner et al., 1994) failed to support this association. Two studies (Calvert et al., 1994, and Jung et al., 1994) included extensive analysis of porphyrin levels on 451 workers with demonstrated or potential exposure to herbicides and TCDD. The studies found no relationship between porphyrin levels and TCDD levels, and no excess of PCT in these cohorts. However, some workers had evidence of increased porphyrins in urine, suggesting that further investigation is warranted. These new reports, combined with the literature reviewed in *VAO*, led the committee to conclude that there is limited/suggestive evidence of an association between PCT and exposure to herbicides and/or TCDD.

Health Outcomes with Inadequate/Insufficient Evidence
to Determine Whether an Association Exists

The scientific data for the remainder of the cancers and other diseases reviewed by the committee were inadequate or insufficient to determine whether an association exists. For cancers in this category, the available studies are of insufficient quality, consistency, or statistical power to permit a conclusion regarding the presence or absence of an association. For example, studies fail to control for confounding or have inadequate exposure assessment. This group includes hepatobiliary cancers, nasal/nasopharyngeal cancer, bone cancer, female reproductive cancers (cervical, uterine, ovarian), breast cancer, renal cancer, testicular cancer, leukemia, and skin cancer. The scientific evidence for each of these cancers is detailed in Chapter 7. Recent published studies contained enough evidence to warrant moving skin cancer from the limited/suggestive evidence of no association category to this categoty. The scientific evidence for two cancers that are of special interest to the DVA—hepatobiliary cancer and nasopharyngeal cancer—will also be summarized here. Because of its public health importance, breast cancer also receives attention.

Several reproductive effects are classified in this category, including spontaneous abortion, birth defects other than spina bifida, neonatal/infant death and stillbirths, low birthweight, childhood cancer in offspring, and abnormal sperm parameters and infertility. The scientific evidence for reproductive effects is detailed in Chapter 9. Neurobehavioral effects that are classified in this category include cognitive and neuropsychiatric disorders, motor/coordination dysfunction, and chronic peripheral nervous system disorders. The scientific evidence for these effects is detailed in Chapter 10. Other health effects that are classified in this category include metabolic and digestive disorders, immune system disorders, circulatory disorders, and respiratory disorders. The scientific evidence for these effects is detailed in Chapter 11.

On the whole, the estimated relative risks for skin cancer are fairly evenly distributed around the null, and in a number of studies the confidence intervals were relatively narrow. This conclusion led the committee responsible for *VAO* to conclude that there was limited/suggestive evidence of no association between skin cancer and exposure to herbicides used in Vietnam. One other recent study (Lynge, 1993), however, found an excess risk of skin cancer. Based on four cases, a statistically significant increase in the risk of melanoma was observed in the subgroup of men who had been employed for at least one year, using a ten-year latency period (SIR = 4.3, CI 1.2-10.9). However, no information is given about the risk in men with less than 10 years of latency and expected numbers for women are not reported so observed elevated risk in the men with 10+ years of latency cannot be put into context. Another study found a significant excess risk in men from the Seveso area (SMR = 3.3), based on only three cases (Bertazzi et al., 1989a,b). The committee felt that these results, while not even suggestive evidence about an association, undermined the evidence of no association in VAO, and thus warranted changing skin cancer to the "inadequate/insufficient evidence to determine whether an association exists" category.

There are relatively few occupational, environmental, and veterans studies of hepatobiliary cancer, and most of these are small in size and have not controlled for lifestyle-related factors. The estimated relative risk in the various studies range from 0.3 to 3.3, usually with broad confidence intervals. Given the methodological difficulties associated with most of these studies, the evidence regarding hepatobiliary cancer is not convincing with regard to either an association or lack of association with herbicides or TCDD. The few studies that have been published since VAO (Asp et al., 1994; Bertazzi et al., 1993; Blair et al., 1993; Collins et al., 1993; and Cordier et al., 1993) do not change the conclusion that there is inadequate evidence to determine whether an association exists between exposure to herbicides and hepatobiliary cancer.

There are only a few occupational studies, one environmental study, and one veterans study of nasal and/or nasopharyngeal cancer, including two recently published studies (Asp et al., 1994, and Bertazzi et al., 1993). The estimated relative risks in the various studies range from 0.6 to 6.7, usually with broad confidence intervals. Thus, there is inadequate/insufficient evidence to determine whether an association exists between exposure to herbicides and nasal/nasopharyngeal cancer.

There have been a few occupational studies, two environmental studies, and two veterans studies of breast cancer among women exposed to herbicides and/or TCDD. These include four recently published studies (Bertazzi et al., 1993; Blair et al., 1993; Dalager et al., 1995; and Kogevinas et al., 1993). Most of these studies reported a relative risk of approximately 1.0 or less, but it is uncertain whether or not the female members of these cohorts had substantial chemical exposure. TCDD appears to exert a protective effect on the incidence of mammary tumors in experimental animals (see Chapter 3), which is consistent with the tendency for the relative risks to be less than 1.0. In summary, however, the committee believes that there is insufficient evidence to determine whether an association exists between exposure to herbicides and breast cancer.

Health Outcomes with Limited/Suggestive Evidence of No Association

In VAO, the committee found a sufficient number and variety of well-designed studies to conclude that there is limited/suggestive evidence of no association between a small group of cancers and exposure to TCDD or herbicides. This group includes gastrointestinal tumors (colon, rectal, stomach, and pancreatic), brain tumors, and bladder cancer. The recent scientific evidence continues to support the classification of these cancers in this category, and it is detailed in Chapter 7. Based on the recent literature, there are no additional diseases that satisfy the criteria necessary for this category.

For outcomes in this category, several adequate studies covering the full range of levels of herbicide exposure that human beings are known to encounter are mutually consistent in not showing a positive association between exposure and health risk at any level of exposure. These studies have relatively narrow confidence intervals. A conclusion of "no association" is inevitably limited to the conditions, level of exposure, and length of observation covered by the available studies. In addition, the possibility of a very small elevation in risk at the levels of exposure studied can never be excluded.

The Relationship Between the Length of Time Since Exposure and the Possible Risk of Cancer Development

The importance of latency effects and other time-related factors in determining cancer risk has long been recognized, and statistical methodologies have been developed to study this issue. A variety of practical difficulties relating to exposure assessment and other data requirements, however, have limited the use of these methods in epidemiological studies of environmental carcinogens. In response to the request from the DVA to explore latency issues related to herbicides used in Vietnam, the committee attempts in Chapter 8 to establish a methodology to address the timing of herbicide exposure and the risk of cancer. This chapter also reviews the literature on herbicide exposure and cancers classified in the "Sufficient Evidence of an Association" and "Limited/Suggestive Evidence of an Association" categories for results that describe how timing of exposure affects the relative risk due to exposure.

For four of the cancers studied—soft-tissue sarcoma, non-Hodgkin's lymphoma, Hodgkin's disease, and multiple myeloma—the committee concluded that there was not enough information in the literature about the timing of exposure and subsequent risk to further discuss latency issues. The committee did find that there was enough information about the timing of exposure and respiratory and prostate cancers, with considerably more information about the former than the latter, to warrant analysis of results. Both of these cancers are in the "Limited/Suggestive Evidence of an Association" category, and this conclusion has not changed after this investigation of time-related factors.

The evidence in the literature suggests that the time from exposure to TCDD to increased risk of respiratory cancer is less than ten years, and that the increase in relative risk continues for somewhat more than 20 years. The available literature does not indicate how long it takes for relative risks to return to one. These conclusions are based primarily on the study conducted by the National Institute for Occupational Safety and Health (Fingerhut, 1991), since this study is the most informative about the changes in risk of respiratory cancer with time since first exposure to TCDD, but the calculations are supported by other studies that have investigated time-related effects. The epidemiological literature was not informative on the effect of the age at which the exposure was received, or whether the carcinogen appeared to act at an early or late stage of the carcinogenic process. The limited data do not indicate any increase in the relative risk of prostate cancer with time since exposure to TCDD. For prostate cancer, the epidemiological literature was not informative on how long the effects of exposure last, the effect of the age at which the exposure was received, or whether the carcinogen acts at an early or late stage of the carcinogenic process.

Increased Risk of Disease in Vietnam Veterans

Although there have been numerous health studies of Vietnam veterans, most have been hampered by relatively poor measures of exposure to herbicides or TCDD, in addition to other methodological problems. Most of the evidence on which the findings in Table 1-1 are based comes from studies of people exposed to dioxin or herbicides in occupational and environmental settings, rather than from studies of Vietnam veterans. The committee found this body of evidence sufficient for reaching the conclusions about statistical associations between herbicides and the health outcomes summarized in Table 1-1; however, the lack of adequate data on Vietnam veterans per se complicates the second part of the committee's charge, which is to determine the increased risk of disease among individuals exposed to herbicides during service in Vietnam. Given the large uncertainties that remain about the magnitude of potential risk from exposure to herbicides in the epidemiologic studies that have been reviewed (Chapters 7, 9, 10, and 11), the inadequate control for important confounders, and the uncertainty about the nature and magnitude of exposure to herbicides in Vietnam (Chapter 5), the necessary information to undertake a quantitative risk assessment is lacking. Thus, in general, it is not possible for the committee to quantify the degree of risk likely to be experienced by veterans because of their exposure to herbicides in Vietnam. The quantitative and qualitative evidence about herbicide exposure among various groups studied suggests that most Vietnam veterans (except for selected groups with documented high exposures, such as participants in Operation Ranch Hand) had lower exposure to herbicides and TCDD than the subjects in many occupational and environmental studies. However, individual veterans who had very high exposures to herbicides could have risks approaching those in the occupational and environmental studies.

REFERENCES

Alavanja MC, Merkle S, Teske J, Eaton B, Reed B. 1989. Mortality among forest and soil conservationists. Archives of Environmental Health 44:94-101.

Asp S, Riihimaki V, Hernberg S, Pukkala E. 1994. Mortality and cancer morbidity of Finnish chlorophenoxy herbicide applicators: an 18-year prospective follow-up. American Journal of Industrial Medicine 26:243-253.

Berkley MC, Magee KR. 1963. Neuropathy following exposure to a dimethylamine salt of 2,4-D. Archives of Internal Medicine 111:133-134.

Bertazzi PA, Zocchetti C, Pesatori AC, Guercilena S, Sanarico M, Radice L. 1989a. Mortality in an area contaminated by TCDD following an industrial incident. Medicina Del Lavoro 80:316-329.

Bertazzi PA, Zocchetti C, Pesatori AC, Guercilena S, Sanarico M, Radice L. 1989b. Ten-year mortality study of the population involved in the Seveso incident in 1976. American Journal of Epidemiology 129:1187-1200.

Bertazzi A, Pesatori AC, Consonni D, Tironi A, Landi MT, Zocchetti C. 1993. Cancer incidence in a population accidentally exposed to 2,3,7,8-tetrachlorodibenzo-*para*-dioxin. Epidemiology 4:398-406.

Blair A, Mustafa D, Heineman EF. 1993. Cancer and other causes of death among male and female farmers from twenty-three states. American Journal of Industrial Medicine 23:729-742.

Boeri R, Bordo B, Crenna P, Filippini G, Massetto M, Zecchini A. 1978. Preliminary results of a neurological investigation of the population exposed to TCDD in the Seveso region. Rivista di Patologia Nervosa e Mentale 99:111-128.

Burmeister LF, Everett GD, Van Lier SF, Isacson P. 1983. Selected cancer mortality and farm practices in Iowa. American Journal of Epidemiology 118:72-77.

Calvert GM, Sweeney MH, Fingerhut MA, Hornung RW, Halperin WE. 1994. Evaluation of porphyria cutanea tarda in U.S. workers exposed to 2,3,7,8-tetrachlorodibenzo-*p*-dioxin. American Journal of Industrial Medicine 25:559-571.

Centers for Disease Control. 1989. Health status of Vietnam veterans. Vietnam Experience Study. Atlanta: U.S. Department of Health and Human Services. Vols. I-V, Supplements A-C.

Collins JJ, Strauss ME, Levinskas GJ, Conner PC. 1993. The mortality experience of workers exposed to 2,3,7,8-tetrachlorodibenzo-*p*-dioxin in a trichlorophenol process accident. Epidemiology 4:7-13.

Cordier S, Le TB, Verger P, Bard D, Le CD, Larouze B, Dazza MC, Hoang TQ, Abenhaim L. 1993. Viral infections and chemical exposures as risk factors for hepatocellular carcinoma in Vietnam. International Journal of Cancer 55:196-201.

Dalager MS, Kang HK, Thomas TL. 1995. Cancer mortality patterns among women who served in the military: the Vietnam experience. Journal of Occupational and Environmental Medicine 37:298-305.

Erickson JD, Mulinare J, Mcclain PW. 1984. Vietnam veterans' risks for fathering babies with birth defects. Journal of the American Medical Association 252:903-912.

Filippini G, Bordo B, Crenna P, Massetto N, Musicco M, Boeri R. 1981. Relationship between clinical and electrophysiological findings and indicators of heavy exposure to 2,3,7,8-tetrachlorodibenzo-*p*-dioxin. Scandinavian Journal of Work, Environment, and Health 7:257-262.

Fingerhut MA, Halperin WE, Marlow DA, Piacitelli LA, Honchar PA, Sweeney MH, Greife AL, Dill PA, Steenland K, Suruda AJ. 1991. Cancer mortality in workers exposed to 2,3,7,8-tetrachlorodibenzo-*p*-dioxin. New England Journal of Medicine 324:212-218.

Flesch-Janys D, Gurn P, Jung D, Konietzke J, Papke O. 1994. First results of an investigation of the elimination of polychlorinated dibenzo-*p*-dioxins and dibenzofurans (PCDD/F) in occupationally exposed persons. Organohalogen Compounds 21:93-99.

Goldstein NP, Jones PH, Brown JR. 1959. Peripheral neuropathy after exposure to an ester of dichlorophenoxyacetic acid. Journal of the American Medical Association 171:1306-1309.

Hill, AB. 1971. Principles of Medical Statistics, 9th ed. New York: Oxford University Press.

Institute of Medicine. 1994. Veterans and Agent Orange Health Effects of Herbicides Used in Vietnam. National Academy of Sciences, National Academy Press: Washington, DC.

Jung D, Konietzko J, Reill-Konietzko G, Muttray A, Zimmermann-Holz HJ, Doss M, Beck H, Edler L, Kopp-Schneider A. 1994. Porphyrin studies in TCDD-exposed workers. Archives of Toxicology 68:595-598.

Kogevinas M, Saracci R, Winkelmann R, Johnson ES, Bertazzi PA, Bueno de Mesquita BH, Kauppinen T, Littorin M, Lynge E, Neuberger M. 1993. Cancer incidence and mortality in women occupationally exposed to chlorophenoxy herbicides, chlorophenols, and dioxins. Cancer Causes and Control 4:547-553.

Lynge E. 1993. Cancer in phenoxy herbicide manufacturing workers in Denmark, 1947-87: an update. Cancer Causes and Control 4:261-272.

Michalek JE, Pirkle JL, Caudill SP, Tripathi RC, Patterson DG, Needham LL. 1996. Pharmacokinetics of TCDD in veterans of Operation Ranch Hand: 10 year follow-up. Journal of Exposure Analysis and Environmental Epidemiology 47:102-112.

Morrison H, Savitz D, Semenciw R, Hulka B, Mao Y, Morison D, Wigle D. 1993. Farming and prostate cancer mortality. American Journal of Epidemiology 137:270-280.

Needham LL, Gerthoux PM, Patterson DG, Brambilla P, Pirkle JL, Tramacere PI, Turner WE, Beretta C, Sampson EJ, Mocarelli P. 1994. Half-life of 2,3,7,8-tetrachlorodibenzo-*p*-dioxin in serum of Seveso adults: interim report. Organohalogen Compounds 21:81-85.

Ott MG, Messerer P, Zober A. 1993. Assessment of past occupational exposure to 2,3,7,8-tetrachlorodibenzo-*p*-dioxin using blood lipid analyses. International Archives of Occupational and Environmental Health 65:1-8.

Pocchiari F, Silano V, Zampieri A. 1979. Human health effects from accidental release of tetrachlorodibenzo-*p*-dioxin (TCDD) at Seveso, Italy. Annals of the New York Academy of Science 320:311-320.

Todd RL. 1962. A case of 2,4-D intoxication. Journal of the Iowa Medical Society 52:663-664.

Verger P, Cordier S, Thuy LT, Bard D, Dai LC, Phiet PH, Gonnord MF, Abenhaim L. 1994. Correlation between dioxin levels in adipose tissue and estimated exposure to Agent Orange in south Vietnamese residents. Environmental Research 65:226-242.

Von Benner A, Edler L, Mayer K, Zober A. 1994. 'Dioxin' investigation program of the chemical industry professional association. Arbeitsmedizin Sozialmedizin Praventivmedizin 29:11-16.

Wolfe WH, Michalek JE, Miner JC, Rahe AJ, Moore CA, Needham LL, Patterson D.G. 1995. Paternal serum dioxin and reproductive outcomes among veterans of Operation Ranch Hand. Epidemiology 6:17-22.

2

Veterans and Agent Orange:
The Initial IOM Report

BACKGROUND

The U.S. Congress enacted Public Law 102-4, referred to as the "Agent Orange Act of 1991," on February 6, 1991. This legislation directed the Secretary of Veterans Affairs to request that the National Academy of Sciences conduct a comprehensive review and evaluation of scientific and medical information regarding the health effects of exposure to Agent Orange, other herbicides used in Vietnam, and their components, including dioxin. In February 1992, the Institute of Medicine (IOM) of the National Academy of Sciences signed an agreement with the Department of Veterans Affairs (DVA) to review and summarize the strength of the scientific evidence concerning the association between herbicide exposure during Vietnam service and each disease or condition suspected to be associated with such exposure. The IOM was also asked to make recommendations concerning the need, if any, for additional scientific studies to resolve areas of continuing scientific uncertainty and to comment on four particular programs mandated in Public Law 102-4.

To carry out the study, the IOM established the Committee to Review the Health Effects in Vietnam Veterans of Exposure to Herbicides. The results of the committee's work were published in 1994 as *Veterans and Agent Orange* (henceforth called *VAO*). In conducting its study, the committee operated independently of the DVA and other government agencies. The committee was not asked to and did not make judgments regarding specific cases in which individual Vietnam veterans have claimed injury from herbicide exposure; this was not part of its congressional charge. Rather, the study provides scientific information for the Secretary of Veterans Affairs to consider as the DVA exercises its responsibilities to Vietnam veterans.

In fulfilling its charge of judging whether each of a set of human health effects is associated with exposure to herbicides or dioxin, the committee primarily concentrated on reviewing and interpreting epidemiologic studies. The committee began its evaluation presuming neither the existence nor the absence of association. It sought to characterize and weigh the strengths and limitations of the available evidence. These judgments have both quantitative and qualitative aspects. They reflect the nature of the exposures, health outcomes, and populations exposed; the characteristics of the evidence examined; and the approach taken to evaluate that evidence. To facilitate independent assessment of the committee's conclusions, Chapter 5 of VAO describes as explicitly as possible the methodological considerations that guided the committee's review and its process of evaluation.

In reviewing the literature, the committee discerned that the existing epidemiologic data base is severely lacking in quantitative measures of individual exposure to herbicides and dioxin. Assessment of the intensity and duration of individual exposures is a key component in determining whether specific health outcomes are associated with exposure to dioxin or other chemicals found in the herbicides used in Vietnam. Although different approaches have been used to estimate exposure in Vietnam veterans and in others exposed occupationally or environmentally, each approach is limited in its ability to determine precisely the degree and level of individual exposure. The problems associated with each of these approaches are discussed in detail in Chapter 6 of VAO. The available quantitative and qualitative evidence about herbicide exposure summarized in that chapter suggests that Vietnam veterans as a group had substantially lower exposure to herbicides and dioxin than the subjects in many occupational studies. The participants in Operation Ranch Hand are an exception to this pattern, and it is likely that others among the approximately 3 million men and woman who served in Vietnam were exposed to herbicides at levels associated with health effects. Thus, in the committee's judgment, a sufficiently large range of exposures may exist among Vietnam veterans to conduct a valid epidemiologic study for certain health outcomes (see research recommendations below).

To obtain additional information pertinent to the evaluation of possible health effects of herbicide exposure, the committee decided to review studies of other groups potentially exposed to the herbicides used in Vietnam and to TCDD, especially phenoxy herbicides, including 2,4-dichlorophenoxyacetic acid (2,4-D) and 2,4,5-T, chlorophenols, and other compounds. These groups include chemical production and agricultural workers, residents of Vietnam, and people possibly exposed heavily to herbicides or dioxins as a result of residing near the site of an accident or certain toxic-waste dumping areas. The committee felt that considering studies of other groups could help address the issue of whether these compounds might be associated with particular health outcomes, even though these results would have only an indirect bearing on the increased risk of disease in veterans themselves. Some of these studies, especially those of workers in chemical production plants, provide stronger evidence about health effects than studies of veterans because exposure was generally more easily quantified and measured. Furthermore, the general level and duration of exposure to the chemicals were greater and the studies were of sufficient size to examine the health risks among those with varying levels of exposure.

Conclusions About Health Outcomes

Chapters 8 through 11 of *VAO* provide a detailed review of the epidemiologic studies evaluated by the committee and their implications for cancer, reproductive problems, neurobehavioral problems, and other health effects. The committee's specific mandate was to determine, if possible,

1. whether there is a statistical association between the suspect diseases and herbicide use, taking into account the strength of the scientific evidence and the appropriateness of the methods used to detect the association;
2. the increased risk of disease among individuals exposed to herbicides during service in Vietnam; and
3. whether there is a plausible biologic mechanism or other evidence of a causal relationship between herbicide exposure and a disease.

The committee addressed the first part of this charge by assigning each of the health outcomes under study into one of the four categories listed in Table 2-1 on the basis of the epidemiologic evidence that it reviewed. The specific rationale for each of the findings summarized in this table is given in Chapters 8 through 11 of *VAO*. The second part of the charge is addressed at the end of this section. The committee's response to the third part of the charge is summarized in general terms in Chapter 4 of *VAO*, and specific findings for each health outcome are also given in Chapters 8 through 11 of *VAO*.

The definitions of the categories and the criteria for assigning a particular health outcome to them are described in Table 2-1. Consistent with the charge to the Secretary of Veterans Affairs in Public Law 102-4, the distinctions between categories are based on "statistical association," not on causality, as is common in scientific reviews. The committee was charged with reviewing the scientific evidence, rather than making recommendations regarding DVA policy, and Table 2-1 does not imply or suggest any policy decisions; these must rest with the Secretary.

Health Outcomes with Sufficient Evidence of an Association

The committee found sufficient evidence of an association with herbicides

TABLE 2-1 Summary of Findings from *Veterans and Agent Orange* (1994) in Occupational, Environmental, and Veterans Studies Regarding the Association between Specific Health Problems and Exposure to Herbicides

Sufficient Evidence of an Association

Evidence is sufficient to conclude that there is a positive association. That is, a positive association has been observed between herbicides and the outcome in studies in which chance, bias, and confounding could be ruled out with reasonable confidence. For example, if several small studies that are free from bias and confounding show an association that is consistent in magnitude and direction, there may be sufficient evidence for an association. There is sufficient evidence of an association between exposure to herbicides and the following health outcomes:

> Soft-tissue sarcoma
> Non-Hodgkin's lymphoma
> Hodgkin's disease
> Chloracne
> Porphyria cutanea tarda (in genetically susceptible individuals)

Limited/Suggestive Evidence of an Association

Evidence is suggestive of an association between herbicides and the outcome but is limited because chance, bias, and confounding could not be ruled out with confidence. For example, at least one high-quality study shows a positive association, but the results of other studies are inconsistent. There is limited/suggestive evidence of an association between exposure to herbicides and the following health outcomes:

> Respiratory cancers (lung, larynx, trachea)
> Prostate cancer
> Multiple myeloma

Inadequate/Insufficient Evidence to Determine Whether an Association Exists

The available studies are of insufficient quality, consistency, or statistical power to permit a conclusion regarding the presence or absence of an association. For example, studies fail to control for confounding, have inadequate exposure assessment, or fail to address latency. There is inadequate or insufficient evidence to determine whether an association exists between exposure to herbicides and the following health outcomes:

> Hepatobiliary cancers
> Nasal/nasopharyngeal cancer
> Bone cancer
> Female reproductive cancers (breast, cervical, uterine, ovarian)
> Renal cancer
> Testicular cancer
> Leukemia
> Spontaneous abortion
> Birth defects
> Neonatal/infant death and stillbirths
> Low birthweight
> Childhood cancer in offspring
> Abnormal sperm parameters and infertility
> Cognitive and neuropsychiatric disorders

TABLE 2-1 Continued

Inadequate/Insufficient Evidence to Determine Whether an Association Exists
(continued)

  Motor/coordination dysfunction
  Peripheral nervous system disorders
  Metabolic and digestive disorders (diabetes, changes in liver enzymes,
    lipid abnormalities, ulcers)
  Immune system disorders (immune modulation and autoimmunity)
  Circulatory disorders
  Respiratory disorders

Limited/Suggestive Evidence of No Association
  Several adequate studies, covering the full range of levels of exposure that human beings
  are known to encounter, are mutually consistent in not showing a positive association
  between exposure to herbicides and the outcome at any level of exposure. A conclusion
  of "no association" is inevitably limited to the conditions, level of exposure, and length
  of observation covered by the available studies. *In addition, the possibility of a very
  small elevation in risk at the levels of exposure studied can never be excluded.* There is
  limited/suggestive evidence of *no* association between exposure to herbicides and the
  following health outcomes:

  Skin cancer
  Gastrointestinal tumors (stomach cancer, pancreatic
    cancer, colon cancer, rectal cancer)
  Bladder cancer
  Brain tumors

NOTE: "Herbicides" refers to the major herbicides used in Vietnam: 2,4-D (2,4-dichlorophenoxyacetic acid); 2,4,5-T (2,4,5-trichlorophenoxyacetic acid) and its contaminant TCDD (2,3,7,8-tetrachlorodibenzo-*p*-dioxin); cacodylic acid; and picloram. The evidence regarding association is drawn from occupational and other studies in which subjects were exposed to a variety of herbicides and herbicide components.

and/or TCDD for three cancers: soft tissue sarcoma, non-Hodgkin's lymphoma, and Hodgkin's disease.   For diseases in this category, a positive association between herbicides and the outcome must be observed in studies in which chance, bias, and confounding can be ruled out with reasonable confidence. The committee regarded evidence from several small studies that are free from bias and confounding, and that show an association that is consistent in magnitude and direction, as sufficient evidence for an association.

    The other two health outcomes for which the committee found sufficient evidence of an association with herbicides or TCDD are chloracne and porphyria cutanea tarda (see Chapter 11 of *VAO*).

Health Outcomes with Limited/Suggestive Evidence of an Association

The committee found limited/suggestive evidence of an association for three other cancers: respiratory cancers, prostate cancer, and multiple myeloma. For diseases in this category, the evidence must be suggestive of an association between herbicides and the outcome, but the association may be limited because chance, bias, or confounding could not be ruled out with confidence. Typically, at least one high-quality study indicates a positive association, but the results of other studies may be inconsistent.

Health Outcomes with Inadequate/Insufficient Evidence to Determine Whether an Association Exists

The scientific data for many of the cancers and other diseases reviewed by the committee were inadequate or insufficient to determine whether an association exists. For diseases in this category, the available studies are of insufficient quality, consistency, or statistical power to permit a conclusion regarding the presence or absence of an association. For example, studies fail to control for confounding or have inadequate exposure assessment.

Health Outcomes with Limited/Suggestive Evidence of No Association

For a small group of cancers, the committee found a sufficient number and variety of well-designed studies to conclude that there is limited/suggestive evidence of *no* association between these cancers and TCDD or the herbicides under study. This group includes gastrointestinal tumors (colon, rectal, stomach, and pancreatic), skin cancer, brain tumors, and bladder cancer. For outcomes in this category, several adequate studies covering the full range of levels of exposure that human beings are known to encounter are mutually consistent in not showing a positive association between exposure to herbicides and the outcome at any level of exposure, and which have relatively narrow confidence intervals. A conclusion of "no association" is inevitably limited to the conditions, level of exposure, and length of observation covered by the available studies. In addition, the possibility of a very small elevation in risk at the levels of exposure studied can never be excluded.

Increased Risk in Vietnam Veterans

Although there have been numerous health studies of Vietnam veterans, most have been hampered by relatively poor measures of exposure to herbicides or TCDD, in addition to other methodological problems. In Table 2-1, most of the evidence on which the findings are based comes from studies of people exposed to dioxin or herbicides in occupational and environmental settings, rather than from studies of Vietnam veterans. The committee found this body of evidence sufficient for reaching the conclusions about statistical associations between herbicides and health outcomes summarized in Table 2-1. However, the lack of adequate data on Vietnam veterans per se complicated the second part of the committee's charge, which is to determine the increased risk of disease among individuals exposed to herbicides during service in Vietnam. To estimate the magnitude of risk for a particular health outcome among herbicide-exposed Vietnam veterans, quantitative information about the dose-time-response relationship for each health outcome in humans, information on the extent of herbicide exposure among Vietnam veterans, and estimates of individual exposure are needed. Given the large uncertainties that remain about the magnitude of potential risk from exposure to herbicides in the studies that have been reviewed (Chapters 8-11 in *VAO*), the inadequate control for important confounders, and the uncertainty about the nature and magnitude of exposure to herbicides in Vietnam (Chapter 6 in *VAO*), none of the ingredients necessary for a quantitative risk assessment is available. Thus, it was not possible for the committee to quantify the degree of risk likely to be experienced by veterans because of their exposure to herbicides in Vietnam. The available quantitative and qualitative evidence about herbicide exposure among various groups studied suggests that most Vietnam veterans (except those with documented high exposures, such as participants in Operation Ranch Hand) had lower exposure to herbicides and TCDD than did the subjects in many occupational and environmental studies. However, individual veterans who had very high exposures to herbicides could have risks approaching those in the occupational and environmental studies.

Research Recommendations

The committee was also asked to make recommendations concerning the need, if any, for additional scientific studies to resolve areas of continuing scientific uncertainty concerning the health effects of the herbicides used in Vietnam. Based on its review of the epidemiologic evidence and a consideration of the quality of exposure information available in existing studies, especially of Vietnam veterans, the committee concluded that a series of epidemiologic studies of veterans could yield valuable information if a new, valid exposure reconstruction model could be developed. The committee also saw value in continuing the existing Ranch Hand study and expanding it to include Army Chemical Corps veterans. The committee's research recommendations emphasized studies of Vietnam veterans, rather than general toxicologic or epidemiologic studies of occupationally or environmentally exposed populations. A substantial amount of research on the toxicology and epidemiology of herbicides and herbicide components is already under way in the United States and abroad. Indeed, many of the studies on which the committee's conclusions are based have been published since 1991. Although this research is not targeted specifically to Vietnam veterans, it probably will also contribute to the knowledge of potential health effects in this population.

IMPACT OF THE REPORT

On July 27, 1993, the Institute of Medicine released *Veterans and Agent Orange: Health Effects of Herbicides Used in Vietnam* to the news media and the public. Immediately following the press conference, the Senate Committee on Veterans Affairs held a hearing on the report. Testifying at the hearing, Secretary of Veterans Affairs Jesse Brown announced that the Department of Veterans Affairs was already compensating Vietnam veterans exposed to herbicides for soft-tissue sarcoma, Hodgkin's disease, and chloracne. Based on the findings of the IOM committee, the DVA decided to begin immediately to compensate Vietnam veterans for non-Hodgkin's lymphoma and porphyria cutanea tarda (Category I diseases) (U.S. DVA, 1994). In September 1993, Secretary Brown announced that the DVA would also begin to compensate Vietnam veterans for respiratory cancers and multiple myeloma (Category II diseases) (U.S. DVA, 1993).

DVA Task Force

In July 1993, the Department of Veterans Affairs established the Agent Orange Task Force to review the IOM's report. In October 1993, the Task Force issued its report, which outlined a comprehensive course of action for the Secretary to take in response to the IOM's recommendations regarding epidemiologic studies of Vietnam veterans (U.S. DVA, 1993). The DVA is now implementing some of the committee's recommendations.

Recommendation 1. The committee endorses continued follow-up of the Air Force Ranch Hand cohort and its comparison group and recommends that members of the Army Chemical Corps and an appropriate comparison group be followed in a similar study. An independent, nongovernmental scientific panel should be established to review and approve a new, expanded research protocol for both study populations and to commission and direct a common analysis of the results. In response to this recommendation, the DVA's Task Force recommended that the Secretary "expand and design an Army Chemical Corps Vietnam Veterans Health Study to collect the necessary information to address the possible relationship between herbicide exposure and particular health outcomes."

Recommendation 2. The Department of Defense and the Department of Veterans Affairs should identify Vietnam service in the computerized index of their records. In response, the Task Force recommended to the Secretary that the DVA "explore the feasibility of accomplishing this recommendation to an acceptable degree by using computerized/automated data bases maintained by the

Defense Manpower Data Center (DMDC) (Department of Defense) and by VA [the Veterans Administration]." The Task Force also recommended that the DVA "attempt to obtain the names of Vietnam veterans who received bonuses offered by individual states for their service in Vietnam (at least 20 states provided these bonuses)" (U.S. DVA, 1993).

Recommendation 3. Biomarkers for herbicide exposure should be developed further. In response, the Task Force recommended that the Secretary "continue to monitor scientific developments on the subject and actively follow key researchers for their research findings, and . . . solicit research proposals from VA research scientists who are engaged in research projects related to toxicokinetics or biomarkers of environmental chemicals in connection with establishment of toxic environmental hazards research/clinical centers in the VA" (U.S. DVA, 1993).

Recommendation 4. A nongovernmental organization with appropriate experience in historical exposure reconstruction should be commissioned to develop and test models of herbicide exposure for use in studies of Vietnam veterans.

Recommendation 5. The exposure reconstruction models developed according to Recommendation 4 should be evaluated by an independent, nongovernmental scientific panel established for this purpose.

Recommendation 6. If the scientific panel proposed in Recommendation 5 determines that a valid exposure reconstruction model is feasible, the Department of Veterans Affairs and other government agencies should facilitate additional epidemiologic studies of veterans.

In response to Recommendation 4, the Task Force recommended that the DVA "request the NAS to develop and test the reconstruction model under a contract with the VA" (U.S. DVA, 1993). Regarding recommendation 5, the Task Force recommended that the DVA "request a professional society (e.g., Society for Epidemiologic Research, American College of Epidemiology, American Public Health Association, International Society of Exposure Analysis, American Industrial Hygiene Association, etc.) to commission a scientific panel to evaluate the proposed models" (U.S. DVA, 1993). And regarding recommendation 6, the Task Force recommended that the DVA "reanalyze the data already collected for the many completed studies of Vietnam veterans using the exposure reconstruction model" (U.S. DVA, 1993).

The DVA has subsequently entered into a contract with the IOM to establish a committee to oversee the development and evaluation of models of herbicide exposure for use in studies of Vietnam veterans, as recommended in *Veterans and Agent Orange*. The committee's first step would be to develop and disseminate a Request for Proposals (RFP). Ultimately, the DVA may request the IOM to: a) evaluate the proposals received in response to the RFP and select one or more academic or other non governmental groups to develop the exposure reconstruction model; b) provide scientific and administrative oversight of the work of the subcontractor(s); and c) evaluate the models developed by the subcontractor(s) and prepare a report to the DVA, which would be published for a broader audience (IOM, 1994).

MILITARY USE OF HERBICIDES IN VIETNAM

Approximately 3 million U.S. military personnel served in or near Vietnam, but the precise number cannot be readily determined from existing military records, since individual service records have not been computerized. Surveys of veterans vary in their estimates because of differences in terminology and sample selection procedures. Existing military records do document assignments of military personnel to units and the location of most units at most times. Individual military experiences of Americans who served in Vietnam varied, as the nature of the war in different areas of the country changed over time. Individual experiences also varied by branch of service, military occupation, rank, and type of military unit.

Between 1962 and 1971, U.S. military forces sprayed nearly 19 million gallons of herbicides over approximately 3.6 million acres in Vietnam. The preparation known as Agent Orange accounted for approximately 11.2 million gallons of the total amount sprayed. Herbicides were used to strip the thick jungle canopy that helped conceal opposition forces, to destroy crops that enemy forces might depend on, and to clear tall grass and bushes from around the perimeters of U.S. base camps and outlying fire support bases. Most large-scale spraying operations were conducted using airplanes and helicopters, but considerable quantities of herbicides were sprayed from boats and ground vehicles, as well as by soldiers wearing back-mounted equipment. Spraying began in 1962 and increased greatly in 1967. After a scientific report in 1969 concluded that one of the primary chemicals used in Agent Orange—namely, 2,4,5-trichlorophenoxyacetic acid (2,4,5-T)—could cause birth defects in laboratory animals, U.S. forces suspended use of this herbicide in 1970 and halted all herbicide spraying in Vietnam the next year.

As the decade wore on, concern about possible long-term health consequences of Agent Orange and other herbicides heightened, fueled in particular by reports from growing numbers of Vietnam veterans that they had developed cancer or fathered handicapped children, which they attributed to wartime exposure to the herbicides. Along with the concerns of Vietnam veterans, public awareness increased because of reports of health concerns surrounding occupational and environmental exposure to dioxin—more specifically, 2,3,7,8-tetrachlorodibenzo-p-dioxin (2,3,7,8-TCDD), informally known as TCDD—a contaminant of 2,4,5-T. Thousands of scientific studies have since been conducted, numerous government hearings have been held, and veterans organizations have pressed for conclusive answers, but the question of the health effects of herbicide exposure in Vietnam remains shrouded in controversy and mistrust. Indeed, some veterans organizations, researchers, and public interest organizations remain skeptical that the issue has received full and impartial consideration by the Department of Veterans Affairs (DVA; formerly the Veterans Administration) and other federal agencies.

FEDERAL GOVERNMENT'S RESPONSE TO CONCERNS OVER THE MILITARY USE OF HERBICIDES IN VIETNAM

The federal government has been involved with international and domestic policy issues related to the healh effects associated with the military use of herbicides, particularly Agent Orange, since the defoliation program began in Vietnam. On December 16, 1974, the U.S. Senate ratified the Geneva Protocol, which broadly sought an international commitment from all governments that they would never use chemical or biological weapons (including herbicides) in war. In April 1975, President Ford issued Executive Order 11850 renouncing future use of herbicides in war.

U.S. Congress

A major focus of the Senate and House Committees on Veterans' Affairs has been to understand better the human health effects of exposure to herbicides, including Agent Orange, during the Vietnam era. Legislation concerning Agent Orange falls primarily into three categories: (1) health care (access to VA medical centers for veterans exposed to Agent Orange during service in Vietnam; (2) scientific research (epidemiologic research on the health effects of exposure to Agent Orange in Vietnam); and (3) compensation issues (for disabilities that might have resulted from exposure to Agent Orange in Vietnam) (U.S. Congress, Senate, 1989). As documented in *VAO*, during the past 20 years congressional committees have held hearings and introduced bills on this topic, and in an attempt to resolve this issue, Congress has passed several laws dealing with the human health effects of exposure to Agent Orange used in Vietnam. This section focuses on congressional action since the release of *VAO*.

Hearings on Agent Orange

Three congressional hearings were held on *VAO*. The first hearing was held by the Senate Committee on Veterans Affairs immediately following the release of the report on July 27, 1993. The IOM's president, the chairman of the committee, and selected committee members were asked to testify. On August 4, 1993, the House Committee on Veterans Affairs requested the IOM's president, the committee's vice-chair, and a committee member to testify at its hearing. On November 2, 1993, the Senate Committee on Veterans Affairs called a hearing (which subsequently turned into a staff forum) on the direction of future research on the health effects of Agent Orange.

Legislation on Agent Orange

In 1970, Congress enacted the first public law dealing with the military use of herbicides. Congress has legislated numerous acts to appropriate funds for Agent Orange research, to provide clarification on payments received from the Agent Orange settlement fund, and to review and evaluate scientific literature regarding associations between diseases and exposure to dioxin and other chemical compounds in herbicides used in Vietnam.

Health Care   Public Law 97-72, enacted on November 3, 1981, expanded eligibility for health care services to include veterans exposed to Agent Orange in Vietnam. The effect of this legislation was to provide health care for Vietnam veterans for conditions requiring treatment that may have resulted from exposure to Agent Orange. Veterans need not demonstrate any direct link with Agent Orange; rather, care is provided unless the condition is shown to be due to something other than exposure, e.g., congenital or developmental conditions or conditions resulting from postservice trauma (Conway, 1993). Public Law 103-452 extended the program through June 30, 1995. [H.R. 1565 has been passed by the House to extend the program through December 31, 1997].

Epidemiologic Studies   Public Law 96-151, enacted on December 20, 1979, ordered the Veterans Administration to conduct an epidemiologic study of the possible health effects in veterans of exposure to dioxin found in the herbicides used in Vietnam. The legislation also required the Office of Technology Assessment to review and approve the protocol for the study. In 1981, Public Law 97-72 expanded the scope of the epidemiologic study to include an evaluation of the impact on the health of Vietnam veterans of other environmental factors that occurred in Vietnam; this study was later transferred from the Veterans Administration to the Centers for Disease Control and is referred to as the "Vietnam Experience Study." On April 7, 1986, Congress enacted Public Law 99-272, directing the VA to conduct an epidemiologic study of the long-term health effects of herbicides on women who served in Vietnam. The Women Veterans Health Programs Act of 1992 expanded the program for women veterans.

Compensation   On October 24, 1984, Congress enacted Public Law 98-542, the Veterans' Dioxin and Radiation Exposure Compensation Standards Act, to address the issue of compensation for disabilities that might have resulted from exposure to Agent Orange in Vietnam. This law "provided for payment, during a two-year interim period from October 1, 1984, to September 30, 1986, of disability and death benefits for Vietnam veterans with chloracne and porphyria cutanea tarda (an uncommon disorder of urinary porphyrin metabolism manifest in patients by thinning and blistering of the skin) which became manifest within one year after service in Vietnam and the survivors of veterans with such conditions" (U.S. Congress, Senate, 1989). Public Law 102-4, the Agent Orange Act of 1991, was enacted on February 6, 1991, to grant disability compensation payments for chloracne, non-Hodgkin's lymphoma, and soft-tissue sarcoma (other than osteosarcoma, chondrosarcoma, Kaposi's sarcoma, or mesothelioma) associated with Agent Orange. This law called for the National Academy of Sciences to conduct a review of the scientific literature concerning the association between herbicide exposure during Vietnam service and each health outcome suspected to be associated with such exposure.

Department of Veterans Affairs

The Department of Veterans Affairs is also responsible for providing health care, compensation, and benefits to veterans of the Vietnam era. For almost 17 years, the DVA has been involved in conducting and assessing research and in monitoring studies on the health effects of Agent Orange.

Health Care

The DVA provides certain health care services to veterans of the Vietnam era (defined as August 5, 1964 through May 7, 1975) who were possibly exposed to herbicides contaminated with dioxin. Prior to receiving the health care services, veterans must provide proof of service in Vietnam. Health care services are limited to hospital and nursing home care and outpatient care in DVA facilities, on a pre- or post-hospitalization basis or to prevent a need for hospitalization (U.S. DVA, 1992). When a veteran requests DVA medical care, he or she undergoes a physical examination and appropriate diagnostic studies, which may serve as the Agent Orange examination (U.S. DVA, 1992).

Research Efforts

The DVA's Environmental Epidemiology Service (EES) has conducted several research studies on Vietnam veterans. The Agent Orange Registry (AOR) serves as a health surveillance data base; it contains records on approximately 10 percent of the entire Vietnam veteran population (self-selected) and is routinely reviewed for changes in health outcomes and mortality patterns. Studies published in 1994 evaluated whether an association exists between posttraumatic stress disorder and the risk of traumatic deaths among Vietnam veterans (Bullman and Kang, 1994), and whether there is an association between Agent Orange exposure and risk of testicular cancer (Bullman et al., 1994). A review article published in 1994 evaluated the effects of military exposure to a number of herbicides, including Agent Orange, on Vietnam veterans (Bullman and Kang, 1994). In 1995, a study of cancer mortality patterns among female Vietnam veterans was published (Dalager et al., 1995).

Compensation and Benefits

The DVA compensates veterans for certain diseases related to exposure to dioxin-containing herbicides during their service in Vietnam. Whenever the Secretary determines that there is sound medical and scientific evidence indicating a positive association between the exposure to an herbicide agent and the occurrence of a disease in humans, the department issues regulations stating that a presumption of service connection is warranted for that disease.

The DVA's compensation policy now provides that the Secretary must take into account reports from the National Academy of Sciences and all other sound medical and scientific information and analysis in making determinations. In evaluating any study, the Secretary must take into consideration whether the results are statistically significant, are capable of replication, and can withstand peer review [38 USC 1116 (b)(2)]. An association between the occurrence of a disease in humans and exposure to an herbicide agent is considered to be positive if the credible evidence for the association is equal to or outweighs the credible evidence against the association [38 USC 1116 (b)(3)]. Proposed regulations regarding compensation or denial of compensation for these diseases are published in the *Federal Register*. The DVA solicits comments from the public before final regulations are issued.

Prior to the release of *VAO*, the Secretary of Veterans Affairs established presumptive service connection in Vietnam (based on exposure to a herbicide containing dioxin) for three diseases: chloracne, non-Hodgkin's lymphoma, and soft-tissue sarcoma (other than osteosarcoma, chondrosarcoma, Kaposi's sarcoma, or mesothelioma) (57 FR, 29107-9, May 19, 1993). After the release of *VAO*, the Secretary established presumptive service connection in Vietnam for Hodgkin's disease and porphyria cutanea tarda (59 FR 5106-07, February 3, 1994), and several months later established presumptive service connection in Vietnam for multiple myeloma and respiratory cancers (lung, bronchus, larynx, and trachea). The DVA stipulated that the diseases have to "become manifest to a degree of 10 percent or more at any time after service, except that chloracne or other acneform disease consistent with chloracne and porphyria cutanea tarda shall have become manifest to a degree of 10 percent or more within a year, and respiratory cancers within 30 years, after the last date on which the veteran was exposed to an herbicide agent during active military, naval, or air service" (59 FR 29724, June 9, 1994).

As of March 1995, the DVA was providing compensation for service-connected diseases to the following numbers of Vietnam veterans:

| | Number of Veterans |
Disease	Compensated
Porphyria Cutanea Tarda	53
Multiple Myeloma	67
Hodgkin's Disease	117
Chloracne	180
Respiratory Cancers	475
Soft-Tissue Sarcoma*	679
Non-Hodgkin's Lymphoma	851

*To be recognized by the DVA as a soft-tissue sarcoma, a tumor must be malignant and must arise from tissue of mesenchymal origin.

Outreach Activities

The DVA's Environmental Agents Service (EAS) is responsible for developing and implementing the national medical policies and procedures regarding exposure of military veterans to possible environmental hazards, including Agent Orange. The EAS maintains the Agent Orange Registry, a computerized index of Agent Orange medical examinations. As of September 1995, there were 246,611 veterans on the registry, whose diagnoses were recorded using ICD codes (Rosenblum, 1995). In addition to diagnostic data, the AOR also contains a variety of self-reported demographic and military characteristics (U.S. DVA, 1992). The registry's participants (all self-selected) receive the *Agent Orange Review*, a newsletter that provides updated information about Agent Orange. The EAS also compiles fact sheets, called *Agent Orange Briefs*, about Agent Orange and related concerns; copies of these briefs are available through the Agent Orange Coordinator at all DVA medical centers.

Department of the Air Force

In 1979, the Air Force began an epidemiologic study of the "Ranch Hand" personnel who participated in the aerial spraying of herbicides in Vietnam. The 20-year Ranch Hand study is designed to determine whether long-term adverse health effects exist and can be attributed to occupational exposure to Agent Orange and other herbicides and dioxins. The health of Ranch Hand personnel is being compared to other Air Force personnel who served in Vietnam but were not exposed to herbicides (U.S. Congress, Senate, 1989). The study consists of mortality and morbidity components, based on follow-up examination results. The following Air Force Ranch Hand reports have been published to date:

- 1982 Baseline Mortality Report (AFHS, 1983)

- Baseline Morbidity Report (AFHS, 1984a)
- 1985 Follow-up Examination Results (AFHS, 1987)
- 1987 Follow-up Examination Results (AFHS, 1990)
- Serum Dioxin Level Follow-up Examination Results (AFHS, 1991b)
- Mortality Updates 1984, 1985, 1986, 1989, 1991 (AFHS, 1984b, 1985, 1986, 1989, 1991a)
- Reproductive Outcomes (AFHS, 1992)
- 1992 Follow-up Examination Results (AFHS, 1995)

The morbidity study followups, conducted in 1985, 1987, and 1992, are comprised of questionnaires, medical record reviews, and physical examinations. Additional follow-up examinations are scheduled for 1997 and 2002 (AFHS, 1995). An evaluation of the relationship between paternal serum dioxin in Ranch Hand veterans and reproductive outcomes was published in 1995 (Wolfe et al., 1995).

Environmental Protection Agency

In 1991, the Environmental Protection Agency (EPA) began a scientific reassessment of the risks of exposure to the dioxin 2,3,7,8-TCDD and chemically similar compounds. The EPA undertook this project in response to newly emerging scientific knowledge about the mechanisms of action of dioxin (U.S. EPA, 1992). The reassessment is part of EPA's efforts to improve the research and scientific base of the agency and incorporate solid research and science into its decisions. In 1994, the EPA released a draft report on the project. It asserted that a wide range of adverse health effects could be attributed to exposure to low levels of dioxin and related compounds by the general population (U.S. EPA, 1994a,b). The report also contended that there is no threshold or level of exposure below which dioxin poses no health risks. Adverse health effects that have been demonstrated in laboratory animals exposed to low levels of dioxin include such diverse conditions as reproductive problems, endometriosis, and cancer. However, the EPA Science Advisory Board, an outside panel of 39 scientists, criticized the agency for failing to give equal weight to all available evidence on the health effects of dioxin exposure. The board cautioned that the EPA's reliance on a single dose-response model to explain the dioxin effects that dioxin triggers after it binds to what is called the aryl hydrocarbon receptor casts doubt on this report's conclusions, because there are other models by which dioxin is thought to exert its effects. The EPA is currently revising its report, and it expects to release a revised draft in 1996.

REFERENCES

Air Force Health Study. 1983. An Epidemiologic Investigation of Health Effects in Air Force Personnel Following Exposure to Herbicides: Baseline Mortality Study Results. Brooks AFB, TX: USAF School of Aerospace Medicine. NTIS AD-A130 793.

Air Force Health Study. 1984a. An Epidemiologic Investigation of Health Effects in Air Force Personnel Following Exposure to Herbicides: Baseline Morbidity Study Results. Brooks AFB, TX: USAF School of Aerospace Medicine. NTIS AD-A138 340.

Air Force Health Study. 1984b. An Epidemiologic Investigation of Health Effects in Air Force Personnel Following Exposure to Herbicides. Mortality Update: 1984. Brooks AFB, TX: USAF School of Aerospace Medicine.

Air Force Health Study. 1985. An Epidemiologic Investigation of Health Effects in Air Force Personnel Following Exposure to Herbicides. Mortality Update: 1985. Brooks, AFB, TX: USAF School of Aerospace Medicine.

Air Force Health Study. 1986. An Epidemiologic Investigation of Health Effects in Air Force Personnel Following Exposure to Herbicides. Mortality Update: 1986. Brooks AFB, TX: USAF School of Aerospace Medicine. USAFSAM-TR-86-43.

Air Force Health Study. 1987. An Epidemiologic Investigation of Health Effects in Air Force Personnel Following Exposure to Herbicides. First Followup Examination Results. Brooks AFB, TX: USAF School of Aerospace Medicine. USAFSAM-TR-87-27. 2 vols.

Air Force Health Study. 1989. An Epidemiologic Investigation of Health Effects in Air Force Personnel Following Exposure to Herbicides. Mortality Update: 1989. Brooks AFB, TX: USAF School of Aerospace Medicine. USAFSAM-TR-89-9.

Air Force Health Study. 1990. An Epidemiologic Investigation of Health Effects in Air Force Personnel Following Exposure to Herbicides. Brooks AFB, TX: USAF School of Aerospace Medicine. USAFSAM-TR-90-2. 2 vols.

Air Force Health Study. 1991a. An Epidemiologic Investigation of Health Effects in Air Force Personnel Following Exposure to Herbicides. Mortality Update: 1991. Brooks AFB, TX: Armstrong Laboratory. AL-TR-1991-0132.

Air Force Health Study. 1991b. An Epidemiologic Investigation of Health Effects in Air Force Personnel Following Exposure to Herbicides. Serum Dioxin Analysis of 1987 Examination Results. Brooks AFB, TX: USAF School of Aerospace Medicine. 9 vols.

Air Force Health Study. 1992. An Epidemiologic Investigation of Health Effects in Air Force Personnel Following Exposure to Herbicides. Reproductive Outcomes. Brooks AFB, TX: Armstrong Laboratory. AL-TR-1992-0090.

Air Force Health Study. 1995. An Epidemiologic Investigation of Health Effects in Air Force Personnel Following Exposure to Herbicides. 1992 Followup Examination Results. Brooks AFB, TX: Epidemiologic Research Division. Armstrong Laboratory. 10 vols.

Bullman TA, Kang HK. 1994. The effects of mustard gas, ionizing radiation, herbicides, trauma, and oil smoke on U.S. military personnel: the results of veteran studies. Annual Review of Public Health 15:69-90.

Bullman TA, Watanabe KK, Kang HK. 1994. Risk of testicular cancer associated with surrogate measures of Agent Orange exposure among Vietnam veterans on the Agent Orange Registry. Annals of Epidemiology 4:11-16.

Conway F. 1993. Memorandum to the Institute of Medicine Committee to Review the Health Effects in Vietnam Veterans of Exposure to Herbicides. Washington: Department of Veterans Affairs. May 18, 1993.

Dalager NA, Kang HK, Thomas TL. 1995. Cancer mortality patterns among women who served in the military: the Vietnam experience. Journal of Occupational and Environmental Medicine 37:298-305.

Hickman J. 1995. Letter to the Institute of Medicine Committee to Review the Health Effects in Vietnam Veterans of Exposure to Herbicides. Washington: U.S. Department of Veterans Affairs, Compensation and Pension Service.

Institute of Medicine. 1994. Veterans and Agent Orange Health Effects of Herbicides Used in Vietnam. National Academy of Sciences, National Academy Press: Washington, DC.

Rosenblum DJ. 1995. Telephone Conversation with Institute of Medicine Committee to Review the Health Effects in Vietnam Veterans of Exposure to Herbicides Staff. Washington: U.S. Department of Veterans Affairs, Environmental Agents Service.

U.S. Congress. Senate. 1989. Committee on Veterans' Affairs. Report on Veterans' Agent Orange Exposure and Vietnam Service Benefits Act of 1989. 101st Cong., 2nd sess. Report 101-82.

U.S. Department of Veterans' Affairs. 1992. Agent Orange Briefs A1-D5. Washington: DVA, Environmental Agents Service.

U.S. Department of Veterans' Affairs. 1993. Report to the Secretary of Veterans' Affairs: VA Agent Orange Task Force. Washington: DVA.

U.S. Department of Veterans' Affairs. 1994. News Release: VA Announces Rules in Place for More Agent Orange-Related Diseases. Washington: DVA, Office of Public Affairs.

U.S. Environmental Protection Agency. 1992. Workshop Review Draft of Health Assessment for 2,3,7,8-tetrachlorodibenzo-*p*-dioxin (TCDD) and Related Compounds. Washington: EPA, Office of Research and Development.

U.S. Environmental Protection Agency. 1994a. Estimating Exposure to Dioxin-Like Compounds. Review Draft. Volumes I-III. Washington: EPA, Office of Research and Development.

U.S. Environmental Protection Agency. 1994b. Health Assessment Document for 2,3,7,8-tetrachlorodibenzo-*p*-dioxin (TCDD) and Related Compounds. Review Draft. Volumes I-III. Washington: EPA, Office of Research and Development.

Wolfe WH, Michalek JE, Miner JC, Rahe AJ, Moore CA, Needham LL, Patterson DGJr. 1995. Paternal serum dioxin and reproductive outcomes among veterans of Operation Ranch Hand. Epidemiology 6:17-22.

3

Toxicology

This chapter is an update of the toxicological information that appeared in Chapter 4 of *Veterans and Agent Orange: Health Effects of Herbicides Used in Vietnam* (IOM, 1994). The chapter begins with a summary of the new information presented and a summary of information presented in the previous report. This is followed by an overview of the toxicological profile updates on 2,4-D; 2,4,5-T; cacodylic acid; picloram; and TCDD. The toxicological profile updates on these five substances are a review of the results of experimental studies published during the period 1992-95 and comprise the remainder of this chapter.

SUMMARY

Introduction

In this section, we summarize information on the following:

• Toxicokinetics: the way in which dioxin and the herbicides enter and leave the bodies of animals; that is, the way these substances are absorbed, distributed, metabolized, and excreted by animals;
• Mechanism of action: the way in which dioxin and the herbicides act on the body to produce a toxic effect; and
• Toxicity: the toxic effects from exposure to dioxin and the herbicides on laboratory animals and nonhuman systems.

Understanding how dioxin and the herbicides affect animals and nonhuman systems allows us to reasonably determine whether these effects can occur in humans.

Toxicokinetics

During the past three years new information was published on the distribution of 2,4-D and 2,4,5-T in the body. There is also new information on the metabolism of cacodylic acid. Both 2,4-D and 2,4,5-T remain in the body for a short period of time—less than two weeks. 2,4-D enters liver cells and binds to protein and lipid molecules; the consequence of this is unknown. Both 2,4-D and 2,4,5-T enter the brain. Cacodylic acid is metabolized to a more toxic and reactive form called the dimethylarsenic radical.

TCDD, unlike the herbicides, stays in the body for a long time. It is removed from the body as it metabolizes to less toxic forms that are more easily excreted than TCDD itself. During the past three years, models have been further developed that provide insight into the complex ways in which TCDD is distributed in the body.

Mechanism of Action

Little is known about the way in which the herbicides produce toxic effects in animals. Tests with 2,4-D and cacodylic acid indicate that these substances are toxic to the body's cells and genetic material. The recent discovery that inorganic arsenicals are metabolized in mammals to dimethylarsenic acid suggests that the toxic effects of 2,4-D may be similar to that produced by cacodylic acid, which is dimethylarsenic acid.

To date, the consensus is that TCDD is not toxic to the body's genetic material and that its ability to cause cancer in animals is due to other events. It may cause cancer by affecting the body's enzymes, the way cells reproduce, and the rate at which cells die.

New tests suggest that TCDD causes chloracne by affecting the development of one of the layers of skin: the epidermis. New tests also indicate that wasting syndrome results from TCDD's preventing glucose uptake by fat cells and by cells in the brain and pancreas.

Most of the tests published during the past three years have examined the molecular mechanisms of TCDD toxicity. The tests confirm earlier findings that the toxic effects of TCDD are caused by the binding of TCDD to a protein called the aryl hydrocarbon (Ah) receptor. The binding of TCDD to this receptor triggers other effects that result in a toxic sequelae. However, some tests also suggest that other events, in addition to the binding of TCDD to the protein receptor, are involved.

Disease Outcomes and Mechanisms of Toxicity

Tests with 2,4-D, 2,4,5-T, cacodylic acid, and picloram indicate that these substances are not very toxic. High concentrations are needed to produce toxic effects in laboratory animals and nonhuman systems. No new information has been published to indicate that these herbicides cause cancer in animals. Nerve damage has been reported in rats given high doses of 2,4-D in food and teratogenic effects have been seen in sea urchin eggs exposed to 2,4,5-T during early development. Cacodylic acid has been shown to produce lesions in the kidneys of rats. TCDD has been reported to produce a number of toxic effects in several different animal species. The toxic effects include carcinogenicity, immunotoxicity, reproductive/developmental toxicity, hepatotoxicity, neurotoxicity, chloracne, and loss of body weight.

Not all these effects are seen in all species. Some are seen in males and not females, and vice versa; some are seen in young animals only. TCDD does cause cancer in animals. Recent tests show that young animals are particularly sensitive to TCDD. The reproductive capability of newborn males exposed to TCDD is adversely affected. Recent studies also show that TCDD can damage animals' nerves, enlarge their livers, and impair the ability of their hearts to contract. Tests using nonhuman systems suggest that TCDD can also affect the cells in the kidney, but these effects have not been shown in live animals. Although TCDD has been shown to cause adverse effects on the immune response in nonhuman systems, the immune response in live animals does not appear to be affected.

SUMMARY OF *VAO*

Multiple chemicals were used for various purposes in Vietnam. Four herbicides documented in military records were of particular concern and were extensively addressed in Chapter 4 of *VAO* (IOM, 1994). These included 2,4-dichlorophenoxyacetic acid (2,4-D); 2,4,5-trichlorophenoxyacetic acid (2,4,5-T); picloram; and cacodylic acid. In addition, the toxicologic properties of 2,3,7,8-tetrachlorodibenzo-*p*-dioxin (TCDD or dioxin), a contaminant of 2,4,5-T, were described. Complete toxicity profiles for each of the five substances were presented. The chapter focused to a large extent on the toxicological effects of TCDD, because considerably more information was available on TCDD than on the herbicides.

As stated in Chapter 4 of *VAO* (IOM, 1994), the primary purpose of reviewing the animal studies on the five substances was to contribute to an understanding of the biologic plausibility of the associations observed in epidemiologic studies that are relevant to herbicide exposure in Vietnam. In examining the individual toxicity profiles of the chemicals, it was recognized that differences in chemical levels, frequency of administration, single or combined exposures, pre-existing health status, genetic factors, and routes of exposure significantly influence toxicity outcomes. Thus, any attempt to extrapolate from experimental studies to human exposure must carefully consider such variables before conclusions are made.

The remainder of this section summarizes what appeared in *VAO* on what was known about the chemistry, toxicokinetics, disease outcomes, and mechanisms of toxicity of the five substances.

Chemistry

2,4-D and 2,4,5-T are called chlorophenoxy acids and are made up of carbon, hydrogen, oxygen, and chlorine. They both dissolve in water and are very similar in structure to a natural plant hormone called auxin. As a result of this similarity, 2,4-D and 2,4,5-T can mimic the action of auxin in some plants, and this activity is thought to account for herbicidal activity.

TCDD forms as a by-product during the manufacture of 2,4,5-T and also contains carbon, hydrogen, oxygen, and chlorine. TCDD dissolves easily in fats and oils, but not in water, and is persistent in the environment. The primary source of TCDD in the environment is combustion and industrial processes. The primary source of human exposure is through food.

Cacodylic acid contains carbon, hydrogen, oxygen, and arsenic and was called Agent Blue. Picloram contains carbon, hydrogen, oxygen, chlorine, and nitrogen. The combination of cacodylic acid and 2,4-D was known as Agent White. Both compounds dissolve in water.

Toxicokinetics

TCDD is ingested by animals through contaminated food. More than 50 percent is absorbed into the body through the gastrointestinal tract. Most of the TCDD breathed in the air is thought to be absorbed through the lungs, but this route of exposure is not well studied. In contrast, TCDD is not absorbed well through the skin. The same pattern of absorption applies for 2,4-D and 2,4,5-T, and probably for picloram and cacodylic acid.

TCDD is distributed primarily to the liver and to body fat. The amount of time that TCDD remains in the liver or fat is different for different species. 2,4-D and 2,4,5-T are distributed widely in the body; the distribution patterns of picloram and cacodylic acid are less well understood. Some cacodylic acid that is absorbed is bound to red blood cells. Although cacodylic acid binds readily to red blood cells in rats, it does not bind to human red blood cells.

TCDD is metabolized by enzymes in the liver to form derivatives that can dissolve in water and thus are more easily eliminated from the body than TCDD itself, which does not dissolve in water. Water-soluble derivatives of TCDD are thought to be much less toxic to animals than TCDD itself. 2,4-D, 2,4,5-T, and cacodylic acid are not metabolized to any significant extent in the body.

Mice and rats eliminate TCDD from the body in both urine and feces, whereas all other species studied eliminate TCDD primarily through feces. Elimination from the body is slow; in humans it may take seven to ten years or more for half of the body burden of TCDD to be removed. 2,4-D, 2,4,5-T, picloram, and cacodylic acid are eliminated rapidly from humans, mostly in the urine. Cacodylic acid that is bound to red blood cells is eliminated as the cells die naturally.

Disease Outcomes and Mechanisms of Toxicity

In this section, we summarize studies that investigated the toxic effects of TCDD and the herbicides. If known, the mechanism of toxicity is also explained.

Carcinogenicity: TCDD

The ability of TCDD to cause cancer in animals has been studied using rats, mice, and hamsters exposed to TCDD for one to two years. The results of these studies were summarized in detail in *VAO*. In these studies, TCDD was fed to animals, applied to their skin, injected under their skin, or injected into their abdominal cavities.

Increased tumor rates have been reported to occur at several different sites in the body. In studies in which liver cancer occurred, other toxic changes in the liver also occurred. Other organs in which increased cancer rates were observed in animals exposed to TCDD include the thyroid and adrenal glands, the skin, and the lungs. Organs in which decreased cancer rates were observed in animals exposed to TCDD include the uterus, the pancreas, and the pituitary, mammary, and adrenal glands.

In addition to increasing cancer rates in animals by itself, TCDD can increase tumor formation by other chemicals. For example, when a single dose of a known carcinogen is applied to the skin of mice and that dose is followed by multiple doses of TCDD over a period of several months, more skin tumors are seen than would be expected from the single dose of carcinogen alone. Similar results are obtained in rat livers when a single dose of a liver carcinogen is followed by multiple doses of TCDD.

In rats, liver tumor formation associated with TCDD exposure is dependent on the presence of ovaries; in other words, only female rats that have not had their ovaries removed can develop liver tumors when they are exposed to TCDD. This observation indicates that complex hormonal interactions are likely to be involved in TCDD-induced carcinogenesis.

Mechanism of Toxicity   TCDD has a wide range of effects on growth regulation, hormone systems, and other factors associated with the regulation of activities in normal cells. These actions of TCDD may affect tumor formation. Understanding how TCDD influences tumor formation in laboratory animals may help us understand whether TCDD affects tumor formation in humans.

It has been shown that TCDD binds to a protein in animal and human cells called the Ah receptor. It is thus possible that TCDD, together with the Ah receptor, can interact with sites on DNA and alter the information obtained from DNA in such a way that a normal liver cell is transformed into a cancerous liver cell. Direct proof of this possibility has not been obtained.

Carcinogenicity: Herbicides

Several studies of the carcinogenicity of 2,4-D, 2,4,5-T, picloram, and cacodylic acid have been performed in laboratory animals. In general, they produced negative results, although some were not performed using rigorous criteria for the study of cancer in animals, and some produced equivocal results that could be interpreted as either positive or negative. These studies and their results were summarized in detail in *VAO*.

2,4-D was administered to rats, mice, and dogs in their food, by injecting it under their skin, or by placing it directly into their stomachs. All the results were negative, except for one study that found an increased rate of brain tumors in male rats, but not female rats, receiving the highest dose. These tumors also occurred in the control group and thus may have occurred spontaneously and not as a result of 2,4-D exposure.

2,4,5-T has been administered to rats and mice in their food, in their drinking water, by injecting it under their skin, or by placing it directly into their stomachs.

Picloram has been tested in rats and mice in their food. Results of all of these studies were uniformly negative, with the exception of one study using picloram in which liver tumors appeared, but were attributed to the presence of a contaminant, hexachlorobenzene.

Cacodylic acid has been tested in a very limited study in mice both in their food and by placing it directly into their stomachs.

Immunotoxicity: TCDD

TCDD was shown to have a number of effects on the immune systems of laboratory animals. Studies in mice, rats, guinea pigs, and monkeys indicated that TCDD suppresses the function of certain components of the immune system in a dose-related manner; that is, as the dose of TCDD increases, its ability to suppress immune function increases. TCDD suppressed the function of cells of the immune system, such as lymphocytes (cell-mediated immune response), as well as the generation of antibodies by B cells (humoral immune response). Increased susceptibility to infectious disease has been reported following TCDD administration. In addition, TCDD increased the number of tumors that formed in mice following injection of tumor cells.

The effects of TCDD on the immune system appear to vary among species.

Mechanism of Toxicity It is likely that the Ah receptor plays a role in some types of immunotoxicity. Some studies indicate that an animal's hormonal status may contribute to its sensitivity to immunotoxicity. The fact that TCDD induces such a wide variety of effects in animals suggests that it is likely to have some effect in humans as well.

Immunotoxicity: Herbicides

The potential immunotoxicity of the herbicides used in Vietnam has been studied to only a very limited extent. Effects on the immune system of mice were reported for 2,4-D administered at doses that were high enough to produce clinical toxicity, but these effects did not occur at low doses. The potential for picloram to act as a contact sensitizer (i.e., to produce an allergic response on the skin) was tested, but other aspects of immunotoxicology were not examined.

Reproductive and Developmental Toxicity: TCDD

TCDD was reported to have a number of effects on the reproductive and developmental functions of laboratory animals. For example, administration of TCDD to male rats, mice, guinea pigs, marmosets, monkeys, and chickens can elicit reproductive toxicity by affecting testicular function, decreasing fertility, and decreasing the rate of sperm production. TCDD has also been found to decrease the levels of hormones such as testosterone in rats. The reproductive systems of adult male laboratory animals are considered to be relatively insensitive to TCDD, because high doses are required to elicit effects. Potential developmental toxicity following exposure of male animals to TCDD has not been studied.

Studies in female animals are limited but demonstrate reduced fertility, decreased ability to remain pregnant throughout gestation, decreased litter size, increased fetal death, impaired ovary function, decreased levels of hormones such as estradiol and progesterone, and increased rates of fetal abnormalities. Most of these effects may have occurred as a result of TCDD's general toxicity to the pregnant animal, however, and not as a result of a TCDD-specific mechanism that acted directly on the reproductive system.

Mechanism of Toxicity Little information is available on the cellular and molecular mechanisms of action that mediate TCDD's reproductive and developmental effects in laboratory animals. Evidence from mice indicates that the Ah receptor may play a role: mice with Ah receptors that have a relatively high affinity for TCDD respond to lower doses than do mice with a relatively low affinity. Other, as-yet-unidentified, factors also play a role, however, and it is

possible that these effects occur only secondarily to TCDD-induced general toxicity. Extrapolating these results to humans is not straightforward, because the
many factors that determine susceptibility to reproductive and developmental
effects vary among species.

Reproductive and Developmental Toxicity: Herbicides

Several studies evaluated the reproductive and developmental toxicity of
herbicides in laboratory animals. Results indicated that 2,4-D does not affect
male or female fertility and does not produce fetal abnormalities, but when pregnant rats or mice are exposed it does reduce the rate of growth of offspring and
increase their rate of mortality. Very high doses were required to elicit these
effects. 2,4,5-T was toxic to fetuses when administered to pregnant rats, mice,
and hamsters. Cacodylic acid is toxic to rat, mouse, and hamster fetuses at high
doses that are also toxic to the pregnant mother. Limited data suggested that
picloram may produce fetal abnormalities in rabbits at doses that are also toxic to
the pregnant animals.

Investigations of the developmental toxicity of the herbicides suggested that
they can be toxic to developing animals, but high doses are required.

Other Toxicities: TCDD

TCDD has been reported to elicit several other kinds of toxicity in laboratory
animals. Effects of TCDD on the liver include increasing the rate at which liver
cells multiply, increasing the rate of other cell death, increasing fat levels in liver
cells, decreasing bile flow, and increasing the levels of protein and of substances
that are precursors to heme synthesis. TCDD also increases the levels of certain
enzymes in the liver, but this effect is not considered toxic. Mice and rats are
susceptible to TCDD-induced liver toxicity, but guinea pigs and hamsters are not.
It is possible that liver toxicity is associated with susceptibility to liver cancer.

Other toxic effects of TCDD that have been reported in laboratory animals
include reduced blood glucose levels and starvation, increased rates at which
cells in the gastrointestinal tract multiply, and changes in skin cells.

Other Toxicities: Herbicides

The herbicides used in Vietnam were reported to elicit adverse effects in a
number of organs in laboratory animals. The liver is a target organ for toxicity
induced by 2,4-D, 2,4,5-T, and picloram, with changes reportedly similar to those
induced by TCDD. Some kidney toxicity was reported in animals exposed to 2,4-
D and cacodylic acid. Exposure to 2,4-D has also been associated with effects on
blood, such as reduced levels of heme and red blood cells.

LITERATURE UPDATE

In this section, the results of experimental studies published during the period 1992-95 are reviewed. The section begins with an overview of the toxicology data on dioxin and the four herbicides. This is followed by updates of the toxicological profiles reviewed in *VAO*. These include 2,4-dichlorophenoxyacetic acid (2,4-D); 2,4,5-trichlorophenoxyacetic acid (2,4,5-T); picloram; and cacodylic acid; as well as the contaminant 2,3,7,8-tetrachlorodibenzo-*p*-dioxin (TCDD). As in *VAO*, this review is intended to summarize the experimental data that provide the scientific basis for the assessment of biologic plausibility of the health outcomes reported in epidemiologic studies. Efforts to establish the biologic plausibility of effects due to herbicide exposure in the laboratory strengthen the evidence for the effects of the herbicides suspected to occur in humans.

Overview

This chapter reviews the results of animal studies published during the past three years that investigated the toxicokinetics, mechanism of action, and disease outcomes of dioxin and the four herbicides employed in Vietnam. These data were used to provide the scientific basis for the assessment of biologic plausibility of the health outcomes in epidemiological studies. In examining the individual toxicity profiles of the chemicals in question, readers must consider that differences in chemical levels, frequency of administration, predetermined health status, genetic factors, and routes of exposure influence toxicity outcomes.

The toxicity of the herbicides used in Vietnam remains poorly studied. In general, 2,4-D, 2,4,5-T, cacodylic acid, and picloram have not been identified as particularly toxic substances, since high concentrations are often required to modulate cellular and biochemical processes. However, some studies reported during the period 1992-95 have observed impairment of motor function in rats administered high single oral doses of 2,4-D. The ability of 2,4,5-T to interfere with calcium homeostasis in vitro was documented and linked to the teratogenic effects of 2,4,5-T on the early development of sea urchin eggs. Cacodylic acid was reported to induce renal lesions in rats. No studies were published pertaining to the toxicity of picloram.

The half-life of 2,4-D and 2,4,5-T is relatively short and does not appear to extend beyond two weeks. 2,4-D binds covalently to hepatic proteins and lipids, but the molecular basis of this interaction and its biologic consequences are unknown. Evidence was presented suggesting that both 2,4-D and 2,4,5-T are capable of gaining access to the central nervous system and that the uptake process is energy-dependent. A series of studies indicates that high concentrations of cacodylic acid result in the formation of a toxic intermediate, the dimethylarsenic radical.

TCDD elicits a diverse spectrum of sex-, strain-, age-, and species-specific effects, including carcinogenicity, immunotoxicity, reproductive/developmental toxicity, hepatotoxicity, neurotoxicity, chloracne, and loss of body weight. To date, the consensus is that TCDD is not genotoxic and that its ability to influence the carcinogenic process is mediated via epigenetic events such as enzyme induction, cell proliferation, apoptosis, and intracellular communication.

Recent studies on the effects of TCDD and related substances on the immune system amplify earlier findings and suggest that these compounds affect primarily the T-cell arm of the immune response. The effects may result from decreased functions of the thymus gland. Direct effects of TCDD on T cells in vitro, however, have not been demonstrated, suggesting that the action of TCDD may be indirect. A number of recent studies suggest that cytokines may play an important role in regulating the immune response. It should be emphasized that very little change to the overall immune competence of the intact animal has been reported. In contrast, a number of animal studies of the reproductive and developmental toxicity of TCDD suggest that developing animals may be particularly sensitive to the effects of TCDD. Specifically, male reproductive function has been reported to be altered following perinatal exposure to TCDD. In addition, experimental studies in rats of the effects of TCDD on the peripheral nervous system suggest that a single low dose of TCDD can cause a toxic polyneuropathy.

Other studies published during the reference period provide evidence that hepatotoxicity of TCDD involves AhR-dependent mechanisms. Specifically, there is evidence that the AhR receptor plays a role in the co-mitogenic action of TCDD with epidermal growth factor and in the induction of liver enzymes involved in the metabolism of xenobiotics. Acute exposures to TCDD have been correlated with effects on intermediary metabolism and hepatomegaly. The myocardium has been shown to be a target of TCDD toxicity; impairment of a cAMP-modulated contraction has been implicated. TCDD has been reported to decrease an acidic type I Keratin involved in epidermal development, leading to keratinocyte hyperproliferation and skin irritations such as chloracne. Recent evidence suggests that the inhibition of glucose transport in adipose tissue, pancreas, and brain may be one of the major contributing factors to the wasting syndrome. Finally, in vitro studies have identified glomerular mesangial cells as sensitive cellular targets. These findings are consistent with epidemiologic reports that aromatic hydrocarbons result in glomerulonephritis.

By far, the majority of the studies identified during the reference period focused on the elucidation of the molecular mechanism of TCDD toxicity. The evidence further supports the concept that the toxic effects of TCDD involve AhR-dependent mechanisms. A better appreciation of the complexity of TCDD effects in target cells has led to the development of refined, physiologically based pharmacokinetic models. These models take into account intracellular diffusion, receptor and protein binding, and liver induction to establish the fractional distribution of the total body burden as a function of the overall body concentration.

The association of TCDD with the cytosolic AhR was shown to require a second protein, known as ARNT, for DNA binding capability and transcriptional activation of target genes. Comparison of the murine and human AhR have demonstrated that the carboxy terminal region involved in transactivation is hypervariable, a feature which may account in part for species differences in TCDD responsiveness. During the referenced period, expression of multiple forms of the AhR was documented suggesting differences in cellular responsiveness to TCDD, and the multiplicity of biological effects may be related to such differences. Evidence has also begun to accumulate suggesting that events in addition to receptor binding also influence the biological response to TCDD. Specifically, there is evidence for ligand-independent activation of the AhR evidence for transcriptional independent responses, and data to support the review that the transcriptional regulation of the AhR-responsive genes is dictated by combinatorial interactions among proteins. It is now also clear that AhR-related signaling influences, and is itself influenced by, other signal transduction mechanisms at low concentrations. Signaling interactions explaining the toxic effects of TCDD may involve growth factors, free radicals, the interaction of TCDD with the estrogen transduction pathway, and protein kinases.

The normal cellular functions of the AhR and its role in cellular homeostasis remain undefined. Dioxin-independent activation of the AhR has now been demonstrated, suggesting that unidentified endogenous ligands are operational in the absence of TCDD. The exciting development of AhR-deficient "knock-out" mice by homologous recombination in embryonic stem cells will likely provide the tools to define the roles of the AhR in mammalian species (Fernandez-Salguero et al., 1995).

Toxic equivalency factors (TEFs) have been used to estimate the potential health risks associated with exposure to TCDD and complex mixtures containing structurally similar chemicals. The approach assumes linearity of the toxic response for TCDD and is based on a receptor-mediated mechanism of action. The TEF approach has come under increasing scrutiny because it disregards potentially significant kinetic interactions, tissue-specific effects, and interactions among chemicals present in complex mixtures. These factors, in addition to dietary factors and interspecies and interindividual differences in sensitivity, may influence TCDD toxicity.

UPDATE OF TOXICITY PROFILES

In this section, we update the toxicological profiles on the five substances discussed in *VAO*: 2,4-dichlorophenoxyacetic acid (2,4-D); 2,4,5-trichlorophenoxyacetic acid (2,4,5-T); picloram; cacodylic acid; and 2,3,7,8-tetrachlorodibenzo-*p*-dioxin (TCDD or dioxin). Each update begins with a summary, which is followed by a review of the experimental studies published during the period

1992-95. This information is organized under the headings of toxicokinetics, mechanism of action, and disease outcomes and mechanisms of toxicity.

Toxicity Profile Update of 2,4-D

Summary

Studies published during the period 1992-95 provide evidence that 2,4-D binds covalently to hepatic proteins and lipids; the molecular basis of this interaction and its biologic consequences are unknown. 2,4-D has also been shown to accumulate in the brain. This process is mediated through an active anion transport system. 2,4-D is not considered to be particularly toxic because high concentrations are often required to modulate cellular and biochemical processes. Impairment of motor functions has been reported in rats orally administered a single high oral dose of 2,4-D.

Toxicokinetics

Measurable amounts of 2,4-D can be detected in the blood and urine of dogs several days after exposure to contaminated lawns under natural conditions (Reynolds et al., 1994). Among 44 dogs potentially exposed to 2,4-D-treated lawns for an average of 10.9 days, 33 dogs (75 percent) had urine concentrations of 2,4-D greater than or equal to 10 µg/l, and 17 dogs (39 percent) had urine concentrations of ≥ 50 µg/l. Among 15 dogs with no known exposure to 2,4-D-treated lawns in the previous 42 days, 4 (27 percent) had 2,4-D in urine, 1 at a concentration of ≥ 50 µg/l. The highest mean concentration of 2,4-D in urine (21.3 mg/l) was found in dogs sampled within two days after application of the herbicide.

The hepatocellular distribution of 2,4-D was examined by Evangelista et al. (1993). The herbicide decreases total lipids, especially phospholipids, both in total liver and in microsomes. 2,4-D crosses the liver plasma membrane and can be detected in all subcellular fractions. 2,4-D binds covalently to hepatic proteins and lipids, with protein binding being ten-fold higher than lipid. The mechanism of and implications for covalent binding of 2,4-D remain to be defined.

2,4-D has been demonstrated to accumulate in the brain without damaging the blood–brain barrier. This accumulation is related to the biochemical properties of 2,4-D, which is a very strong acid and is partially soluble in water. Recent experiments have demonstrated that the mechanism that mediates the accumulation of 2,4-D in the brain is the saturation of an active organic anion transport system in the choroid plexus (Kim et al., 1988; Kim et al., 1994). The brain depends on the active transport of organic anions by the choroid plexus to keep potentially toxic anions, including foreign chemicals, as 2,4-D and endogenous neurotransmitter metabolites, at low concentrations in the central nervous system. Levels of endogenous anionic brain metabolites of dopamine and serotonin increase when elevated levels of organic anions, such as 2,4-D, are present in the serum (Kim et al., 1988).

No other studies pertaining to the absorption, distribution, metabolism, and excretion of 2,4-D were identified.

Mechanism of Action

The mechanisms underlying the toxic effects of 2,4-D may involve alterations in mitochondrial bioenergetics, effects on the metabolism of xenobiotics, and/or inhibition of protein synthesis. Mechanistic studies investigating these effects are summarized below.

Jover et al. (1994) completed an extensive series of in vitro toxicity studies in which the toxic effects of several chemicals, including 2,4-D, were examined in human and rat cultured hepatocytes and in two established cell lines (HepG2 and 3T3). 2,4-D elicited a basal cytotoxic effect at high concentrations but was not considered to be particularly hepatotoxic or to exert species-specific toxicity. Palmeira et al. (1994a) reported that cytotoxicity involves alterations in mitochondrial bioenergetics. Concentration-dependent decreases in mitochondrial membrane potential and in repolarization rate were observed in isolated mitochondria. Tripathy et al. (1993) reported that 2,4-D is genotoxic in somatic and germ-line cells of Drosophila at high concentrations. The relevance of the findings in Drosophila to humans is uncertain.

2,4-D appears to modulate hepatocyte function and to influence biochemical pathways involved in drug metabolism. Palmeira et al. (1994a) reported that 2,4-D induces cell death in isolated rat hepatocytes by decreasing cellular glutathione and depleting adenine and pyridine nucleotide contents. These results are in opposition to those reported by Evangelista et al. (1993), in which fertilized hen eggs were topically treated with 3.1 mg of the 2,4-D butyl ester before starting incubation. The microsomal and cytosolic glutathione S-transferase activities remained unchanged. No significant change in reduced glutathione content between control and treated livers was observed. However, the catalase activity doubled and the glucose-6-phosphatase activity decreased by 46 percent, suggesting that the ester but not the parent compound may have effects on the metabolism of xenobiotics. Despite different effects on cellular glutathione levels, studies conducted by Palmeira et al. (1994a,b) and Evangelista et al. (1993) suggest that 2,4-D appears to modulate hepatocyte function and to influence the biochemical pathways involved in the metabolism of xenobiotics.

A significant decrease in total lipids, especially phospholipid content, was observed. In vivo studies did not reveal any changes in glutathione-S-transferase activity, although in vitro a decrease in enzymatic activity was observed. Catalase levels increased two-fold, while glucose-6-phosphatase activity decreased 46 percent. Although the relevance of the findings in chickens to humans is unknown, these data provide additional support that 2,4-D may influence the biochemical pathways involved in the metabolism of xenobiotics.

The effect of 2,4-D on the in vitro synthesis of proteins was studied in Chinese hamster ovary cells by Rivarola et al. (1992), who reported marked inhibition of protein synthesis in cells treated with 1 Mm of 2,4-D for 24 hours. Interestingly, this effect could be reversed by the addition of 0.1 Mm of putrescine, spermidine, or spermine, suggesting that alterations in polyamine metabolism mediate the ability of 2,4-D to interfere with protein synthesis. In a recent study, fertilized hen eggs were externally treated with a single 3.1 mg of 2,4-D (de Moro et al., 1993). The herbicide was shown to induce hypomyelination even before the period of active myelination. The DNA content in brain was increased from the fourteenth embryonic day to the first day of hatching. It is not clear if similar changes occur in mammalian species.

Disease Outcomes and Mechanisms of Toxicity

In this section, we summarize studies that investigated the toxic effects of 2,4-D. The mechanism of toxicity, if known, is also explained.

Carcinogenicity   Data prior to 1993 suggest that, in general, 2,4-D produced negative results in carcinogenicity bioassays. In support of this, Edwards et al. (1993) found no association between 2,4-D exposure and mutation of C-N-ras in the dog, suggesting that oncogenic activation of this gene does not occur.

Neurotoxicity   Case reports of human poisonings and studies in cats and dogs administered high doses of 2,4-D have demonstrated several central nervous system effects, including general sedation, tenseness, loss of righting reflex, motor incoordination, and coma. The animal studies suggest that the primary site of action is the cerebral cortex or the reticular formation (Dési et al., 1962a,b; Arnold et al., 1991).

The acute effects of 2,4-D on the central nervous system were recently studied in male Wistar rats (Oliveira and Palermo-Neto, 1993). Behavioral, neuroanatomical, and neurochemical studies were performed. The rats were given single oral doses of 2,4-D ranging from 10 mg/kg of body weight to 300 mg/kg. These doses were chosen because they were high enough to induce sedation and impairment of motor functions but were lower than the calculated LD_{50} for Wistar rats (945 mg/kg). Single doses of 2,4-D were able to decrease rearing frequencies, decrease locomotion, and increase the deviation of immobility in an open-field test. The neuroanatomical and neurochemical results suggested that 2,4-D modified the functional activities of serotonergic systems within the central nervous system.

Other Toxicities   No other studies were identified that implicated other health outcomes in laboratory animals.

Toxicity Profile Update of 2,4,5-T

Summary

Only one toxicokinetic study and one developmental toxicity study were published on 2,4,5-T during the period 1992-95. Evidence was presented suggesting that 2,4,5-T gains access to the central nervous system and that the uptake process is energy-dependent. The ability of this herbicide to interfere with calcium homeostasis in vitro was also documented and linked to the teratogenic effects of 2,4,5-T on the early development of sea urchin eggs. The relevance of this finding to humans is not known.

Toxicokinetics

Kim and Pritchard (1993) examined the transport of 2,4,5-T across the blood–cerebrospinal fluid barrier using the isolated choroid plexus of the adult rabbit in vitro and ventriculocisternal perfusion in vivo. In vitro transport was effective at tissue concentrations 20 times those found in the medium after only five min of incubation with 1 μM 2,4,5-T. Uptake was energy-dependent and inhibited by ouabain, phloridzin, and several organic anions, suggesting that 2,4,5-T is a suitable substrate for the organic anion transport system of the rabbit choroid plexus. These data suggest that 2,4,5-T can gain access to the central nervous system.

No other studies were identified pertaining to the absorption, distribution, metabolism, and excretion of 2,4,5-T.

Disease Outcomes and Mechanisms of Toxicity

In this section, we summarize studies that investigate the toxic effects of 2,4,5-T. The mechanism of toxicity, if known, is also explained.

Developmental Toxicity   The effects of 2,4,5-T on the early development of sea urchin eggs were investigated by Graillet and Girard (1994). Concentrations lower than 5×10^{-4} M were shown to delay the first cleavages and produce a teratogenic effect characterized by a large spectrum of structural malformations at the pluteus stage. The relevance of these findings to humans is not known.

Mechanism of Toxicity   2,4,5-T has been shown to increase plasmalemmal calcium permeability of unfertilized sea urchin eggs by opening voltage-dependent calcium channels. Calcium permeability was also increased after fertilization of eggs. ATP-dependent intracellular sequestration of calcium in cortices in vivo was inhibited, suggesting that the teratogenic potency of 2,4,5-T in sea urchin eggs is associated with delay in first cleavages and alterations in calcium homeostasis.

Other Toxicities   No other studies were identified that implicated other health outcomes in laboratory animals.

Toxicity Profile Update of Cacodylic Acid

Summary

During the reference period, cacodylic acid was reported to induce renal lesions in rats. A series of studies indicates that high concentrations of cacodylic acid result in the formation of a toxic intermediate: the dimethylarsenic radical.

Toxicokinetics

No studies were identified pertaining to the absorption, distribution, metabolism, and excretion of cacodylic acid.

Mechanism of Action

In a series of studies conducted by Yamanaka and colleagues (1993, 1994a, 1994b), results indicated that cacodylic acid induces lung DNA damage in mice and that this effect involves formation of the dimethylarsenic peroxyl radical during metabolic processing of cacodylic acid. DNA damage was hypothesized to result from the radical's ability to induce single-strand breaks and DNA-protein crosslinks. These results were later reproduced in a human embryonic alveolar epithelial cell line where alkali-labile sites in DNA were shown to precede the formation of DNA single-strand breaks and DNA-protein crosslinks (Yamanaka et al., 1994b). However, the relevance of these data has been questioned, because the changes have only been observed at high concentrations of the parent compound.

Disease Outcomes and Mechanisms of Toxicity

In this section, we summarize studies that investigate the toxic effects of cacodylic acid. The mechanism of toxicity, if known, is also explained.

Renal Toxicity   Only one study examined the toxicological effects of cacodylic acid. In 1993, Murai et al. reported that cacodylic acid induces renal lesions in F344/DuCrj rats following oral administration. Male and female rats were administered 57, 85, and 113 mg/kg of cacodylic acid for four weeks. Chemical treatment was associated with dose-related decreases in body weight and survival rates in both sexes. Mortality was higher and appeared more quickly in females than males. Histopathological analysis revealed proximal tubular degeneration and necrosis, as well as papillary necrosis, and hyperplasia of the epithelium covering the papillae. Since extensive proximal tubular necrosis was only found in dead animals of both sexes, these investigators concluded that death was indeed mediated by nephrotoxicity.

Other Toxicities No other studies were identified that implicated other health outcomes in laboratory animals.

Toxicity Profile Update of Picloram

No studies were identified during the period 1992-1995 pertaining to the toxicokinetics, mechanism of action, or toxicity of picloram.

Toxicity Profile Update of TCDD

Summary

TCDD elicits a diverse spectrum of sex-, strain-, age-, and species-specific effects, including carcinogenicity, immunotoxicity, reproductive/developmental toxicity, hepatotoxicity, neurotoxicity, chloracne, loss of body weight, and numerous biological responses, such as the induction of phase I and phase II drug-metabolizing enzymes and the modulation of hormone systems and factors associated with the regulation of cellular differentiation and proliferation.

TCDD is slowly removed from the body. It is metabolized by liver enzymes to water-soluble derivatives that are more easily eliminated from the body than TCDD itself. The development of refined, physiologically based pharmacokinetic models provides insight into the complexity of TCDD effects in target cells. These models take into account intracellular diffusion, receptor and protein binding, and liver enzyme induction to establish the fractional distribution of the total body burden as a function of the overall body concentrations.

The evidence to date continues to support the notion that the biologic effects of TCDD are often mediated by the aryl hydrocarbon receptor (AhR), a member of the ligand-activated transcription factor superfamily. The AhR requires a second protein, known as ARNT, for DNA binding capability and transcriptional activation. Cloning of the AhR and ARNT proteins have identified them as bHLH proteins. Comparisons of the murine and human AhR have demonstrated that the N-terminal but not the C-terminal region of both proteins is highly conserved. The carboxy terminal region involved in transactivation is hypervariable, a feature that may account in part for the species differences in TCDD responsiveness.

Evidence is beginning to accumulate that both the expression of multiple forms of the AhR in target tissues and events other than receptor binding influence the biological response to TCDD. With respect to the latter, there is evidence for ligand-independent activation of the AhR, for transcriptional independent responses (e.g., modulation of cellular kinase activities and calcium homeostasis), and data to support the view that the transcriptional regulation of the AhR-responsive genes is dictated by combinatorial interactions among proteins.

It is clear that AhR-related signaling influences, and is itself influenced by, other signal transduction mechanisms at low concentrations. Signaling interactions explaining the toxic effects of TCDD may involve growth factors, free radicals, the interaction of TCDD with the estrogen transduction pathway, and protein kinases. It appears that PKC is responsible for the phosphorylation of the active complex, but it appears unlikely that PKC phosphorylation is required for ligand binding and transformation. The biologic significance of phosphorylation-related events is not yet fully understood, but it is interesting to note that intracellular protein tyrosine kinase phosphorylation is a more sensitive index of TCDD exposure than hepatic EROD induction.

Toxic equivalency factors (TEFs) have been used to estimate the potential health risks associated with exposure to TCDD and complex mixtures containing structurally similar chemicals. The approach assumes linearity of the toxic response for TCDD and is based on a receptor-mediated mechanism of action. The TEF approach has come under increasing scrutiny, because it disregards potentially significant kinetic interactions, tissue-specific effects, and interactions among chemicals present in complex mixtures. These factors, in addition to dietary factors and interspecies and interindividual differences in sensitivity, may influence TCDD toxicity.

Studies published during the reference period have focused primarily on the mechanisms of toxicity of TCDD. To date, the consensus is that TCDD is not genotoxic and that its ability to influence the carcinogenic process is mediated via epigenetic events such as enzyme induction, cell proliferation, apoptosis, and intracellular communication.

Recent studies on the effects of TCDD and related substances on the immune system amplify earlier findings and suggest that these compounds affect primarily the T-cell arm of the immune response. The effects may result from decreased functions of the thymus gland. Direct effects of TCDD on T cells in vitro, however, have not been demonstrated, suggesting that the action of TCDD may be indirect. A number of recent studies suggest that cytokines may play an important role in regulating the immune response. It should be emphasized that very little change to the overall immune competence of the intact animal has been reported. In contrast, a number of animal studies of the reproductive and developmental toxicity of TCDD suggest that developing animals may be particularly sensitive to the effects of TCDD. Specifically, male reproductive function has been reported to be altered following perinatal exposure to TCDD. In addition, experimental studies in rats of the effects of TCDD on the peripheral nervous system suggest that a single low dose of TCDD can cause a toxic polyneuropathy.

Other studies have focused on the mechanism of hepatotoxicity, cardiovascular toxicity, wasting syndrome, chloracne, and renal toxicity. There is evidence that hepatotoxicity of TCDD involves AhR-dependent mechanisms. Specifically, there is evidence that the AhR receptor plays a role in the co-mitogenic action of TCDD with epidermal growth factor and in the induction of liver enzymes involved in the metabolism of xenobiotics. Acute exposures to TCDD have been correlated with effects on intermediary metabolism and hepatomegaly. The myocardium has been shown to be a target of TCDD toxicity; impairment of a cAMP-modulated contraction has been implicated. TCDD has been reported to decrease an acidic type I Keratin involved in epidermal development, leading to keratinocyte hyperproliferation and skin irritations such as chloracne. Recent evidence suggests that the inhibition of glucose transport in adipose tissue, pancreas, and brain may be one of the major contributing factors to the wasting syndrome. Finally, in vitro studies have identified glomerular mesangial cells as sensitive cellular targets. These findings are consistent with epidemiologic reports that aromatic hydrocarbons result in glomerulonephritis.

Toxicokinetics

Physiologically based pharmacokinetic models for the tissue distribution and enzyme-induction properties of dioxin have recently been proposed by Anderson et al. (1993) and Carrier et al. (1995a, 1995b). In the most recent model, Carrier et al. (1995a) describes the distribution kinetics of polychlorinated dibenzodioxins (PCDDs) and polychlorinated dibensofurans (PCDFs) in mammalian species. The model was designed to take into account intracellular diffusion, receptor and protein binding, and liver enzyme induction to establish the fractional distribution of the total body burden between liver and adipose tissues as a function of the overall body concentrations at any one time. In this model, the distribution in rats, monkeys, and humans was shown to follow a nonlinear pattern. In a companion study (Carrier et al., 1995b), it was shown that the liver fraction of the total body burden decreases as overall body concentration decreases, leading to lower global elimination rates and longer half-lives. The study also concluded that for a given body burden of PCDDs and PCDFs, the adipose tissue concentration is inversely proportional to the mass of the adipose tissue.

A recent study by Geyer et al. (1993) concluded that total body fat content for lipophilic chemicals, including TCDD, correlates inversely with lethality and in some instances serves as a detoxication mechanism by which TCDD is removed from sites of action. This interpretation is consistent with the conclusions reached for veterans of Operation Ranch Hand (Wolfe et al., 1994). The extent to which fat mobilization influences TCDD toxicity has not been completely defined but is likely to be of toxicological significance. The wasting syndrome may influence the disposition of TCDD (Weber et al., 1993), with TCDD concentrations in tissue increasing only when the relative tissue volumes decrease more rapidly than the whole body elimination rate (Roth et al., 1994).

TCDD is removed slowly from the body. In humans it takes seven to ten years or more for half of the body burden to be removed (Wolfe et al., 1994). TCDD is metabolized by enzymes in the liver to form water-soluble derivatives that are more easily eliminated from the body than TCDD itself. Due to their more rapid elimination, the water-soluable derivatives of TCDD are also thought to be much less toxic to animals than TCDD itself.

Mechanism of Action

The mechanism by which TCDD elicits its effects is thought to be mediated by the aryl hydrocarbon receptor (AhR), a member of the ligand-activated transcription factor superfamily. The studies summarized below discuss the structural and functional aspects of the AhR, its DNA binding capability and transcriptional activation, and the biological consequences associated with the activation. This is followed by a discussion of the body of accumulating evidence (see Inconsistencies in the Receptor Model) suggesting that multiple forms of the AhR, as well as events in addition to receptor binding, influence the biological response to TCDD. This section ends with a discussion of the method used to estimate the potential health risk associated with exposure to TCDD and the factors influencing TCDD toxicity (e.g., tissue specificity, interspecies and interindividual differences in sensitivity, chemical interaction).

Structural and Functional Aspects of the AhR   A cDNA encoding the murine Ah receptor (Ahb-1 allele) was first isolated and characterized from wild type Hepa-1c1c7 cells (Burbach et al., 1992; Ema et al., 1992). Sequence analysis revealed three domains: a basic helix-loop-helix (BHLH) motif; a region that exhibits sequence homology with Per (a Drosophilia circadian rhythm protein) and Sim (a regulatory protein that participates in Drospholia central nervous system development), termed the "PAS" region; and a "glutamine-rich" region. The BHLH region is believed to be involved in heterodimerization and DNA binding, the PAS region in ligand binding (Dolwick et al., 1993), and the "glutamine-rich" region in activiation (Whitlock, 1993). With respect to the BHLH region, of particular significance is the fact that the AhR itself does not bind strongly to DNA but requires another protein, the AhR nuclear translocator (ARNT) protein, for DNA binding capability and transcriptional activation (Reyes et al., 1992).

The AhR locus encodes the structural gene for the AhR and has recently been localized to human chromosome 7, band p21 (Le Beau et al., 1994; Ema et al., 1994). Recent studies have characterized a cDNA encoding a human AhR and shown that this protein shares many of the same structural and functional regions as the murine AhR (Dolwick et al., 1993). Comparison of the murine and human receptors has demonstrated that the amino terminal halves of these proteins are highly conserved. This high degree of homology is consistent with the region's role in ligand binding, DNA recognition, and dimerization. A number of conserved phosphorylation sites are also present in the amino terminal half of the protein and a consensus nuclear localization sequence in the center of the PAS region. In contrast, the "glutamine-rich" carboxy end of the proteins is poorly conserved and referred to as a hypervariable region (Dolwick et al., 1993). This region is believed to participate in receptor transformation to a high DNA affinity conformation and transcriptional activation and thus may account for the variability often reported within and across species.

The cDNA for mouse and human ARNT have been recently cloned (Reisz-Porszasz et al., 1994; Li et al., 1994). The human ARNT cDNA encodes an 86 kDa protein which, like the AhR, contains a BHLH domain and a domain homologous to Per and Sim. ARNT itself does not bind TCDD or DNA (Whitelaw et al., 1993), but the AhR:ARNT heterodimer functions as a transcriptional enhancer of a number of genes. This is described in more detail below (see DNA Binding Capability and Transcriptional Activation).

In mice, four receptor alleles have been identified that encode for the AhR (Poland et al., 1994). These alleles differ by a few point mutations in the open reading frame and by additional sequences in their carboxy ends. The AhR[b-1], AhR[b-2], and AhR[b-3] alleles encode proteins of 95, 104, and 105 kDa, respectively. The Ah[b-1] receptor is more thermostable than the Ah[b-2] and is not as easily activated in vitro (Poland et al., 1994). The fourth allele, referred to as AhR[d], encodes a 104 kDa protein that has a ten-fold lower affinity for agonist relative to other alleles; thus mice harboring the Ahr[d] allele are much less susceptible to the biological effects of receptor ligands. A polymerase chain reaction approach has been used to determine the AhR mRNA content in several tissues of C57BL/6J and DBA/2J mice (Li et al., 1994). The highest mRNA level was found in lung, followed by heart, liver, thymus, brain, and placenta. Low levels were found in spleen, kidney, and muscle. No significant differences in mRNA levels were found between the two mouse strains.

The normal cellular functions of the AhR and its role in cellular homeostasis have remained elusive for the past 20 years. The AhR binds aromatic hydrocarbons and in this manner serves as a sink for highly lipophilic molecules. This, however, is not likely to be the primary function of the protein under normal conditions. In support of this suggestion is the demonstration that loss of the AhR is associated with immune deficiency and lymphocyte loss (Fernandez-Salguero et al., 1995).

The exciting development of AhR-deficient "knock-out" mice by homologous recombination in embryonic stem cells will likely provide the tools to define the roles of the AhR in mammalian species (Fernandez-Salguero et al., 1995). The data in this highly publicized study implicate the AhR in the regulation of liver and immune system development. Decreased accumulation of lymphocytes in spleen and lymph node, but not in thymus, was observed in these animals. The livers of these mice were reduced in size by 50 percent and exhibited bile duct fibrosis.

DNA Binding Capability and Transcription Activation   The molecular mechanism of AhR-mediated responses has primarily been defined based on studies of TCDD-induced cytochrome P450-IA1 (CYP1A1) gene expression. The unbound AhR appears to be a multimeric cytosolic complex that undergoes a process of transformation following binding of a ligand, such as TCDD, to the AhR complex. Recent immunofluorescence studies have confirmed the cytosolic localization of the unoccupied AhR and the nuclear translocation after ligand binding (Pollenz and Poland, 1993). Although the molecular events associated with the transformation process have yet to be fully defined, transformation involves dissociation of two molecules of heat shock protein 90 (Hsp90). Hsp90 itself is composed of two separate gene products, hsp86 and hsp84 (Perdew et al., 1993). Hsp90 represses the intrinsic DNA binding ability of the AhR and preserves the conformation of the AhR (Pongratz et al., 1992). The dissociation of Hsp90 allows the transformed ligand-bound receptor to form a heterodimer with ARNT (Whitelaw et al., 1993).

The TCDD-transformed AhR complex binds to xenobiotic responsive sequences (XREs) in the 5′ flanking region of downstream genes, resulting in initiation of transcription. Analysis of the murine TCDD-responsive domain of CYP1A1 indicates that enhancer activity results from the sum of the activities of as many as six xenobiotic responsive elements (XREs), which can function independently and coordinately (Wu and Whitlock, 1993). Both components of the transformed AhR complex (the AhR and ARNT) directly contact DNA. It is interesting to note that the XRE recognized by the AhR/ARNT heterodimer differs from the recognition sequence for nearly all other BHLH proteins, such as MyoD, a protein known to influence determination and differentiation of muscle cells. As with other DNA binding proteins, the primary interaction of the ligand/ AhR complex occurs within the core sequence, but nucleotides adjacent to the core also contribute to XRE binding (Lusska et al., 1993). Analysis of mutant XREs have revealed that substitution within the four-base-pair core sequence 5′- CGTG-3′ results in loss of binding of the ligand/AhR complex. The three base pairs immediately flanking each end of the essential domain are thought to contribute less strongly to receptor binding (Shen and Whitlock, 1992). The mechanism by which the AhR complex influences transcription is still unclear, but the AhR has been reported to influence DNA bending (Elferink and Whitlock, 1990), chromatin structure (Durrin and Whitlock, 1989), and nucleosome displacement (Morgan and Whitlock, 1992) and to increase promoter accessibility (Wu and Whitlock, 1992).

Biological Consequences of Activation The ability of TCDD to regulate the expression of growth-related genes has recently been shown. This association is not surprising, in view of the similarities that exist between the AhR/ARNT heterodimer and the Myc/Max or MyoD/E2A growth regulatory heterodimers. TCDD induces the expression of c-jun and c-fos in Hepa-1 cells, although this effect may be cell- type-specific (Puga et al., 1992). Binding of the AhR complex to a XRE has been correlated with induction of c-Ha-ras and c-myc expression (Sadhu et al., 1993). XREs have also been identified in the human estrogen receptor (White and Gasiewicz, 1993); thus it is likely that TCDD interacts in a significant manner with the estrogen signal transduction pathway. Evidence consistent with this suggestion has recently been published (Krishnan et al., 1994). In their studies, TCDD was shown to inhibit 17-β estradiol-induced cathepsin D gene expression by targeted interaction of the nuclear AhR with imperfect XREs strategically located within the estrogen receptor-Sp1 enhancer sequence of this gene. While all of the molecular features of AhR-mediated effects have not been fully elucidated, structure activity studies using ligands of varying receptor affinity continue to support the view that most of the biologic actions of TCDD are mediated through interaction with the AhR.

Inconsistencies in the Receptor Model Evidence is beginning to accumulate that multiple forms of the AhR and events in addition to receptor binding influence the biological response to TCDD. These are discussed below.

Multiple Forms of AhR The expression of multiple forms of the AhR in target tissue has long been suspected, but concrete evidence in support of this view has been lacking. In 1992, Denison reported the presence of two distinct forms of the AhR, alpha and beta, in similar concentrations in cytosolic extracts of rat liver. The binding of ligand to the alpha form requires the receptor to be in its oligomeric conformation (8-10S). In contrast, ligand binding to the beta form can occur with the dissociated species (5-6S). The addition of molybdate to cytosol during homogenization stabilizes alpha against salt-dependent inactivation and subunit dissociation but does not appear to influence the overall amount of TCDD/AhR complex bound to its specific DNA recognition site. These results suggest that alpha, but not beta, is unable to transform or, alternatively, to bind to the XRE with high affinity, which raises interesting questions regarding the heterogeneity of the response to AhR ligands.

Combinatorial Interactions Two DNA-binding proteins have been identified in cytosolic and nuclear extracts of mouse Hepa-1 cells, which overlap the

DNA-binding specificities to the AhR (Carrier et al., 1994). One of these proteins has an apparent mass of 35-40 kDa and only binds to XRE3, one of six DNA binding sites in the promoter region of the CYP1A1 gene. This protein was tentatively identified as a member of the c/EBP family of transcription factors. The second protein, purified by DNA-affinity chromatography, has an apparent molecular mass of 95 kDa and binds to a larger DNA motif that includes the XRE sequence, in XRE3 and XRE5 but not in XRE1 and XRE2. This protein is not likely to be AhR or ARNT, since it was found in receptorless and nuclear-translocation-deficient cells, as well as in cells not exposed to TCDD. In vivo methylation protection assays indicated that two G residues flanking XRE3, one of which is required for binding of the 95 kDa protein, may be protected from methylation in uninduced cells and become exposed upon TCDD treatment, suggesting that the 95 kDa protein may be constitutively bound to XRE3 and displaced by binding of the AhR complex. These results lend support to the view that the transcriptional regulation of the Ah battery of genes, and perhaps other genes influenced by TCDD, could be modulated by combinatorial interactions of the AhR complex with other transcription factors. In addition, an inhibitory factor has been identified in rat thymus; this factor interferes with the binding of the cytosolic AhR to the XRE (Kurl, 1994). Using guinea pig hepatic AhR, Swanson et al. (1993) identified four TCDD-inducible protein-DNA complexes and two distinct heteromeric DNA-binding forms. These findings are in agreement with a recent report by Okino et al. (1993).

Ligand-independent Activation　　Evidence for the ligand-independent activation of the AhR has recently been presented by Lesca et al. (1995). Their studies were conducted to determine whether ligand-independent activation of the AhR mediates the induction of CYP1A1 by benzimidazole derivatives, agents that do not appear to bind the AhR directly. Benzimidazoles were shown to bind early and transiently to an unknown protein and to deplete the AhR in a time- and dose-dependent manner, and only in cells that express low-affinity forms of the AhR, such as those present in rabbit and human cells. In contrast, benzimidazoles were unable to induce CYP1A1 mRNA in mouse Hepa-1 cells and to deplete the high-affinity AhR form from these cells. These data are intriguing and provide evidence that the effects of AhR ligands can be influenced at multiple levels.

Transcriptional-independent Responses　　The view that not all of the biological responses elicited by TCDD involve a transcriptional component has become increasingly accepted. This is particularly true for the ability of TCDD at low concentrations to modulate cellular kinase activities (Enan and Matsumura, 1995) and calcium homeostasis (Puga et al., 1992). However, the extent to which transcriptional independent events are mediated through the AhR or directed by receptor-independent mechanisms remains unclear. One of the first observable effects of TCDD in cultured murine hepatoma cells is a rapid, transient increase in Ca^{2+} influx and a minor, but significant, elevation of activated, membrane-bound protein kinase C (PKC) (Puga et al., 1992). Increased PKC is associated with induction of several immediate early proto-oncogenes, including c-fos, jun-B, c-jun, and jun-D, and large increases in AP-1 transcription factor activity. Induction of proto-oncogene expression in hepatoma cells by TCDD is independent of AhR or ARNT (Puga et al., 1992).

AhR Signaling Interactions An interesting correlation was recently established between the induction of the multidrug resistance (MDR) gene product, P-glycoprotein, and AhR signaling in primary human hepatocyte cultures (Schuetz et al., 1995). In these studies, induction profiles of *mdr* mRNA were compared to those for CYP1A1 mRNA. Induction of CYP1A1 mRNA was observed in hepatocyte cultures from 15 different individuals treated with TCDD or 3-methylcholanthrene. However, induction of *mdr* mRNA was only observed in half of the preparations treated with TCDD, suggesting that TCDD regulates *mdr* in humans by a mechanism distinct from the classical AhR pathway.

There is a growing body of evidence that AhR-related signaling influences, and is itself influenced by, other signal transduction mechanisms at low concentrations. The toxic effects of TCDD involve disruption of various signal transduction pathways. Signaling interactions explaining the toxic effects of TCDD are discussed below. These involve growth factors and their corresponding receptors, free radicals, protein kinases, and the interaction of TCDD with the estrogen transduction pathway.

Growth Factor In vivo and in vitro evidence suggests that TCDD influences epidermal growth factor (EGF), transforming growth factor (TGF) α_, TGF β_, interleukin (IL) 1β, and tumor necrosis factor (TNF), among others. TGFβ1 exerts an inhibitory effect of TCDD-induced EROD activity in cultured cells (Vogel et al., 1994). Likewise, IL-1β interferes with TCDD induction of CYP1A1 and CYP1A2 via a transcriptional mechanism (Barker et al., 1992). Down-regulation of TCDD-induced CYP1A1 activity has also been demonstrated for other cytokines or growth factors (Jeong et al., 1993). In non-transformed human keratinocytes treated with 10 nM TCDD prior to confluence, TCDD altered both the mRNA and protein concentrations of TGFα, TGFβ2, plasminogen activator inhibitor (PAI)-2, and IL-1β, regulatory proteins known to influence the cellular programming of growth and differentiation in these cells (Gaido and Maness, 1994). However, the effects of TCDD on the signal transduction cascades triggered by these factors are strongly influenced by cell type and by the degree of cellular differentiation and hormonal status. For instance, TCDD decreases binding of EGF in the livers of intact female rats but not in ovariectomized rats, suggesting that the response is dependent on estrogen action (Kohn et al., 1993).

Free Radicals   Several investigators have suggested that oxidative stress plays a critical role in TCDD toxicity (Enan and Matsumura, 1995). Although the contribution of the AhR to the oxidative stress response elicited by TCDD continues to be debated, recent evidence suggests that the response is mediated by the AhR complex (Alsharif et al., 1994). In some studies, congenic mice differing at the Ah locus were administered TCDD (5-125 μg/kg) as a single oral dose, and these studies showed dose-dependent increases in superoxide anion production by macrophages from the TCDD-responsive C57BL/6J (bb) mice relative to control cells. Only the highest dose of TCDD produced a significant increase in superoxide anion formation in C57BL/6J (dd) mice. The acute toxic effects of TCDD may involve TNFα, a cytokine which sensitizes and activates phagocytic cells to agents that elicit release of reactive oxygen species (Alsharif et al., 1994). TNFα may act as an amplifying loop in TCDD-induced oxidative stress, as suggested by the ability of anti-TNFα to reduce oxidative stress.

Protein Kinases   The interaction of AhR signaling with protein kinase C (PKC)-dependent signal transduction has received the most attention during the past two years (Carrier et al., 1992; Okino et al., 1992; Berghard et al., 1993; Weber et al., 1994). The interaction of proteins with DNA with each other, or with other transcription factors is influenced at the posttranscriptional level. For instance, the AhR is phosphorylated on both serine and threonine residues (Perdew, 1992), and dephosphorylation of the ligand/AhR complex by phosphatase acid decreases the DNA binding ability of both cytosolic and nuclear AhR preparations (Pongratz et al., 1991). Mahon and Gasiewicz (1995) have recently confirmed the suggestion that the AhR itself is a phosphoprotein and further demonstrated that phosphorylation sites are also present in the C-terminal half of the protein, a region within or adjacent to a DNA-binding repressor domain. In their study, total AhR phosphorylation was not altered by transformation, but phosphorylation was implicated in the formation of the active complex that associates with cis-acting regulatory elements. The DNA-binding ability of the dephosphorylated AhR can be restored by addition of a PKC inhibitor-sensitive cytosolic factor (Berghard et al., 1993). Co-administration of TCDD and TPA to C57BL/6J mice inhibits the accumulation of TCDD-inducible liver CYP1A1 mRNA, and this effect is paralleled by a reduction in DNA binding of the AhR complex to the XRE secondary to loss of nuclear AhR levels (Okino et al., 1992). In addition, TPA significantly decreases EROD activity in human MCF-7 breast cancer cells (Moore et al., 1993).

Carrier et al. (1992) have shown that 2-aminopurine, an inhibitor of protein kinase activity, inhibits induction of CYP1A1 mRNA and corresponding enzymatic activity by TCDD. In their studyies formation of DNA/AhR complexes was also inhibited by this agent. Hepa-1 cells treated with staurosporine prior to induction with TCDD were unable to form active complexes, while depletion of PKC by prolonged treatment with PMA suppressed CYP1A1 induction by TCDD.

These data were interpreted to suggest that phosphorylation is necessary for the formation of a transcriptional complex and for activation of the CYP1A1 gene. In agreement with this view, pretreatment of mouse hepatocyte cultures and hepatoma cells with staurosporine inhibited TCDD-activated transactivation of CYP1A1 in a dose-dependent manner (Chun et al., 1994). Tyrphostin AG213, a specific tyrosine kinase inhibitor, had no effects on TCDD-induced CYP expression, further supporting the view that PKC is the kinase involved in this process. However, the effects of TCDD on PKC and inositol phosphate metabolism in primary cultures of rat hepatocytes exhibit markedly different profiles from phorbol esters, suggesting that these tumor promoters modulate hepatocyte signal transduction via distinct mechanisms (Wolfle et al., 1993). Thus, it remains to be determined with certainty whether PKC is involved in phosphorylation of the ligand/AhR complex or whether phosphorylation of the AhR occurs subsequent to ligand binding and transformation. This issue was addressed by Schafer et al. (1993), who examined the role of PKC on the functionality of the hepatic cytosolic Ah receptor. In these experiments, two nonspecific PKC inhibitors, H7 and staurosporine, and one specific PKC inhibitor, calphostin c, were employed in assays of Ah receptor transformation and DNA binding. AhR transformation and DNA binding occurred in hepatic cytosol despite the absence of detectable kinase activity. Functional PKC activity was not required for ligand-dependent transformation or DNA binding of the Ah receptor complex. An interesting finding in their studies was that staurosporine, a nonspecific kinase inhibitor, formed an AhR/DNA complex that co-migrates with that produced by TCDD and can effectively compete with TCDD for DNA binding. Although some controversy remains, it appears that phosphorylation events occur early in the process of AhR complex formation in the absence of ligand binding. Phosphorylation may influence the stability of the AhR protein and/or DNA binding.

The biological significance of TCDD-induced changes in protein phosphorylation remains to be defined. TCDD modulates PKC as well as other kinases in somatic cells at low concentrations, and these effects can influence the physiology of the cells. For instance, a dose-dependent increase in tyrosine phosphorylation of five hepatic intracellular proteins has been reported in TCDD-treated C57BL/6J female mice (Ma et al., 1992). TCDD induces a rapid rise in protein phosphorylation activities in the extranuclear fraction (i.e., cytosol and cellular membranes) of the adipose tissue from male guinea pigs (Enan and Matsumura, 1994). This effect occurs both in vivo and in vitro and is not abolished by actinomycin D, an inhibitor of transcription. However, inhibition of protein synthesis by cycloheximide partially suppresses the effect of TCDD. These responses correlate with a quick rise in ras GTP binding activity, as well as phosphorylation of nuclear c-myc protein. In view of the lack of inhibition by actinomycin D and the short time required for TCDD to induce phosphorylation, it has been suggested that stimulation of protein phosphorylation activities by TCDD is not mediated via a transcriptional process. In support of this interpretation is the finding that TCDD activates protein phosphorylation activity under cell-free conditions and in the absence of nuclear protein. The ability of TCDD to influence protein phosphorylation is seen in cells of varying embryologic origin and at different stages of differentiation. For instance, the ability of TCDD to influence PKC may involve cell-cycle-related events, became TCDD and its structural analogs decrease PKC activity in G_o-synchronized cell populations (Weber et al., 1994) but increase activity in cycling cells (Weber et al., 1995b). Exposure of immature thymocytes to TCDD transiently increased detergent-extractable PKC activity. At later time points, PKC activity returned to control values (DePetrillo and Kurl, 1993). TCDD induces an increase in protein-tyrosine kinases in pancreas at early stages of poisoning (Ebner et al., 1993). Most critical to this discussion is the finding that alterations in intracellular protein tyrosine kinase phosphorylation is a more sensitive indicator of TCDD exposure than EROD induction (Ma et al., 1992).

Anti-Estrogenicity TCDD has been shown to interact with the estrogen signal transduction pathway. Harper et al. (1994) have recently demonstrated that AhR ligands can inhibit estrogen-induced responses in MCF-7 human breast cancer cells. TCDD inhibited 17β-estradiol (E2)-induced progesterone receptor (PR) binding, immunoreactive protein, nuclear PR formation, and PR mRNA levels. Scatchard analysis of PR binding demonstrated that TCDD decreased the number of E2-induced PR binding sites, but not the binding affinity for promegestrone. For a series of halogenated aromatics including TCDD, 2,3,7,8- and 1,2,7,8-tetrachlorodibenzofuran, 1,3,7,8-TCDD, and 6-methyl-1,3,8-trichlorodibenzofuran, their rank order of potency for inhibiting E2-induced PR binding paralleled their rank order for binding to the AhR, suggesting a role for the receptor in the antiestrogenic activity of polynuclear and halogenated aromatic hydrocarbons.

The antiestrogenic effects of TCDD on 17β-estradiol-induced pS2 expression has recently been examined in several cell types, including MCF-7, ZR-75, HeLa, and Hepa-1c1c7 wild-type and mutant cells (Zacharewski et al., 1994). The responses to TCDD were compared to a weaker AhR congener, 2,8-dichlorodibenzo-*p*-dioxin, and to the well-established antiestrogens ICI 164,384 and tamoxifen. Their results implicated a role for the Ah receptor in TCDD-mediated suppression of E2-induced pS2 expression and suggested that antiestrogenicity required sequences within the pS2 promoter other than the estrogen response element. These results are particularly significant became since pS2 has been proposed as a prognostic marker for breast cancer (Koerner et al., 1992).

The effects of E2 alone or in combination with TCDD have recently been evaluated in weanling female S-D rats (White et al., 1995). In this species, TCDD did not influence E2-induced responses including uterine weight and keratinization of the vaginal epithelium, suggesting that the antiestrogenic effects of TCDD may exhibit species-, strain-, and age-dependence.

Estimating Potential Health Risk and Factors Influencing Toxicity

TEF Approach   Toxic equivalency factors (TEFs) have been proposed to estimate the potential health risk associated with exposure to dibenzo-p-dioxins, dibenzofurans, and polyhalogenated biphenyls and to complex mixtures containing these chemicals (Safe, 1990). This approach assumes linearity of the toxic response for TCDD and related chemicals and is based on a receptor-mediated mechanism of action. The TEF approach has come under increasing scrutiny, because the relative inductive potency of these chemicals may be tissue-specific (De Vito et al., 1993) and may be influenced by additive and negative interactions among the chemicals present in complex mixtures (Van den Berg et al., 1994); the approach also disregards potentially significant kinetic interactions. As such, estimates of TEFs based on hepatic ethoxyresorufin-O-deethylase (EROD) may not accurately reflect the potency of these chemicals in nonhepatic tissue or the chronic toxicity of the agents in question. Clearly, additional research is needed to begin to resolve this controversy.

Interspecies and Interindividual Differences in Sensitivity   Species differences in susceptibility to TCDD toxicity are best exemplified by differences in LD_{50} values. The large differences in LD_{50} values between species and strains was previously discussed and depicted in Table 4-1 of Chapter 4 of the NAS 1994 publication of *Veterans and Agent Orange*. The suggestion has been made that humans are less sensitive to the toxic effects of TCDD than other species employed (Dickson and Buzik, 1993). Studies conducted by Fan and Rozman (1995) demonstrate that Long Evans rats are less susceptible to TCDD toxicity than are Sprague-Dawley rats (Fan and Rozman, 1995). Subtle differences in the regulation of intermediary metabolism between these two rat strains appear to be responsible for strain differences in susceptibility to TCDD. Hepatic phosphoenol pyruvate carboxy kinase (PEPCK) activity is decreased in a dose-dependent manner in Long Evans and in Sprague-Dawley rats, indicating inhibition of gluconeogenesis. This is an early and reversible effect of TCDD (Fan and Rozman, 1995). Inhibition of feed intake appeared to be secondary to elevated serum tryptophan levels. Hepatic gamma-glutamyl transferase was also reduced in a dose-dependent fashion. Dose-dependent responses in Long Evans rats occurred in a higher dose range than those required for the reduction of PEPCK activity, thus providing an explanation for the decreased susceptibility of the Long-Evans rats to TCDD relative to Sprague-Dawley rats. While such pharmacogenetic differences have been defined in laboratory species, we are only beginning to gain an appreciation of such differences in human populations, as evidenced by cytochrome P450 polymorphisms (Landi et al., 1994).

The relative toxic potency of four chlorinated dibenzo-p-dioxins (CDDs) in two species with different sensitivities (guinea pig, Sprague-Dawley rat) was reviewed by Rozman et al. (1993). These investigators defined a dissociation between AhR-mediated enzyme induction and acute toxicity in these two species and suggested that AhR-mediated effects cannot be fundamental to the mechanism of acute toxicities of CDDs. Of perhaps more significance was the finding that the relative toxic potencies for CDDs in rats were similar for acute, subchronic, and chronic doses, suggesting that multiplicity of effects reflects different time-dependent adaptive responses of the organism.

Tissue Specificity A recent study by Thomas and Gallo (1994) demonstrated that the polyamines putrescine, spermidine, and spermine induce changes in the sedimentation profile and DNA binding of the AhR. Spermidine and spermine caused the precipitation of the 9S oligomeric receptor, with a gradual decrease in receptor peak during density gradient sedimentation. RNase A treatment transformed the 9S AhR to a 6S form, and DNA binding increased by twofold. Following partial purification of transformed AhR, it lost the ability to bind to DNA, but addition of spermidine increased DNA binding in a concentration-dependent manner, suggesting that polyamines modulate the structure and DNA binding of the AhR. These data raise the intriguing possibility that polyamine levels are important in the tissue-specific toxicity and the cell-cycle-specific effects of TCDD in somatic cells.

Significant Interactions *Dietary Interactions* Significant interactions between TCDD toxicity and dietary intake have long been suspected. Chou et al. (1993) have recently shown that caloric restriction alters the activities of several xenobiotic metabolizing enzymes, including CYP1A1-dependent EROD and AHH activities and CYP1B1 dependent pentoxyresorufin-O-dealkylase (PROD) in DBA/2J or C57BL/6N mice. The nature of the interaction was not clear, since cytosolic AhR binding in both strains of mice was not increased and hepatic cytochrome CYP1A1 activity was increased in DBA/2J mice, a strain lacking normal AhR binding. The effects of caloric restriction, sex, and strain on CYP1A1 induction by TCDD are greater in females than in males of both strains, whereas the CYP isozymes induced in male DBA mice had less specificity toward 7-ethoxyresorufin than in C57BL/6N mice. TCDD induction was potentiated by caloric restriction in the DBA strain, indicating the interactive involvement of different regulatory mechanisms. In other studies, dietary fiber was shown to stimulate the fecal excretion of polychlorinated dibenzofurans (PCDF) and polychlorinated dibenzo-*p*-dioxins (PCDD) in rats (Morita et al., 1993).

Chemical Interactions De Jongh et al. (1993) have presented evidence that toxicokinetic interactions occur in mixtures of PCDDs, PCDFs, and PCBs. In their studies, C57BL/6J mice were given single oral doses of 1,2,3,7,8-pentachlorodibenzo-*p*-dioxin (PnCDD), 1,2,3,6,7,8-hexachloro-dibenzo-*p*-dioxin (HxCDD), or 2,3,4,7,8-pentachlorodibenzofuran (PnCDF) (1.5-10.6 nmol/kg) as single compounds or in combination with 300 µmol/kg 2,2′,4,4′,5,5′-hexachlorobiphenyl (HxCB). Two other groups of mice received a mixture of the first three compounds, either with or without HxCB. The hepatic deposition and elimination of the compounds and their CYP1A1-dependent EROD activity were studied for 175 days. Interactive effects on the hepatic deposition of PnCDD were observed in most of the mixed-dose groups. For HxCDD and PnCDF, interactive effects were either very small or absent. No interactive effects were observed on the hepatic elimination rates of PnCDD, HxCDD, or PnCDF. Collectively, these data support the view that chemical interactions play critical roles in the disposition of chemical mixtures.

In related studies, the hexachlorobiphenyl (HxCB) deposition in the livers of mothers and offspring was shown to be doubled in the presence of TCDD (DeJongh et al., 1994). HxCB co-administration did not influence hepatic TCDD deposition, suggesting that the mechanisms of interactions are different for both groups of compounds.

Weber et al. (1992) have completed comparative toxicity studies in which male Sprague-Dawley rats were treated with an LD_{20}, an LD_{50}, and an LD_{80} of TCDD, 1,2,3,7,8-pentachlorodibenzo-p-dioxin (penta-CDD), 1,2,3,4,7,8-hexachlorodibenzo-p-dioxin (hexa-CDD), 1,2,3,4,6,7,8,-heptachlorodibenzo-p-dioxin (hepta-CDD), respectively, and a mixture of the four homologues representing one-fourth of the previously established LD_{20}, LD_{50}, and LD_{80} for each hydrocarbon. While plasma tryptophan levels increased in a dose-dependent manner, EROD activity and liver weights in CDD-treated animals did not. These data suggest that a poor correlation exists between plasma tryptophan levels, a biomarker of acute toxicity, and EROD activity, a biomarker of AhR-mediated enzyme induction. It is clear that future studies must attempt to define the extent to which the presence of multiple chemicals in complex mixtures influences short-term versus long-term toxicity outcomes.

Disease Outcomes and Mechanisms of Toxicity

In this section, we summarize studies published during the period 1992-95 that investigated the toxic effects of TCDD. The mechanism of toxicity, if known, is also explained.

Carcinogenicity   Since relatively little data are available on carcinogenicity of TCDD in human populations with known TCDD body burdens, results from chronic feeding studies of laboratory animals continue to be used as the basis for human risk assessment. The results from animal bioassays were summarized in VAO. Recent investigations have focused on the mechanisms of carcinogenicity. These studies are summarized below.

Mechanism of Toxicity   The sex specificity of TCDD-induced hepatocellular carcinoma, along with the reduced tumor incidences of the pituitary, uterus, mammary gland, pancreas and adrenals in female relative to male rats, emphasize the view that hormonal control modulates TCDD carcinogenicity (Kociba et al., 1978). In addition to its ability to increase cancer rates in animals, TCDD can act as a promoter of tumor formation following initiation by other chemicals. To date, the consensus is that TCDD is not genotoxic and that its ability to influence the carcinogenic process is mediated via epigenetic events such as enzyme induction, cell proliferation, apoptosis, and intracellular communication. Studies investigating the epigenetic effects of TCDD are summarized below.

Enzyme Induction   The ability of TCDD to induce xenobiotic-metabolizing enzymes which can metabolize chemicals to reactive intermediates that are capable of causing injury has received considerable attention as a predictable biomarker of human exposures and/or carcinogenicity. The profiles of enzyme induction in experimental systems in vivo and in vitro often correlates with the patterns observed in human populations. Particular attention has been given to the induction of CYP1A1 and CYP1A2, and more recently to the newly characterized CYP1B1. The induction of CYP1A1 and CYP1A2, along with increases in phosphorylated forms of pp 32, 34, and 38, have been proposed as sensitive indicators of TCDD exposure (De Vito et al., 1994). In mice, the Ah gene battery also includes NAD(p)H:menadione oxidoreductase, aldehyde dehydrogenase, UDP-glucuronosyltransferase, and glutathione transferase, enzymes involved in phase II metabolism (Dunn et al., 1993; Takimoto et al., 1992; Vasiliou et al., 1992; Puga et al., 1992). The ability of TCDD to regulate the transcription of these genes is believed to occur via a receptor-mediated mechanism and is not restricted to the liver (Vasilou et al., 1993).

The CYP1A1 gene is not inducible in certain cell types due to the presence of a putative repressor(s) that competes with the ligand/AhR complex for the responsive element or which otherwise precludes AhR/Arnt activity. Mechanistic studies with both wild-type and mutant cell lines have revealed a putative repressor of TCDD-dependent induction of CYP1A1 (Watson and Hankinson, 1992) that appears to be encoded by one of the Ah loci (Karenlampi et al., 1988). Basal levels of CYP1A1 transcription are controlled by a negative regulatory protein (Puga et al., 1992; Boucher et al., 1993; Sterling et al., 1993; Ou and Ramos, 1995), but this effect exhibits considerable species-specificity. For instance, three NRE binding proteins have been identified by electrophoretic mobility shift assays (EMSA) to participate in the negative regulation of the human CYP1A1 gene (Boucher et al., 1993). Normal human fibroblast nuclear extracts contain two constitutive protein-DNA complexes, which appear to be immunochemically distinct from the AhR (Gradin et al., 1993). Collectively, these data suggest that species- or cell-specific differences in responsiveness to TCDD and related chemicals involve interactions of multiple signals in the regulation of gene expression and raise important questions regarding heterogeneity of disease outcomes following herbicide exposures.

Another complicating factor regarding the inducibility of CYP isozymes is recent data regarding the non-AhR inducibility of some of these enzymes. Daujat et al. (1992) showed that omeprazole, a benzimidazole derivative, induces both CYP1A1 and CYP1A2 in human liver via a nonreceptor mechanism. However, Quattrochi and Tukey (1993) have published a report that omeprazole does initiate AhR activation and that induction of the human CYP1A1 gene is indeed receptor-dependent.

Cell Proliferation   The effects of TCDD on hepatic epidermal growth factor receptor (EGFR) levels in a two-stage initiation/promotion model were recently investigated by Sewall et al. (1993). The doses employed encompassed the range used in bioassays to assess cancer potency for human health risk assessment. TCDD was administered bi-weekly by gavage to female Sprague-Dawley rats for 30 weeks following initiation by a single dose of diethylnitrosamine (DEN). Consistent with previous data, TCDD induced a decrease in EGFR in intact but not ovariectomized animals. A significant dose-dependent decrease in plasma membrane EGFR binding capacity was observed in initiated and non-initiated rats. The decrease in plasma membrane EGFR determined by equilibrium binding was confirmed by measurements of EGFR autophosphorylation and by immunohistochemical detection. Collectively, these results demonstrate that decreases of the EGFR by TCDD is ovarian-dependent and is a sensitive effect induced at dose levels associated with TCDD hepatocarcinogenicity in rodent bioassays.

TCDD and HCDD had no effects on the proliferation of normal hepatocytes, but the labeling indices of enzyme-altered liver lesions were slightly enhanced by chemical treatment (Buchmann et al., 1994). Whether the selective, albeit moderate, increase in proliferation of enzyme-altered liver cells is sufficient to explain the promoting activity of dioxin, or whether additional factors such as effects of apoptosis are also important, remains to be established.

Apoptosis   Apoptosis (programmed cell death) has long been recognized as a normal process during organogenesis. More recently, apoptosis has been implicated as a key regulatory event in disorders of growth and differentiation, such as cancer. Selective apoptosis, in concert with cell-specific replication, may explain the unique promoting effects of different carcinogens such as TCDD, because an undesirable population of cells may be afforded a growth advantage (Marsman and Barrett, 1994). Studies to test this hypothesis will be useful in defining the role of apoptosis in TCDD-induced carcinogenesis.

Intracellular Communication   TCDD and two co-planar PCBs caused a rapid and sustained dose-dependent inhibition of intracellular communication in Hepa-1 cells (De Hann et al., 1994). The time course of inhibition of intracellular communication paralleled that of EROD induction, although the onset of communication inhibition preceded changes in EROD. A role for the AhR in the inhibition of intracellular communication was proposed based on the lack of inhibition in AhR-defective cells and the observation that α-naphthoflavone, an AhR antagonist, greatly reduced the TCDD effect.

Immunotoxicity   Extensive evidence has been published that halogenated aromatic hydrocarbons, including TCDD, polychlorinated dibenzofurans (PCDFs), polychlorinated biphenyls (PCBs), and polybrominated polyphenols (PBBs) exert toxic effects on the immune system (Kerkvliet and Burleson, 1994). The evidence is based on numerous studies of various animal species, including nonhuman primates, mice, rats, guinea pigs, rabbits, and chickens.

A major target of halogenated aromatic hydrocarbons on the immune system appears to be the T-cell arm of the immune response. The finding that TCDD administration may result in thymic atrophy supports the concept that the immunotoxic effects are primarily mediated through the T cell (Kerkvliet and Burleson, 1994). Direct effects of TCDD on T cells in vitro, however, have not been demonstrated, suggesting that the action of TCDD and related chemicals may be indirect. A number of recent studies have focused on the interactions of halogenated aromatic hydrocarbons and cytokines. These soluble mediators are important in regulating the immune response.

Based on its effect on the generation of T cells, it is reasonable to conclude that TCDD will increase susceptibility of experimental animals to challenge by pathogenic microorganisms that interact primarily with cell-mediated immunity. In support of this, it has been shown that TCDD exposure increases the susceptibility of mice and rats to challenge with intracellular pathogens such as *Salmonella*, *Listeria*, herpes virus, influenza virus, and *Plasmodium*. Similarly, growth of certain transplanted tumors is enhanced in mice treated with TCDD. On the other hand, T cells are usually required for antibody production. Increased susceptibility of mice to challenge by *Streptococcus pneumoniae*, an extracellular pathogen, may relate to impaired antibody production due to loss of T-cell help. In addition, investigations conducted by Neubert et al. (1994) indicate that TCDD under certain conditions appears to have no deleterious effect on the induced immune response. These investigators studied the proliferative capacity of marmoset lymphocytes during a secondary immune response following a tetanus vaccination. The animals were given an additional injection three months or one year following initial immunization. During this period, a proliferative response of lymphocytes to tetanus toxoid was documented. The investigators then studied the effect of TCDD on the booster response. Lymphocyte responses of four marmosets treated with TCDD were, in fact, greater than in control animals at the time of the second (one-year) booster. Summarized below are recent animal studies, conducted in a variety of species, that support the finding that TCDD exposure can result in thymic atrophy and that this effect is primarily mediated through the T cell. In vitro evidence that this action of TCDD may be an indirect effect of TCDD on T cells is also summarized.

Rice et al. (1995) treated female Fischer 344 rats with a single intraperitoneal dose of 0.3, 3.0, or 30 μg/kg TCDD or corn oil and examined cytotoxic T-cell activities 24 days after treatment. Syngeneic in vivo tumor-specific CTLs were generated that model cell-mediated immune reactions against neoplastically transformed self antigens. RT2, a virally-induced Fischer 344 rat glioma, and D74, an ethylnitrosurea-induced Fischer 344 rat glioma were used as targets. This immunological parameter was compared to body, thymic, and liver weights as well as liver ethoxyresorufin deethylase (EROD) activity on day 24 post-TCDD treatment. They found that Fischer 344 rats are very sensitive to TCDD. Immunotoxicity, indicated by severe thymic atrophy, was evident and dose-dependent. In contrast, there was no significant, consistent suppression of cytotoxic T-cell activity in a number of tumor targets, even at the highest dose tested (30 μg/kg dose). TCDD was reported to induce an increase in cytochrome P4501A1 (CYP1A1) activity at all doses tested.

Earlier reports that low doses of TCDD (4 ng/kg/week) in the mouse suppressed the production of cytotoxic T cells were also not confirmed by Hanson and Smialowicz (1994). They did, however, find decreased thymic weight and cellularity at doses of 1.0 and 3.0 μg/kg/week. Similarly, suppression of antibody production was observed only at the higher doses.

De Waal et al. (1993) exposed juvenile male Wistar rats to 150 μg/kg TCDD by oral intubation and killed them four or ten days later. TCDD was shown to retard the differentiation of the thymic epithelium. Specifically, a relative shift from immature to more mature cortical epithelial cells, as judged by electron microscopy, suggested an arrest in orderly cellular differentiation. In TCDD-induced thymic atrophy, the epithelial framework of the cortex becomes more compact, with focal aggregation of epithelial cells. These alterations in epithelial development and architecture may be responsible for defective intrathymic T-cell processing.

Oughton et al. (1995) exposed female C57BL/6 mice to TCDD in a long-term study. Age- and TCDD-related changes in the phenotypes of splenic, thymic, and peripheral blood lymphocytes were investigated. When changes due to age were taken into account, TCDD treatment had no discernible effect on the total number of circulating T cells, B cells, and macrophages. There was, however, a small but statistically significant decrease in the frequency of the sub-population of CD8+ cytotoxic T cells in the spleen following TCDD treatment. These changes were reflected by a significant decrease in the frequency of CD8+ T cells in the blood. Chronic exposure resulted in a small, statistically significant increase in the frequency of CD4CD8- thymic cells. These double negative cells probably represent immature T cells. A small but significant increase in γδ T-cell receptor-bearing thymocytes was observed. TCDD also induced liver CYP1A1 microsomal enzymes.

In conclusion, TCDD has been shown to suppress both cell-mediated immunity (CMI) and humoral immunity (HI) (Lundberg et al., 1992). TCDD prevents the maturation of the thymocytes to mature T cells by inducing differentiation of thymic epithelial cells (Vanden Heuvel and Lucier, 1993). The suppression of CMI is most apparent in young animals (Faith, 1979). Suppression of HI occurs in older animals exposed to TCDD and results in an inhibition of B-lymphocyte differentiation into antibody-producing cells (Lundberg et al., 1992).

Mechanism of Toxicity   Studies indicate that the immunotoxic effects of TCDD and related substances are mediated through binding to the Ah receptor. This conclusion is based on reports that genetic variation at the Ah locus results in differing susceptibilities to TCDD immunotoxicity. Similarly, as demonstrated by Fernandez-Salguero et al. (1995), strains of mice lacking the Ah receptor are relatively resistant to TCDD-induced immunosuppression. By homologous recombination, the investigators constructed mice that were deficient in the Ah receptor. Almost half of the mice died shortly after birth. The survivors showed decreased accumulation of lymphocytes in the spleen and lymph nodes, but not in the thymus. The livers of the "knock-out" Ah-receptor-deficient mice were reduced in size. These mice were unresponsive to TCDD induction of genes encoding P450 enzymes that catalyze the metabolism of foreign compounds. Thus, the Ah receptor appears to play an important role in mediating the immunotoxic effects of TCDD and in promoting the normal development of the immune system.

The effect of TCDD on interleukin-mediated modulation of the immune response in (C57BL/6×C3H)F$_1$ mice was studied by Karras, Conrad and Holsapple (1995). They hypothesized that the immunosuppression mediated by direct exposure of TCDD to B cells in vitro is due to an IL-4-like biological activity. Therefore, they studied the ability of TCDD to mimic the responses of B cells to IL-4, including upregulation of the major histocompatibility complex antigens of class II type, increases in the expression of the Fc receptor for IgE (CD23), and induction of immunoglobulin class switching. At concentrations that readily suppress B cell-proliferative and antibody-forming cell responses, TCDD failed to demonstrate any of the activities of IL-4. Furthermore, when TCDD was preincubated with B cells before addition of IL-4, no evidence of increased IL-4 activity was observed. In fact, TCDD preincubation resulted in decreased secretion of IgG$_1$ and IgE from B cells stimulated to undergo immunoglobulin class switch by LPS and IL-4. Thus, it appears that TCDD inhibits the formation of fully differentiated B cells capable of secreting antibody and has no effects on class-switching events as such. It also appears that the observed immunosuppressive effects of TCDD on B-cell function cannot be explained by biological mimicry of the actions of IL-4.

Takenaka et al. (1995) prepared cell cultures of peripheral blood monocytic cells and tonsil cells from healthy human donors between the ages of 21 and 48 years. They produced B-cell-rich populations by depleting T cells. The B cells were then stimulated by addition of IL-4 plus CD40, and the amount of IgE synthesized was measured. In 3/3 experiments when TCDD was added on the second day, an increase in IgE synthesis was observed. The investigators attributed this effect on IgE production to the direct activity of the Ah receptor on nuclear processes.

Kurl (1994) has described an inhibitory factor in the rat thymus that interferes with binding of the AhR to the XRE. The role of this inhibitor in the thymotoxic effects of TCDD is still unclear.

Reproductive/Developmental Toxicity The literature summarized in *VAO* suggested that exposure to TCDD was associated with a number of reproductive and developmental abnormalities. Adult male reproductive functions, including alterations in hormone levels, spermatogenesis, and fertility, were usually reported at toxic dose levels. Exposure of females resulted in reduced fertility. Developmental toxicity after prenatal exposure to TCDD included cleft palate, hydronephrosis, and other effects. There were few data on male-mediated developmental toxicity—that is, exposure of the adult male to herbicides, leading to abnormalities in the offspring.

A number of animal studies of the reproductive and developmental toxicity of herbicides, specifically TCDD, were published during the reference period. This research suggests that developing animal systems may be particularly sensitive to the effects of TCDD. Specifically, male reproductive function has been reported to be altered following perinatal exposure to TCDD. The research concerning the effects of TCDD on both male and female reproduction and development is summarized below.

Reproductive Toxicity It has been shown that TCDD exposure to adult male animals decreases testis weight, affects testicular morphology, decreases spermatogenesis, and reduces fertility (Moore et al., 1985; Chahoud et al., 1989; Chahoud et al., 1992). These effects have generally been observed at dose levels that reduce feed intake and body weight. At lower doses, TCDD induces androgenic deficiencies. This may be explained by a reduction in the number and size of Leydig cells, resulting in a reduction in total volume of Leydig cells per testis (Johnson et al., 1992, 1994). In terms of relative sensitivity, the current data suggest that perinatal TCDD exposure induces a wide range of effects on male offspring at much lower dose levels than does exposure of the adult male animal. For example, decreased spermatogenesis occurs in adult male rats exposed to a dose as low as 3 µg/kg in comparison to an in utero dose of only 0.064 µg/kg (Chahoud et al., 1992; Mably et al., 1992a). In the context of the potential health effects due to herbicide exposure among Vietnam veterans, the majority of whom were adult men, this new research is of limited relevance.

The major effects of TCDD on female reproduction are reduced fertility, inability to maintain pregnancy, and decreased litter size (Murray et al., 1979; Kociba et al., 1978; Scheutz, 1979). Some of these effects were seen at dose levels that did not induce maternal toxicity. A recent study by Rier et al. (1993) reported that long-term daily exposure of Rhesus monkeys to 5 or 25 ppt of TCDD led to the development of endometriosis in a dose-response fashion. Further research is needed to confirm this finding in experimental animals and to evaluate the potential risk in highly exposed human populations, such as the Seveso residents (Bois and Eskenazi, 1994).

Mechanism of Toxicity   It has been postulated that the adverse reproductive effects observed in female mice and rats is due to an antiestrogenic effect following TCDD exposure. TCCD exposure may alter circulating female hormone levels, although the effects may be species-, age-, and dose-dependent. Recent evidence indicates that the antiestrogenic effects may be due to a decrease in estrogen receptor number and/or an increase in estrogen metabolism mediated by P450-1A1 (Spink et al., 1992; Zacharewski et al., 1992).

Developmental Toxicity   Recent evidence has indicated that the male reproductive system is a sensitive target of in utero and lactational TCDD exposure. Effects can be detected at dose levels much below those required for alterations in adult male reproductive parameters. The specific effects seen after perinatal TCDD exposure include decreased ventral prostate, seminal vesicle, testis, and epididymis weights; decreased anogenital distance; delays in testis descent and puberty; decreased spermatogenesis; feminized regulation of gonadotrophin secretion; and demasculinized and feminized sexual behavior in adulthood (Mably et al., 1992a,b; Bjerke and Peterson, 1994; Gray et al., 1995). The lowest effective maternal dose for most effects was either 0.16 or 0.064 µg TCDD/kg given on day 15 of gestation. The results were obtained using two species of rats and Syrian hamsters (Mably et al., 1992a,b; Gray et al., 1995). Generally, TCDD had no effect on the fertility of in utero-exposed males, or survival and growth of their offspring, except at higher doses (Mably et al., 1992a,b; Gray et al., 1995). In addition, the relevance of these effects to herbicide exposure among Vietnam veterans, the majority of whom were adult men, is questionable.

A recent study reported that for most male reproductive endpoints, both the in utero and lactational TCDD exposure routes produced the same effects, although some effects were seen only after exposure via a specific route (Bjerke and Peterson, 1994). For example, only in utero exposure decreased daily sperm counts, whereas, only lactational exposure resulted in feminized sexual behavior.

Adverse reproductive effects on perinatally-exposed females have also been reported (Gray et al., 1993). The female rat offspring had severe clefting of the clitoris and abnormal vaginal openings. No effects on the estrous cycle were found.

Mechanism of Toxicity   Several hormone-mediated mechanisms have been proposed to explain these adverse effects on exposed male offpsring. These include the reduction in circulating testosterone levels, "imprinting" of androgen receptors by TCDD, and antiestrogenic action. Gray and colleagues have suggested that TCDD may act to alter morphological sex differentiation by modifying levels of growth factors and their receptors involved in cell proliferation and differentiation in the urogenital system (Gray et al., 1995).

TCDD is known to induce cleft palate and hydronephrosis in several strains of mice (Abbott et al., 1994). The ability of TCDD to cause cleft palate in mice may be linked to interactions with another cleft palate teratogen, retinoic acid (RA). Concomitant treatment of mice with TCDD and RA has been associated with induction of palatal clefts in 100 percent of the offspring of mothers at doses considerably below those that induce clefting by either agent alone (Couture et al., 1990). This synergy strongly supports the suggestion by others that there is a convergence in the developmental pathways influenced by these agents. The effects of TCDD on induction of the type II cellular retinoic acid binding protein (CRABP-II) and the retinoic acid receptor b (RARb) by RA in murine embryonic palate mesenchyme cells was recently examined by Weston et al. (1995). While TCDD alone had no effect on basal levels of expression of either gene, the induction of both genes by RA was strongly inhibited by TCDD, suggesting a direct molecular interaction between the RA and TCDD-related signal transduction pathways.

It is interesting to note that the glucocorticoid hydrocortisone (HC) shares with TCDD the ability to induce cleft palate (Abbott et al., 1994). However, the morphology and etiology of the lesions are different because with HC there is formation of small palatal shelves, while TCDD modulates epithelial cell differentiation and proliferation. TCDD treatment in vivo downregulates the Ah receptor and upregulates glucocorticoid receptor expression, whereas HC exerts the opposite effect. Combined treatments increased expression of both receptors collectively. These data demonstrate that these receptor systems can be cross-regulated, but the role of down- versus up-regulation in teratogenesis remains obscure.

Hepatoxicity   TCDD is a potent liver tumor promoter in rats, with females being more sensitive than males.

Mechanism of Toxicity   Evidence published during the reference period provides support that the hepatotoxicity of TCDD (i.e., its role as a potent liver tumor promoter) involves AhR-dependent mechanisms. Specifically, the role of the AhR receptor in the co-mitogenic action of TCDD with epidermal growth factor and in the induction of liver enzymes involved in the metabolism of xenobiotics has been investigated.

TCDD is known to interact with multiple growth-related signal transduction pathways in hepatocytes. The role of the AhR in the co-mitogenic action of TCDD with epidermal growth factor (EGF) was recently examined in hepatocytes isolated from male congenic mice (C57BL/6J) with high affinity (Ah^bAh^b) or low affinity (Ah^dAh^d) for the AhR (Schrenk et al., 1994). In both cell types, TCDD did not stimulate DNA synthesis in the absence of EGF. When added together with EGF, TCDD exhibited opposing effects on DNA synthesis, where increased EGF-stimulated DNA synthesis was observed in Ah^bAh^b cells, but not in Ah^dAh^d cells treated with 3×10^{-14} M at a plating density of 35,000 cells/cm^2. In hepatocytes from Ah^dAh^d mice, 3×10^{-12} M TCDD was required to elicit a similar co-mitogenic response. At a lower density (10,000 cells/cm^2), 3×10^{-12} M TCDD had a pronounced inhibitory effect on EGF-stimulated DNA synthesis in Ah^bAh^b cells but not in Ah^dAh^d cells. These findings demonstrate that TCDD can enhance or antagonize EGF-stimulated DNA synthesis in mouse hepatocytes in a density-dependent fashion. The different concentration-response relationships in hepatocytes from both strains suggest that the Ah receptor regulates both responses.

The ability of TCDD and related aromatic hydrocarbons to induce enzymes involved in the metabolism of xenobiotics has been investigated by Vanden Heuvel et al. (1994). These investigations completed a comprehensive examination of dose-response relationships for hepatic induction of mRNAs following a single injection of TCDD to rats. The induction of CYP1A1 mRNA was compared to UDP glucuronyl transferase (UGT1), plasminogen activator inhibitor (PAI)-2, and TGFα. The induction of CYP1A1 mRNA proved to be extremely sensitive to TCDD and was highly correlated with increased EROD activity. UGT1 mRNA was increased over control, but it required higher TCDD doses than CYP1A1. PAI-2 and TGFα mRNA were not increased in rat liver. These results further support the view that the ability of TCDD to modulate gene expression exhibits differences in sensitivity that involve tissue-, cell-, and species-specific components.

Human CYP1A1 appears to be co-expressed with CYP1B1 (also referred to as P450EF) in MCF-7 cells (Christou et al., 1994). Of potential significance to risk assessment has been the finding that the human gene exhibits differences in positional selectivity for DMBA metabolism relative to animal counterparts. The mouse cytochrome P450-EF has recently been identified as a representative member of the new 1B subfamily of cytochrome P450s (Savas et al., 1994; Sutter et al., 1994). This enzyme represents a novel benz[a]anthracene and TCDD-inducible cytochrome P450. The deduced amino acid sequence (543 amino acids), the longest of any known cytochrome P450, exhibits 41 percent and 38 percent identity to mouse CYP1A1 and CYP1A2, respectively, and less but substantial similarity (30-33 percent identity) to many members of the CYP2 family. Interestingly, CYP1B1 inducibility in Sprague-Dawley rats is sex-dependent (Walker et al., 1995). In this study, the female rats exhibited inducible IB1 in response to TCDD, a response that correlates with the female specificity of tumor formation in Sprague-Dawley rats following aromatic hydrocarbon exposure (Randerath et al., 1988).

The release of normal human epithelial cell from cell-substratum and/or cell-cell adhesion generates cellular signals that induce the expression of CYP1A1 in the absence of xenobiotics. Sadek and Allen-Hoffmann (1994) have recently shown that suspension of wild-type Hepa-1c1c7 cells leads to nuclear localization and activation of the Ah receptor to a DNA-binding form. Suspension of wild-type Hepa-1c1c7 cells for four hours led to an induction of steady-state levels of CYP1A1 mRNA, similar to that obtained following treatment of adherent cells with 10^{-9} M TCDD. Mutants of the Hepa-1c1c7 cells that were defective in different aspects of the Ah receptor signal transduction pathway exhibited negligible or no suspension-mediated induction of CYP1A1 mRNA.

Neurotoxicity Sirkka and colleagues (1992) studied a series of neurological end points in male Han/Wistar rats given 1,000 µg/kg of TCDD intraperitoneally. This dose level is equivalent to one-third of the intraperitoneal LD_{50} for this strain of rat. Their results indicated no significant neurological impairment in animals that developed significant decreases in body weight following TCDD exposure.

The first experimental studies of the effects of TCDD on the peripheral nervous system have recently been published (Grahmann et al., 1993; Grehl et al., 1993). Electrophysiologic studies were performed in 80 adult male Wistar rats after an intraperitoneal injection of a single low dose of TCDD (8.8, 6.6, 4.4 or 2.2 µg/kg) dissolved in corn oil. Twenty control animals received corn oil only. The typical wasting syndrome of high-dose TCDD intoxication was not observed. Motor and sensory nerve conduction velocities in the right sciatic nerve showed dose-dependent and statistically significant slowing in TCDD-exposed rats as compared to controls. Ten months after the administration of TCDD, peripheral nerves showed a progressive, proximally accentuated neuropathy. The extent of changes, however, differed remarkably between individual animals. These results appear to be the first experimental evidence that a single low dose of TCDD can cause a toxic polyneuropathy in rats.

There have been no recent experimental studies that have focused primarily on the effect of TCDD on the central nervous system.

Other Toxicities

Acute Toxicity Weber et al. (1995a) have correlated the effect of acute exposures to TCDD on intermediary metabolism in male C57BL/6J (C57) and DBA/2J (DBA) mice. In these studies, C57 mice were given 0.03 to 235 µg/kg by gavage, while DBA mice were given 1 to 3,295 µg/kg. Hepatomegaly developed at doses above 3 and 97.5 µg/kg in C57 and DBA mice, respectively. EROD activity was induced in liver with an ED_{50} of 1.1 and 16 µg/kg and in kidney with an ED_{50} of 65 and 380 µg/kg, respectively. The activity of phosphoenolpyrate carboxykinase (PEPCK) in livers of both mouse strains was reduced over the entire dose range, displaying a plateau in the dose response at the onset of acute toxicity of TCDD. The liver enzyme activity was decreased by as much as 80 percent at lethal doses, while PEPCK activity in kidney was not affected. Serum glucose concentration was significantly reduced over the entire dose range, but the reduction was significant only at doses in which glucose-6-phosphatase (G-6-Pase) activity was affected. Tryptophan 2,3-dioxygenase activity was not lowered at any dose of TCDD in either mouse strain, and no increase in serum tryptophan levels was observed. Serum levels of thyroxine (T4) and triiodothyronine (T3) were decreased in a dose-dependent fashion over most of the dose range administrated, with T3 levels exactly paralleling T4 levels in both mouse strains.

Mechanism of Toxicity   The acute toxicity in both C57 and DBA/2J mice appeared to be related to severe reduction of gluconeogenesis, but, unlike in rats, it does not involve changes in tryptophan homeostasis.

Cardiovascular Toxicity   The myocardium has been implicated as a target of TCDD toxicity. Using the chick embryo model system, studies have been conducted to examine the effects of TCDD on ventricular muscle contraction and on cardiac myocyte intracellular calcium content (Canga et al., 1993). The relevance of these findings to humans is unknown. TCDD caused an evolving sequence of contractile defects, independent of changes in diet. Impairment of cAMP-modulated contraction was observed after 48 hours and responses to extracellular calcium within seven days. These responses appeared to be specific for TCDD and were not seen with other inducers of cytochrome P450, such as phenobarbital.

Mechanism of Toxicity   Canga et al. (1993) demonstrated that TCDD also depressed inotropic responses to theophylline and forskolin, indicating that biochemical interference involves a post-beta-adrenergic receptor effect on cAMP action.

Dermal Toxicity   TCDD has been shown to induce chloracne in humans as well as in animals (Jones and Krizek, 1962).

Mechanism of Toxicity   The mechanism of TCDD-induced chloracne remains unknown. Recent studies have suggested that TCDD and tumor promoters such as 12-O-tetradecanoylphorbol-13-acetate (TPA) decrease an acidic type I Keratin involved in epidermal development, leading to keratinocyte hyperproliferation and skin irritations, such as chloracne (Molloy and Laskin, 1992).

Wasting Syndrome   TCDD-induced wasting syndrome has been observed in several different species (Kelling et al., 1985).

Mechanism of Toxicity   Recent evidence suggests that the inhibition of glucose transport in adipose tissue, pancreas, and brain may be one of the major contributing factors to the wasting syndrome. Loss of glucose transport may result in elevated blood glucose levels and a wasting syndrome (Enan et al. 1992a, 1992b). Alternatively, TCDD may decrease PEPCK levels in rat livers, and this may block glucose synthesis by rendering the PEPCK gene nonresponsive to its physiological stimuli, thus resulting in weight loss due to a loss in feeding sensation (Stahl et al., 1993).

Renal Toxicity Although studies examining the effects of TCDD in the kidney have been mostly limited to the investigation of TCDD-induced renal teratogenicity, data implicating TCDD and related congeners as potential nephrotoxicants in vitro have been published (Bowes and Ramos, 1994). These studies demonstrated that renal cortical tubular epithelial cells are resistant to aromatic hydrocarbons, but glomerular mesangial cells were identified as a sensitive cellular target for these chemicals within the kidney. These in vitro studies are consistent with epidemiologic reports that human environmental and occupational exposures to certain aromatic hydrocarbons, including petroleum based substances, naphthas, and toluene, result in glomerulonephritis (Hotz, 1994).

REFERENCES

Abbott BD, Perdew GH, Birnbaum LS. 1994. Ah receptor in embryonic mouse palate and effects of TCDD on receptor expression. Toxicology and Applied Pharmacology 126:16-25.

Alsharif NZ, Lawson T, Stohs SJ. 1994. Oxidative stress induced by 2,3,7,8-tetrachlorodibenzo-p-dioxin is mediated by the aryl hydrocarbon (Ah) receptor complex. Toxicology 92:39-51.

Anderson YB, Jackson JA, Birnbaum LS. 1993. Maturational changes in dermal absorption of 2,3,7,8-tetrachlorodibenzo-p-dioxin (TCDD) in Fischer 344 rats. Toxicology and Applied Pharmacology 119:214-20.

Arnold EK, Beasley VR, Parker AJ, Stedelin JR. 1991. 2,4-D toxicosis II: a pilot study of clinical pathologic and electroencephalographic effects and residues of 2,4-D in orally dosed dogs. Veterinary and Human Toxicology 33:446-449.

Barker CW, Fagan JB, Pasco DS. 1992. Interleukin-1beta suppresses the induction of P4501A1 and P4501A2 messenger RNAs in isolated hepatocytes. Journal of Biological Chemistry 267:8050-8055.

Berghard A, Gradin K, Pongratz I, Whitelaw M, Poellinger L. 1993. Cross-coupling of signal transduction pathways: the dioxin receptor mediates induction of cytochrome P-450IA1 expression via a protein kinase C-dependent mechanism. Molecular and Cellular Biology 13:677-689.

Bjerke DL, Peterson RE. 1994. Reproductive toxicity of 2,3,7,8-tetrachlorodibenzo-p-dioxin in male rats: different effects of in utero versus lactational exposure. Toxicology and Applied Pharmacology 127:241-249.

Bois FY, Eskenazi B. 1994. Possible risk of endometriosis for Seveso, Italy, residents: an assessment of exposure to dioxin. Environmental Health Perspectives 102:476-477.

Boucher PD, Ruch RJ, Hines RN. 1993. Characterization of the tri-partite negative regulatory element on the human CYP1A1 gene. Toxicologist 13:432.

Bowes RC, and Ramos KS. 1994. Assessment of cell-specific cytotoxic responses of the kidney to selected aromatic hydrocarbons. Toxicology Vitro 8:1151-1160.

Buchmann A, Stinchcombe S, Korner W, Hagenmaier H, Bock KW. 1994. Effects of 2,3,7,8-tetrachloro- and 1,2,3,4,6,7,8-heptachlorodibenzo-p-dioxin on the proliferation of preneoplastic liver cells in the rat. Carcinogenesis 15:1143-1150.

Burbach KM, Poland A, Bradfield CA. 1992. Cloning of the Ah-receptor cDNA reveals a distinctive ligand-activated transcription factor. Proceedings of the National Academy of Sciences (USA) 89:8185-8189.

Canga L, Paroli L, Blanck TJ, Silver RB, Rifkind AB. 1993. 2,3,7,8-tetrachlorodibenzo-p-dioxin increases cardiac myocyte intracellular calcium and progressively impairs ventricular contractile responses to isoproterenol and to calcium in chick embryo hearts. Molecular Pharmacology 44:1142-1151.

Carrier F, Owens RA, Nebert DW, Puga A. 1992. Dioxin-dependent activation of murine CYP1A-1 gene transcription requires protein kinase C-dependent phosphorylation. Molecular and Cellular Biology 12:1856-1863.

Carrier F, Chang CY, Duh JL, Nebert DW, Puga A. 1994. Interaction of the regulatory domains of the murine CYP1A1 gene with two DNA-binding proteins in addition to the Ah receptor and the Ah receptor nuclear translocator (ARNT). Biochemistry and Pharmacology 48:1767-1778.

Carrier G, Brunet RC, Brodeur J. 1995a. Modeling of the toxicokinetics of polychlorinated dibenzo-p-dioxins and dibenzofurans in mammalians, including humans. I. Nonlinear distribution of PCDD/PCDF body burden between liver and adipose tissues. Toxicology and Applied Pharmacology 131:253-266.

Carrier G, Brunet RC, Brodeur J. 1995b. Modeling of the toxicokinetics of polychlorinated dibenzo-p-dioxins and dibenzofurans in mammalians, including humans. II. Kinetics of absorption and disposition of PCDDs/PCDFs. Toxicology and Applied Pharmacology 131:267-276.

Chahoud I, Krowke R, Schimmel A, Merker HJ, Neubert D. 1989. Reproductive toxicity and pharmacokinetics of 2,3,7,8-tetrachlorodibenzo-p-dioxin. 1. Effects of high doses on the fertility of male rats. Archives of Toxicology 63:432-439.

Chahoud I, Hartmann J, Rune GM Neubert D. 1992. Reproductive toxicity and toxicokinetics of 2,3,7,8-tetrachlorodibenzo-p-dioxin. 3. Effects of single doses on the testis of male rats. Archives of Toxicology 66:567-572.

Chou MW, Pegram RA, Turturro A, Holson R, Hart RW. 1993. Effect of caloric restriction on the induction of hepatic cytochrome P-450 and Ah receptor binding in C57BL/6N and DBA/2J mice. Drug and Chemical Toxicology 16:1-19.

Christou M, Savas U, Spink DC, Gierthy JF, Jefcoate CR. 1994. Co-expression of human CYP1A1 and a human analog of cytochrome P450-EF in response to 2,3,7,8-tetrachloro-dibenzo-p-dioxin in the human mammary carcinoma-derived MCF-7 cells. Carcinogenesis 15:725-732.

Chun YJ, Koh WS, Yang KH. 1994. Suppression of TCDD-induced cytochrome P450 IA1 activity by staurosporine in mouse primary hepatocyte cultures and hepatoma cells. Biochemistry and Molecular Biology International 32:1023-1031.

Couture LA, Abbott BD, Birnbaum LS. 1990. A critical review of the developmental toxicity and teratogenicity of 2,3,7,8-tetrachlorodibenzo-p-dioxin: recent advances toward understanding the mechanism. Teratology 42:619-627.

Daujat M, Peryt B, Lesca P, Fourtanier G, Domergue J, Maurel P. 1992. Omeprazole, an inducer of human CYP1A1 and 1A2, is not a ligand for the Ah receptor. Biochemical and Biophysical Research Communications 188:820-825.

De Duffard AME, De Peretti AF, De Cantarini SC, Duffard R. 1993. Effects of 2,4-dichlorophenoxyacetic acid butyl ester on chick liver. Archives of Environmental Contamination and Toxicology 25:204-211.

De Haan LH, Simons JW, Bos AT, Aarts JM, Denison MS, Brouwer A. 1994. Inhibition of intercellular communication by 2,3,7,8-tetrachlorodibenzo-p-dioxin and dioxin-like PCBs in mouse hepatoma cells (Hepa-1c1c7): involvement of the Ah receptor. Toxicology and Applied Pharmacology 128:283-293.

De Jongh J, Bawman C, Nieboer R, Seinen W, Van den Berg M. 1994. Toxicokinetic mixture between 2,3,7,8-tetrachlorodibenzo-*p*-dioxin and 2, 2′, 4,4′,5,5′-hexachlorobiphenyl in the liver of neonatal rats after pre- and postnatal exposure. Chemosphere 28:1581-1588.

De Jongh J, Nieboer R, Schroders I, Seinen W, Van den Berg M. 1993. Toxicokinetic mixture interactions between chlorinated aromatic hydrocarbons in the liver of the C57BL/6J mouse: 2. Polychlorinated dibenzo-*p*-dioxins (PCDds), dibenzofurans (PCDFs) and biphenyls (PCBs). Archives of Toxicology 67:598-604.

De Moro GM, Duffard RO, De Duffard AME. 1993. Neurotoxicity of 2,4-dichlorophenoxyacetic butyl ester in chick embryos. Neurochemical Research 18:353-359.

De Vito MJ, Maier WE, Diliberto JJ, Birnbaum LS. 1993. Comparative ability of various PCBs, PCDFs and TCDD to induce cytochrome P450 1A1 and 1A2 activity following 4 weeks of treatment (short communication). Fundamental and Applied Toxicology 20:125-130.

De Vito MJ, Ma X, Babish JG, Menache M, Birnbaum LS. 1994. Dose-response relationships in mice following subchronic exposure to 2,3,7,8-tetrachlorodibenzo-*p*-dioxin: CYP1A1, CYP1A2, estrogen receptor, and protein tyrosine phosphorylation. Toxicology and Applied Pharmacology 124:82-90.

De Waal EJ, Rademakers LH, Schuurman HJ, Van Loveren H, Vos JG. 1993. Ultrastructure of the cortical epithelium of the rat thymus after in vivo exposure to 2,3,7,8-tetrachlorodibenzo-*p*-dioxin (TCDD). Archives of Toxicology 67:558-564.

Denison MS. 1992. Heterogeneity of rat hepatic Ah receptor: identification of two receptor forms which differ in their biochemical properties. Journal of Biochemical Toxicology 7:249-256.

DePetrillo PB, Kurl RN. 1993. Stimulation of protein kinase C by 2,3,7,8-tetrachlorodibenzo-*p*-dioxin (TCDD) in rat thymocytes. Toxicology Letters 69:31-36.

Dési I, Sos J, Olasz J, Sule F, Markus V. 1962a. Nervous system effects of a chemical herbicide. Archives of Environmental Health 4:95-102.

Dési I, Sos J, Nikolits I. 1962b. New evidence concerning the nervous site of action of a chemical herbicide causing professional intoxication. Acta Physiologica Academiae Scientiarum Hungaricae 22:73-80.

Dickson LC, Buzik SC. 1993. Health risks of "dioxins": a review of environmental and toxicological considerations. Veterinary and Human Toxicology 35:68-77.

Dolwick KM, Swanson HI, Bradfield CA. 1993. In vitro analysis of Ah receptor domains involved in ligand-activated DNA recognition. Proceedings of the National Academy of Sciences (USA) 90:8566-8570.

Dunn RT 2d, Ruh TS, Ruh MF. 1993. Binding of the Ah receptor to receptor binding factors in chromatin. Biochemical Pharmacology 45:1121-1128.

Durrin LK, Whitlock JP Jr. 1989. 2,3,7,8-tetrachlorodibenzo-*p*-dioxin-inducible aryl hydrocarbon receptor-mediated change in CYP1A1 chromatin structure occurs independently of transcription. Molecular and Cellular Biology 9:5733-5737.

Ebner K, Matsumura F, Enan E, Olsen H. 1993. 2,3,7,8-tetrachlorodibenzo-*p*-dioxin (TCDD) alters pancreatic membrane tyrosine phosphorylation following acute treatment. Journal of Biochemical Toxicology 8:71-81.

Edwards MD, Pazzi KA, Gumerlock PH, Madewell BR. 1993. c-N-ras is activated infrequently in canine malignant lymphoma. Toxicology and Pathology 21:288-291.

Elferink CJ, Whitlock JP Jr. 1990. 2,3,7,8-tetrachlorodibenzo-*p*-dioxin-inducible, Ah receptor-mediated bending of enhancer DNA. Journal of Biological Chemistry 265:5718-5721.

Ema M, Sogawa K, Wanatabe N, Chujoh Y, Matsushita N, Gotch O, Funae Y, Fujii-Kuriyama Y. 1992. cDNA cloning and structure of mouse putative Ah receptor. Biochemical and Biophysical Research Communications 184:246-253.

Ema M, Matsushita N, Sogawa K, Ariyama T, Inazawa J, Nemoto T, Ota M, Oshimura M, Fujii-Kuriyama Y. 1994. Human arylhydrocarbon receptor: functional expression and chromosomal assignment to 7p21. Journal of Biochemistry (Tokyo) 116:845-851.

Enan E, Liu PC, Matsumura F. 1992a. 2,3,7,8-tetrachlorodibenzo-*p*-dioxin causes reduction of glucose transporting activities in the plasma membranes of adipose tissue and pancreas from the guinea pig. Journal of Biological Chemistry 267:19785-19791.

Enan E, Liu PC, Matsumura F. 1992b. TCDD (2,3,7,8-tetrachlorodibenzo-*p*-dioxin) causes reduction in glucose uptake through glucose transporters on the plasma membrane of the guinea pig adipocyte. Journal of Environmental Science and Health 27:495-510.

Enan E, Matsumura F. 1994. Significance of TCDD-induced changes in protein phosphorylation in the adipocyte of male guinea pigs. Journal of Biochemical Toxicology 9:159-170.

Enan E, Matsumura F. 1995. Evidence for a second pathway in the action mechanism of 2,3,7,8-tetrachlorodibenzo-*p*-dioxin (TCDD). Significance of Ah-receptor mediated activation of protein kinase under cell-free conditions. Biochemical Pharmacology 49:249-261.

Esser C, Welzel M. 1993. Ontogenic development of murine fetal thymocytes is accelerated by 3,3',4,4'-tetrachlorobiphenyl. International Journal of Immunopharmacology 15:841-852.

Evangelista D, de Duffard AM, Fabra de Peretti A, Castro de Cantarini S, Duffard R. 1993. Effects of 2,4-dichlorophenoxyacetic acid butyl ester on chick liver. Archives of Environmental Contamination and Toxicology 25:204-211.

Faith RE. 1979. Investigations on the effects of TCDD on parameters of various immune functions. Annals of the New York Academy of Sciences 320:564-571.

Fan F, Rozman KK. 1995. Short- and long-term biochemical effects of 2,3,7,8-tetrachlorodibenzo-*p*-dioxin in female Long-Evans rats. Toxicology Letters 75:209-216.

Fernandez-Salguero P, Pineau T, Hilbert DM, McPhail T, Lee SST, Kimura S, Nebert DW, Rudikoff S, Ward JM, Gonzalez FJ. 1995. Immune system impairment and hepatic fibrosis in mice lacking the dioxin-binding Ah receptor. Science 268:722-726.

Gaido KW, Maness SC. 1994. Regulation of gene expression and acceleration of differentiation in human keratinocytes by 2,3,7,8-tetrachlorodibenzo-*p*-dioxin. Toxicology and Applied Pharmacology 127:199-208.

Geyer HJ, Scheunert I, Rapp K, Gebefugi I, Steinberg C, Kettrup A. 1993. The relevance of fat content in toxicity of lipophilic chemicals to terrestrial animals with special reference to dieldrin and 2,3,7,8-tetrachlorodibenzo-*p*-dioxin (TCDD). Ecotoxicology and Environmental Safety 26:45-60.

Gradin K, Wilhelmsson A, Poellinger L, Berghard A. 1993. Nonresponsiveness of normal human fibroblasts to dioxin correlates with the presence of a constitutive xenobiotic response element-binding factor. Journal of Biological Chemistry 268:4061-4068.

Grahmann F, Claus D, Grehl H, Neundorfer B. 1993. Electrophysiologic evidence for a toxic polyneuropathy in rats after exposure to 2,3,7,8-tetrachlorodibenzo-*p*-dioxin (TCDD). Journal of the Neurological Sciences 115:71-75.

Graillet C, and Girard JP. 1994. Embryotoxic potency of 2,4,5-trichlorophenoxyacetic acid on sea urchin eggs: association with calcium homeostasis. Toxicology Vitro 8:1097-1105.

Gray LE Jr, Ostby J, Kelce W, Marshall R., Diliberto JJ, Birnbaum LS. 1993. Perinatal TCDD exposure alters sex differentiation in both female and male LE hooded rats. Abstracts of the 13th International Symposium on Dioxins and Related Compounds 13:337-340.

Gray LE Jr, Kelce WR, Monosson E, Ostby JS, Birnbaum LS. 1995. Exposure to TCDD during development permanently alters reproductive function in male Long Evans rats and hamsters: reduced ejaculated and epididymal sperm numbers and sex accessory gland weights in offspring with normal androgenic status. Toxicology and Applied Pharmacology 131:108-118.

Grehl H, Grahmann F, Claus D, Neundorfer B. 1993. Histologic evidence for a toxic polyneuropathy due to exposure to 2,3,7,8-tetrachlorodibenzo-*p*-dioxin (TCDD) in rats. Acta Neurologica Scandinavica 88:354-357.

Hanson CD, Smialowicz RJ. 1994. Evaluation of the effect of low-level 2,3,7,8-tetrachlorodibenzo-*p*-dioxin exposure on cell mediated immunity. Toxicology 88:213-224.

Harper N, Wang X, Liu H, Safe S. 1994. Inhibition of estrogen-induced progesterone receptor in MCF-7 human breast cancer cells by aryl hydrocarbon (Ah) receptor agonists. Molecular and Cellular Endocrinology 104:47-55.

Hotz P. 1994. Occupational hydrocarbon exposure and chronic nephropathy. Toxicology 90:163-283.

Institute of Medicine. 1994. Veterans and Agent Orange Health Effects of Herbicides Used in Vietnam. Washington: National Academy of Sciences.

Jeong HG, Jeong TC, Yang KH. 1993. Mouse interferon gamma pretreated hepatocytes conditioned media suppress cytochrome P-450 induction by TCDD in mouse hepatoma cells. Biochemistry and Molecular Biology International 29:197-202.

Johnson L, Dickerson R, Safe SH, Nyberg CL, Lewis RP, Welsh TH Jr. 1992. Reduced Leydig cell volume and function in adult rats exposed to 2,3,7,8-tetrachlorodibenzo-p-dioxin without a significant effect on spermatogenesis. Toxicology 76:103-118.

Johnson L, Wilker CE, Safe SH, Scott B, Dean DD, White PH. 1994. 2,3,7,8-Tetrachlorodibenzo-p-dioxin reduces the number, size, and organelle content of Leydig cells in adult rat testes. Toxicology 89:49-65.

Jones EL, Krizek HA. 1962. A technic for testing acnegenic potency in rabbits applied to the potent acnegen 2,3,7,8-tetrachlorodibenzo-p-dioxin. Journal of Investigative Dermatology 39:511-517.

Jover R, Ponsoda X, Castell JV, Gomez-Lechon MJ. 1994. Acute cytotoxicity of ten chemicals in human and rat cultured hepatocytes and in cell lines: correlation between in vitro data and human lethal concentrations. Toxicology Vitro 8:47-54.

Karenlampi SO, Legraverend C, Gudas JM, Carramanzana N, Hankinson O. 1988. A third genetic locus affecting the Ah (dioxin) receptor. Journal of Biological Chemistry 263:10111-10117.

Karras JG, Conrad DH, Holsapple MP. 1995. Effects of 2,3,7,8-tetrachlorodibenzo-p-dioxin (TCDD) on interleukin-4-mediated mechanisms of immunity. Toxicology Letters 75:225-233.

Kelling CK, Christian BJ, Inhorn SL, Peterson RE. 1985. Hypophagia-induced weight loss in mice, rats, and guinea pigs treated with 2,3,7,8-tetrachlorodibenzo-p-dioxin. Fundamental and Applied Toxicology 5:700-712.

Kerkvliet N, Burleson GR. 1994. Immunotoxicity Of TCDD And Related Halogenated Aromatic Hydrocarbons. In: Dean JH et al. (ed.). Target Organ Toxicology Series: Immunotoxicology and Immunopharmacology, Second Edition. Raven Press, New York: pp. 97-121.

Kim CS, Keizer RF, Pritchard JB. 1988. 2,4-Dichlorophenoxyacetic acid intoxication increases its accumulation within the brain. Brain Research 440:216-226.

Kim CS, Pritchard JB. 1993. Transport of 2,4,5-trichlorophenoxyacetic acid across the blood-cerebrospinal fluid barrier of the rabbit. Journal of Pharmacology and Experimental Therapy 267:751-757.

Kim, CS, Gargas ML, Andersen ME. 1994. Pharmacokinetic modeling of 2,4-dichlorophenoxyacetic acid (2,4-D) in rat and in rabbit brain following single dose administration. Toxicology Letters 74:189-201.

Kociba RJ, Keys DG, Beyer JE, Careon RM, Wade CE, Dittenber DA, Kalnins RP, Frauson LE, Park CN, Barnar SD, Hummel RA, Humiston CG. 1978. Results of a two-year chronic toxicity and oncogenicity study of 2,3,7,8-tetrachlorodibenzo-p-dioxin in rats. Toxicology and Applied Pharmacology 46:279-303.

Koerner FC, Goldberg DE, Edgerton SM, Schwartz LH. 1992. P52 protein and steroid hormone receptors in invasive breast carcinomas. International Journal of Cancer 52:183-188.

Kohn MC, Lucier GW, Clark GC, Sewall C, Tritscher AM, Portier CJ. 1993. A mechanistic model of effects of dioxin on gene expression in the rat liver. Toxicology and Applied Pharmacology 120:138-154.

Krishnan V, Wang X, Ramamurthy P, Safe S. 1994. Effect of 2,3,7,8-tetrachlorodibenzo-p-dioxin (TCDD) on formation of estrogen-induced ER/Sp1 complexes on the cathespsin-D promoter. Society of Toxicology 33rd Annual Meeting. 13-17 Mar 1994. Dallas, TX (USA).

Kurl RN. 1994. An inhibitory factor in rat thymus which interferes with binding of cytosol Ah receptor to xenobiotic responsive element. Biochemistry and Molecular Biology International 34:55-66.

Landi MT, Bertazzi PA, Shields PG, Clark G, Lucier GW, Garte SJ, Cosma G, Caporaso NE. 1994. Association between CYP1A1 genotype, mRNA expression and enzymatic activity in humans. Pharmacogenetics 4:242-246.

Le Beau MM, Carver LA, Espinosa R 3rd, Schmidt JV, Bradfield CA. 1994. Chromosomal localization of the human Ahr locus encoding the structural gene for the Ah receptor to 7p21—>p15. Cytogenetics and Cell Genetics 66:172-176.

Lesca P, Peryt B, Larrieu G, Alvinerie M, Galtier P, Daujat M, Maurel P, Hoogenboom L. 1995. Evidence for the ligand-independent activation of the Ah receptor. Biochemical and Biophysical Research Communications 209:474-482.

Li W, Donat S, Dohr O, Unfried K, Abel J. 1994. Ah receptor in different tissues of C571L/6J and DBA/2J mice: use of competitive polymerase chain reaction to measure Ah-receptor mRNA expression. Archives of Biochemistry and Biophysics 315:279-284.

Lorr NA, Sinclair JF, Sinclair PR, Bloom SE. 1994. Detection and localization of 3,3',4,4'-tetrachlorobiphenyl-induced P4501A protein in avian primary immune tissues. International Journal of Immunopharmacology 16:875-885.

Lundberg K, Dencker L, Gronvik KO. 1992. 2,3,7,8-tetrachlorodibenzo-p-dioxin (TCDD) inhibits the activation of antigen-specific T-cells in mice. International Journal of Immunopharmacology 14:699-705.

Lusska A, Shen E, Whitlock JP Jr. 1993. Protein-DNA interactions at a dioxin-responsive enhancer. Journal of Biological Chemistry 268:6575-6580.

Ma X, Mufti NA, Babish JG. 1992. Protein tyrosine phosphorylation as an indicator of 2,3,7,8-tetrachloro-p-dioxin exposure in vivo and in vitro. Biochemical and Biophysical Research Communications 189:59-65.

Mably TA, Moore RW, Goy RW, Peteron RE. 1992a. In utero and lactational exposure of male rats to 2,3,7,8-tetrachlorodibenzo-p-dioxin. 1. Effects of high doses on the fertility of male rats. Toxicology and Applied Pharmacology 114:97-107.

Mably TA, Moore RW, Goy RW, Peterson RE. 1992b. In utero and lactational exposure of male rats to 2,3,7,8-tetrachlorodibenzo-p-dioxin. 2. Effects on sexual behavior and the regulation of luteinizing hormone secretion in adulthood. Toxicology and Applied Pharmacology 114:108-117.

Mahon MJ, Gasiewicz TA. 1995. Ah receptor phosphorylation: localization of phosphorylation sites to the C-terminal half of the protein. Archives of Biochemistry and Biophysics 318:166-174.

Marsman DS, Barrett JC. 1994. Apoptosis and chemical carcinogenesis. Risk Analysis 14:321-326.

Molloy CJ, Laskin JD. 1992. Altered expression of a mouse epidermal cytoskeletal protein is a sensitive marker for proliferation induced by tumor promoters. Carcinogenesis 13:963-968.

Moore M, Narasimhan TR, Steinberg MA, Wang X, Safe S. 1993. Potentiation of CYP1A1 gene expression in MCF-7 human breast cancer cells cotreated with 2,3,7,8-tetrachlorodibenzo-p-dioxin and 12-O-tetradecanoylphorbol-13-acetate. Archives of Biochemistry and Biophysics 305:483-488.

Moore RW, Potter CL, Theobald HM, Robinson JA, Peterson RE. 1985. Androgenic deficiency in male rats treated with 2,3,7,8-tetrachlorodibenzo-p-dioxin. Toxicology and Applied Pharmacology 79:99-111.

Morgan JE, Whitlock JP Jr. 1992. Transcription-dependent and transcription-independent nucleosome disruption induced by dioxin. Proceedings of the National Academy of Sciences (USA) 89:11622-11626.

Morita K, Hirakawa H, Matsueda T, Iida T, Tokiwa H. 1993. [Stimulating effect of dietary fiber on fecal excretion of polychlorinated dibenzofurans (PCDF) and polychlorinated dibenzo-p-dioxins (PCDD) in rats]. Fukuoka Igaku Zasshi 84:273-281.

Murai T, Iwata H, Otoshi T, Endo G, Horiguchi S, Fukushima S. 1993. Renal lesions induced in F344/DuCrj rats by 4-weeks oral administration of dimethylarsenic acid. Toxicology Letters 66:53-61.

Murray FJ, Smith FA, Nitschke KD, Humiston CG, Kociba RJ, Schwetz BA. 1979. Three generations study of rats given 2,3,7,8-TCDD in the diet. Toxicology and Applied Pharmacology 50:241-252.

Neubert R, Helge H, Neubert D. 1994. Proliferative capacity of marmoset lymphocytes after tetanus vaccination and lack of 2,3,7,8-tetrachlorodibenzo-*p*-dioxin to reduce a booster effect. Life Sciences 56:437-444.

Okino ST, Pendurthi UR, Tukey RH. 1992. Phorbol esters inhibit the dioxin receptor-mediated transcriptional activation of the mouse Cyp1a-1 and Cyn1a-s genes by 2,3,7,8-tetrachlorodibenzo-*p*-dioxin. Journal of Biological Chemistry 267:6991-6998.

Okino ST, Pendurthi UR, Tukey RH. 1993. 2,3,7,8-Tetrachlorodibenzo-*p*-dioxin induces the nuclear translocation of two XRE binding proteins in mice. Pharmacogenetics 3:101-109.

Oliveira GH, Palermo-Neto J. 1993. Effects of 2,4-dichlorophenoxyacetic acid (2,4-D) on open-field behavior and neurochemical parameters of rats. Pharmacology and Toxicology 73:79-85.

Ou X, Ramos KS. 1995. Regulation of cytochrome P4501A1 gene expression in vascular smooth muscle cells through aryl hydrocarbon receptor-mediated signal transduction requires a protein synthesis inhibitor. Archives of Biochemistry and Biophysics 316:116-122.

Oughton JA, Pereira CB, DeKrey GK, Collier JM, Frank AA, Kerkvliet N.I. 1995. Phenotypic analysis of spleen, thymus, and peripheral blood cells in aged C57BL/6 mice following long-term exposure to 2,3,7,8-tetrachlorodibenzo-*p*-dioxin. Fundamental and Applied Toxicology 25:60-69.

Palmeira CM, Moreno AJ, Madeira VM. 1994a. Interactions of herbicides 2,4-D and dinoseb with liver mitochondrial bioenergetics. Toxicology and Applied Pharmacology 127:50-57.

Palmeira CM, Moreno AJ, Madeira VMC. 1994b. Metabolic alterations in hepatocytes promoted by the herbicides paraquat, dinoseb and 2,4-D. Archives of Toxicology 68:24-31.

Perdew GH. 1992. Chemical cross-linking of the cytosolic and nuclear forms of the Ah receptor in hepatoma cell line 1c1c7. Biochemical and Biophysical Research Communications 182:55-62.

Perdew GH, Hord N, Hollenback CE, Welsh MJ. 1993. Localization and characterization of the 86- and 84-kDa heat shock proteins in Hepa-1c1c7 cells. Experimental Cell Research 209:330-336.

Poland A, Palan D, Glover E. 1994. Analysis of the four alleles of the murine aryl hydrocarbon receptor. Molecular Pharmacology 46:915-921.

Pollenz RS, Poland AP. 1993. Immunological analysis of the Ah receptor and Ah receptor nuclear transporter protein in Hepa-1 cell lines (meeting abstract). Proceedings of the Annual Meeting of the American Association of Cancer Researchers 34:A873.

Pongratz I, Stromstedt PE, Mason GGF, Poellinger L. 1991. Inhibition of the specific DNA binding activity of the dioxin receptor by phosphatase treatment. Journal of Biological Chemistry 266:16813-16817.

Pongratz I, Mason GGF, Poellinger L. 1992. Dual roles of the 90-kDa heat shock protein hsp90 in modulating functional activities of the dioxin receptor. Journal of Biological Chemistry 267:13728-13734.

Puga A, Nebert DW, Carrier F. 1992. Dioxin induces expression of c-fos and c-jun proto-oncogenes and a large increase in transcription factor AP-1. DNA Cell Biology 11:269-281.

Quattrochi LC, Tukey RH. 1993. Nuclear uptake of the Ah (dioxin) receptor in response to omeprazole: transcriptional activation of the human CYP1A1 gene. Molecular Pharmacology 43:504-508.

Randerath K, Lu L, Li D. 1988. A comparison between different types of covalent DNA modifications (I-compounds, persistent carcinogen adducts and 5-methylcytosine) in regenerating rat liver. Carcinogenesis 9:1843-1848.

Reisz-Porszasz S, Probst MR, Fukunaga BN, Hankinson O. 1994. Identification of functional domains of the aryl hydrocarbon receptor nuclear translocator protein (ARNT). Molecular and Cellular Biology 14:6075-6086.

Reyes H, Reisz-Porszasz S, Hankinson O. 1992. Identification of the Ah receptor nuclear translocator protein (ARNT) as a component of the DNA binding form of the Ah receptor. Science 256(5060):1193-1195.

Reynolds PM, Reif JS, Ramsdell HS, Tessari JD. 1994. Canine exposure to herbicide-treated lawns and urinary excretion of 2,4-dichlorophenoxyacetic acid. Cancer Epidemiology Biomarkers Prevention 3:233-237.

Rice CD, Merchant RE, Jeong TC, Karras JB, Holsapple MP. 1995. The effects of acute exposure to 2,3,7,8-tetrachlorodibenzo-*p*-dioxin on glioma-specific cytotoxic T-cell activity in Fischer 344 rats. Toxicology 95:177-185.

Rier SE, Martin DC, Bowman RE, Dmowski WP, Becker JL. 1993. Endometriosis in rhesus monkeys (Macaca mulatta) following chronic exposure to 2,3,7,8-tetrachlorodibenzo-*p*-dioxin. Fundamental and Applied Toxicology 21:433-441.

Rivarola V, Mori G, Balegno H. 1992. 2,4-dichlorophenoxyacetic acid action on in vitro protein synthesis and its relation to polyamines. Drug and Chemical Toxicology 15:245-257.

Roth WL, Ernst S, Weber LW, Kerecsen L, Rozman KK. 1994. A pharmacodynamically responsive model of 2,3,7,8-tetrachlorodibenzo-*p*-dioxin (TCDD) transfer between liver and fat at low and high doses. Toxicology and Applied Pharmacology 127:151-162.

Rozman K, Roth WL, Greim H, Stahl BU, Doull J. 1993. Relative potency of chlorinated dibenzo-*p*-dioxins (CDDs) in acute, subchronic and chronic (carcinogenicity) toxicity studies: implications for risk assessment of chemical mixtures. Toxicology 77:39-50.

Sadek CM, Allen-Hoffmann BL. 1994. Suspension-mediated induction of Hepa-1c1c7 CYP1A-1 expression is dependent on the Ah receptor signal transduction pathway. Journal of Biological Chemistry 269:31505-31509.

Sadhu DN, Merchant M, Safe SH, Ramos K. 1993. Modulation of protooncogene expression in rat aortic smooth muscle cells by benzo(a)pyrene. Archives of Biochemistry and Biophysics 300:124-131.

Safe S. 1990. Polychlorinated biphenyls (PCBs), dibenzo-*p*-dioxins (PCDDs), dibenzofurans (PCDFs), and related compounds; environmental and mechanistic considerations which support the development of toxic equivalency factors (TEFs). CRC Critical Reviews in Toxicology 21:51-88.

Savas U, Bhattacharyya KK, Christou M, Alexander DL, Jefcoate CR. 1994. Mouse cytochrome P-450EF, representative of a new 1B subfamily of cytochrome P-450s. Cloning, sequence determination, and tissue expression. Journal of Biological Chemistry 269:14905-14911.

Schafer MW, Madhukar BV, Swanson HI, Tullis K, Denison MS. 1993. Protein kinase C is not involved in Ah receptor transformation and DNA binding. Archives of Biochemistry and Biophysics 307:267-271.

Scheutz BA. 1979. Three-generation reproduction study of rats given TCDD in the diet. Applied Pharmacology 50:241-252.

Schrenk D, Schafer S, Bock KW. 1994. 2,3,7,8-tetrachlorodibenzo-*p*-dioxin as growth modulator in mouse hepatocytes with high and low affinity Ah receptor. Carcinogenesis 15:27-31.

Schuetz EG, Schuetz JD, Thompson MT, Fisher RA, Madariage JR, Strom S.C. 1995. Phenotypic variability in induction of P-glycoprotein mRNA by aromatic hydrocarbons in primary human hepatocytes. Molecular Carcinogenesis 12:61-65.

Sewall CH, Lucier GW, Tritscher AM, Clark GC. 1993. TCDD-mediated changes in hepatic epidermal growth factor receptor may be a critical event in the hepatocarcinogenic action of TCDD. Carcinogenesis 14:1885-1893.

Shen ES, Whitlock JP Jr. 1992. Protein-DNA interactions at a dioxin responsive enhancer: Mutatutional analysis of the DNA binding site for the liganded Ah receptor. Journal of Biological Chemistry 267:6815-6819.

Sirkka U, Pohjanvirta R, Nieminen SA, Tuomisto J, Ylitalo P. 1992. Acute neurobehavioural effects of 2,3,7,8-tetrachlorodibenzo-p-dioxin (TCDD) in Han/Wistar rats. Pharmacology and Toxicology 71:284-288.

Spink DC, Eugster HP, Lincoln DW, Schuetz JD, Schuetz EG, Johnson JA, Kaminsky LS, Gierthy JF. 1992. 17b-Estradiol hydroxylation catalyzed by human cytochrome P4501A1: a comparison of the activities induced by 2,3,7,8-tetrachlorophenol-p-dioxin in MCF-7 cells with those from heterologous expression of the cDNA. Archives of Biochemistry and Biophysics 293:342-348.

Stahl BU, Beer DG, Weber LW, Rozman K. 1993. Reduction of hepatic phosphoenolpyruvate carboxykinase (PEPCK) activity by 2,3,7,8-tetrachlorodibenzo-p-dioxin (TCDD) is due to decreased mRNA levels. Toxicology 79:81-95.

Sterling K, Weaver J, Ho KL, Xu LC, Bresnick E. 1993. Rat CYP1A1 negative regulatory element: biological activity and interaction with a protein from liver and hepatoma cells. Molecular Pharmacology 44:560-568.

Sutter TR, Tang YM, Hayes CL, Wo YY, Jabs EW, Li X, Yin H, Cody CW, Greenlee WF. 1994. Complete cDNA sequence of a human dioxin-inducible mRNA identifies a new gene subfamily of cytochrome P450 that maps to chromosome 2. Journal of Biological Chemistry 269:13902-12909.

Swanson HI, Tullis K, Denison MS. 1993. Binding of transformed Ah receptor complex to a dioxin responsive transcriptional enhancer: evidence for two distinct heteromeric DNA-binding forms. Biochemistry 32:12841-12849.

Takenaka H, Zhang K, Diaz-Sanchez D, Tsien A, Saxon A. 1995. Enhanced human IgE production results from exposure to the aromatic hydrocarbons from diesel exhaust: direct effects on B-cell IgE production. Journal of Allergy and Clinical Immunology 95:103-115.

Takimoto K, Lindahl R, Pitot HC. 1992. Regulation of 2,3,7,8-tetrachlorodibenzo-p-dioxin-inducible expression of aldehyde dehydrogenase in hepatoma cells. Archives of Biochemistry and Biophysics 298:493-497.

Thomas T, Gallo MA. 1994. Polyamine-induced changes in the sedimentation profile and DNA binding of aryl hydrocarbon receptor. Toxicology Letters 74:35-49.

Tripathy NK, Routray PK, Sahu GP, Kumar AA. 1993. Genotoxicity of 2,4-dichlorophenoxyacetic acid tested in somatic and germ-line cells of drosophila. Mutation Research 319:237-242.

Van den Berg M, De Jongh J, Poiger H, Olson JR. 1994. The toxicokinetics and metabolism of polychlorinated dibenzo-p-dioxins (PCDDs) and dibenzofurans (PCDFs) and their relevance for toxicity. Critical Reviews in Toxicology 24:1-74.

Vanden Heuvel JP, Lucier G. 1993. Environmental toxicology of polychlorinated dibenzo-p-dioxins and polychlorinated dibenzofurans. Environmental Health Perspectives 100:189-200.

Vanden Heuvel JP, Clark GC, Kohn MC, Tritscher AM, Greenlee WF, Lucier GW, Bell DA. 1994. Dioxin-responsive genes: examination of dose-response relationships using quantitative reverse transcriptase-polymerase chain reaction. Cancer Research 54:62-68.

Vasiliou V, Puga A, Nebert DW. 1992. Negative regulation of the murine cytosolic aldehyde dehydrogenase-3 (Aldh-3c) gene by functional CYP1A1 and CYP1A2 proteins. Biochemical and Biophysical Research Communications 187:413-419.

Vasiliou V, Reuter SF, Kozak CA, Nebert DW. 1993. Mouse dioxin-inducible cytosolic aldehyde dehydrogenase-3: AHD4 cDNA sequence, genetic mapping, and differences in mRNA levels. Pharmacogenetics 3:281-290.

Vogel C, Doehr O, Abel J. 1994. Transforming growth factor beta SUB 1 inhibits TCDD-induced cytochrome P450IA1 expression in human lung cancer A549 cells. Archives of Toxicology 68:303-307.

Walker NJ, Gastel JA, Costa LT, Clark GC, Lucier GW, Sutter TR. 1995. Rat CYP1B1: an adrenal cytochrome P450 that exhibits sex-dependent expression in livers and kidneys of TCDD-treated animals. Carcinogenesis 16:1319-1327.

Watson AJ, Hankinson O. 1992. Dioxin-dependent and Ah-receptor-dependent protein binding to xenobiotic responsive elements and G-rich DNA studied by in vivo footprinting. Journal of Biological Chemistry 267:6874-6878.

Weber LW, Lebofsky M, Stahl BU, Kettrup A, Rozman K. 1992. Comparative toxicity of four chlorinated dibenzo-*p*-dioxins (CDDs) and their mixture. Part III: Structure-activity relationship with increased plasma tryptophan levels, but no relationship to hepatic ethoxyresorufin o-deethylase activity. Archives of Toxicology 66:484-488.

Weber LW, Ernst SW, Stahl BU, Rozman K. 1993. Tissue distribution and toxicokinetics of 2,3,7,8-tetrachlorodibenzo-*p*-dioxin in rats after intravenous injection. Fundamental and Applied Toxicology 21:523-534.

Weber TJ, Ou X, Merchant M, Wang X, Safe SH, Ramos KS. 1994. Biphasic modulation of protein kinase C (PKC) activity by polychlorinated dibenzo-*p*-dioxins (PCDDs) in serum-deprived rat aortic smooth muscle cells. Journal of Biochemical Toxicology 9:113-120.

Weber LW, Lebofsky M, Stahl BU, Smith S, Rozman KK. 1995a. Correlation between toxicity and effects on intermediary metabolism in 2,3,7,8-tetrachlorodibenzo-*p*-dioxin-treated male C57BL/6J and DBA/2J mice. Toxicology and Applied Pharmacology 131:155-162.

Weber TJ, Fan YY, Chapkin RS, Davidson LA, Ramos KS. 1995b. The isoform specific expression of PKCs during individual phases of the cell cycle in vascular smooth muscle cells is disrupted. The Toxicologist 15:236.

Weston WM, Nugent P, Greene RM. 1995. Inhibition of retinoic-acid-induced gene expression by 2,3,7,8-tetrachlorodibenzo-*p*-dioxin. Biochemical and Biophysical Research Communications 207:690-694.

White TE, Gasiewicz TA. 1993. The human estrogen receptor structural gene contains a DNA sequence that binds activated mouse and human Ah receptors: a possible mechanism of estrogen receptor regulation by 2,3,7,8-tetrachlorodibenzo-*p*-dioxin. Biochemistry and Biophysics Research Communications 193:956-962.

White TE, Rucci G, Liu Z, Gasiewicz TA. 1995. Weanling female Sprague-Dawley rats are not sensitive to the antiestrogenic effects of 2,3,7,8-tetrachlorophenol-p-dioxin (TCDD). Toxicology and Applied Pharmacology 133:313-320.

Whitelaw M, Pongratz I, Wilhelmsson A, Gustafsson J-A, Poellinger L. 1993. Ligand-dependent recruitment of the ARNT coregulatory determines DNA recognition by the dioxin receptor. Molecular and Cellular Biology 13:2504-2514.

Whitlock JP Jr. 1993. Mechanistic aspects of dioxin action. Chemical Research in Toxicology 6:754-763.

Wolfe WH, Michalek JE, Miner JC, Pirkle JL, Caudill SP, Patterson DG Jr, Needham LL. 1994. Determinants of TCDD half-life in veterans of Operation Ranch Hand. Journal of Toxicology and Environmental Health 41:481-488.

Wolfle D, Schmutte C, Marquardt H. 1993. Effects of 2,3,7,8-tetrachlorodibenzo-*p*-dioxin on protein kinase C and inositol phosphate metabolism in primary cultures of rat hepatocytes. Carcinogenesis 14:2283-2287.

Wu L, Whitlock JP Jr. 1992. Mechanism of dioxin action: Ah receptor mediated increase in promoter accessibility in vivo. Proceedings of the National Academy of Sciences (USA) 89:4811-4815.

Wu L, Whitlock JP Jr. 1993. Mechanism of dioxin action: receptor-enhancer interactions in intact cells. Nucleic Acids Research 21:119-125.

Yamanaka K, Tezuka M, Kato K, Hasegawa A, Okada S. 1993. Crosslink formation between DNA and nuclear proteins by in vivo and in vitro exposure of cells to dimethylarsinic acid. Biochemical and Biophysical Research Communications 191:1184-1191.

Yamanaka K, Okada S. 1994a. Induction of lung-specific DNA damage by metabolically methylated arsenics via the production of free radicals. Environmental Health Perspectives 102:37-40.

Yamanaka K, Hayashi H, Kato K, Hasegawa A, Tezuka M, Hanioka KI, Oku N, Okada S. 1994b. Gene damage in human pulmonary cultured cells induced by dimethylarsenics. Japanese Journal of Toxicology and Environmental Health 40:37.

Zacharewski T, Harris M, Biegel L, Morrison V, Merchant M, Safe S. 1992. 6-methyl-1,3,8-trichlorodibenzofuran (MCDF) as an antiestrogen in human and rodent cancer cell lines: evidence for the role of the Ah receptor. Toxicology and Applied Pharmacology 12:311-318.

Zacharewski TR, Bondy KL, McDonell P, Wu ZF. 1994. Antiestrogenic effect of 2,3,7,8-tetrachlorodibenzo-*p*-dioxin on 17 beta-estradiol-induced pS2 expression. Cancer Research 54:2707-2713.

4

Methodologic Considerations in
Evaluating the Evidence

QUESTIONS TO BE ADDRESSED

The committee was charged with the task of summarizing the strength of the scientific evidence concerning the association between herbicide exposure during Vietnam service and each of a set of diseases or conditions suspected to be associated with such exposure. For each disease, the committee has determined, to the extent that available scientific data permit meaningful determinations,

1. whether a statistical association with herbicide exposure exists, taking into account the strength of the scientific evidence and the appropriateness of the statistical and epidemiologic methods used to detect the association;
2. the increased risk of each disease among those exposed to herbicides during Vietnam service; and
3. whether there exists a plausible biologic mechanism or other evidence of a causal relationship between herbicide exposure and the disease.

The law establishing the committee did not provide a specific list of diseases and conditions suspected to be associated with herbicide exposure. The committee staff and members developed such a list based on the diseases and conditions that had been mentioned in the scientific literature or in legal documents that came to their attention through extensive literature searches. The committee's first step efforts was a comprehensive search of relevant computerized data bases. Sixteen data bases covering biomedical, toxicological, chemical, historical, and regulatory information were accessed. The majority of the data bases searched were bibliographic, providing citations to scientific literature. Factual data bases were also searched to provide toxicological and chemical information. Committee staff examined the reference lists of major review articles, books, and reports for relevant citations. Reference lists of individual articles were also scanned for additional relevant references. Literature identification continued through July 31, 1995. The input received both in written and oral form from veterans and other interested persons at the public hearing served as a valuable source of additional information.

This first biennial update concentrates on evaluating the evidence published following the completion of work on *VAO*. For each disease, the new evidence is evaluated, and conclusions are based on the totality of the accumulated evidence, not just on the recently published studies. In other words, the new evidence is not interpreted alone but is put into the context of the previous evidence addressed in *VAO*.

In addition to bringing the earlier work up to date, the committee has addressed several specific areas of concern identified by the Department of Veterans Affairs (DVA). Specifically, the committee was asked:

1. To evaluate the relationship between exposure to herbicides and the development of acute and subacute peripheral neuropathy that arives at the time of exposure. This is in contrast to and in addition to the focus in *VAO* on chronic peripheral neuropathy (see Chapter 10).

2. To pay particular attention to the relationship between exposure to herbicides and the subsequent development of prostate cancer, hepatobiliary cancer, and nasopharyngeal cancer. In addition to addressing these specific cancers, the committee has devoted attention in this report to respiratory cancers and multiple myeloma, both of which appeared in the "limited or suggestive" category of evidence in *VAO*. Attention has also been devoted to breast cancer, because of its public health importance and the publication of new studies that evaluate its association with exposure to herbicides.

3. To discuss the possible relationships between the length of time since exposure to herbicides and possible increases and decreases in the risks of specific cancers. The committee also devoted attention to issues related to estimating of levels of exposure and the potential for assessing the relationship between exposure levels and the magnitude of increased risk (i.e., the "dose-response" relationship). The discussion of dose-response appears in Chapter 5.

The committee's judgments have both quantitative and qualitative aspects, and they reflect both the evidence examined and the approach taken to evaluate it. In *VAO*, the committee described more fully how it approached its task, so that readers would be able to assess and interpret the committee's findings. By offering this information, the committee wished to make the report useful to those seeking to update its conclusions as new information is obtained. Much of this detail has been omitted from the present volume. This chapter outlines the types of evidence that the committee identified; the approaches used in evaluating published reports, both singly and collectively; and the nature of the committee's conclusions. Details of the analysis and specific conclusions concerning each health effect appear in subsequent chapters. Detailed descriptions of methodology and specific information on how the committee interpreted the questions being addressed may be found in Chapter 5 of *VAO*.

Are Herbicides Statistically Associated with the Health Outcome?

The committee necessarily focused on a pragmatic question: what is the nature of the relevant evidence for or against a statistical association between exposure and disease? The evidentiary base that the committee found to be most helpful derived from epidemiologic studies of populations—that is, investigations in which large groups of people are studied to determine the association between the occurrence of particular diseases and exposure to the substances at issue. To determine whether an association exists, epidemiologists estimate the magnitude of an appropriate quantitative measure (such as the relative risk or the odds ratio) that describes the relationship between exposures and disease in defined populations or groups. Usage of "relative risk," "odds ratio," or "estimate of relative risk" is not consistent in the literature reviewed and cited in this report. In its own usage, the committee intends *relative risk* to refer to the results of cohort studies, and *odds ratio* (an estimate of relative risk) to refer to the results of case-control studies. Values of relative risk greater than 1 may indicate a positive or direct association—that is, a harmful association—and are emphasized in this chapter. Values between 1 and 0 may indicate a negative or inverse association—that is, a protective association. The term "statistical significance" is used to desribe an increased risk that is sufficiently greater than 1 to minimize the possibility that the apparent association is due to chance.

Determining whether an observed statistical association between exposure and disease is "real" requires additional scrutiny, because there may be alternative explanations, other than exposure, for the observed association. These include errors in the design, conduct, or analysis of the investigation; bias, or a systematic tendency to distort the measure of association from representing the true relation between exposures and outcomes; confounding, or distortion of the measure of association because another factor, related to both exposures and outcomes, has not been recognized or taken into account in the analysis; and chance, the effect of random variation, producing spurious associations that can, with a known probability, sometimes depart widely from the truth.

Therefore, in deciding whether associations between herbicides and particular outcomes exist, the committee has had to judge in each instance whether there is evidence of an association from the available studies. If an association appears to exist, the committee judged whether it is direct or inverse, and whether it may be due to error, bias, confounding, or chance, or most likely represents a true association between herbicides and the outcome.

In pursuing the question of statistical association, the committee recognized that an absolute conclusion about the *absence* of association may never be attained. As in science generally, studies of health outcomes following herbicide exposure are not capable of demonstrating that the purported effect is impossible or could never occur. Any instrument of observation, including epidemiologic studies, has a limit to its resolving power. Hence, in a strict technical sense, the committee could not prove the absolute absence of a health outcome associated with herbicide exposure. Nevertheless, for some outcomes examined, there was limited or suggestive evidence consistent with *no* association. The committee was able to conclude in some cases that, *within the limits of the current resolving power of the existing studies,* there is no association with herbicide exposure.

What Is the Increased Risk of the Disease in Question Among Those Exposed to Herbicides in Vietnam?

This question, which is pertinent principally (but not exclusively) if there is evidence for an association between exposure and disease, concerns the likely magnitude of the exposure-disease association in Vietnam veterans exposed to herbicides. The most desirable evidence in answering this type of question involves knowledge of the rate of occurrence of the disease in those Vietnam veterans who were actually exposed to herbicides, the rate in those who were not exposed (the "background" rate of the disease in the population of Vietnam veterans), and the degree to which any other differences between exposed and unexposed groups of veterans influence the difference in rates. When exposure levels among Vietnam veterans have not been adequately determined, as has been the case in most studies, this question becomes difficult to answer. The committee found the available evidence sufficient for drawing conclusions about association between herbicides and a number of health outcomes. However, the lack of good data on Vietnam veterans per se, especially with regard to their exposure, complicated the assessment of the increased risk of disease among individuals exposed to the herbicides during service in Vietnam. By considering the magnitude of the association observed in other cohorts, the quality and results of studies that have been made of veterans, and other principles of epidemiologic research discussed in *VAO*, the committee formulated a qualitative judgment regarding the risk of disease among Vietnam veterans. Indeed, most of the evidence on which the findings in this report are based comes from studies of people exposed to dioxin or herbicides in occupational and environmental settings rather than from studies of Vietnam veterans.

When the available data do not permit a meaningful statement regarding risk among Vietnam veterans, no conclusion is stated, and the reader is referred to the appropriate section in *VAO* for additional discussion.

Is There a Plausible Biologic Mechanism?

Chapter 3 details the basic experimental evidence accumulated during the period 1992-95 that provides the basis for the assessment of biologic plausibility; that is, the extent to which a statistical association is consistent with existing biological or medical knowledge. The likelihood that a given chemical exposure-disease relationship reflects a true association in humans is often defined based on evidence of tumorigenicity in animal studies evidence of an association between exposure and disease occurrence in humans and/or evidence that a given outcome is associated with occupational/environmental chemical exposures. It must be recognized, however, that given the limitations of existing biological and medical knowledge, lack of data in support of a plausible biologic mechanism does not rule out the possibility that a causal relationship does exist.

ISSUES IN EVALUATING THE EVIDENCE

Experimental Studies

A valid surrogate animal model for the study of a human disease must reproduce with some degree of fidelity the manifestations of the disease in humans. Whole animal studies or animal-based experimental systems continue to be used to study herbicide toxicity because they allow for rigid control of chemical exposures and for close monitoring of health outcomes. Because many of the chemical exposures presently associated with cancer in humans are confirmed in experimental studies (Huff, 1993; Huff et al., 1994), data derived from experimental studies are generally accepted as a valuable guide in the assessment of biological plausibility.

As discussed in Chapter 3, many of the toxic effects of the herbicides used in Vietnam have been ascribed to TCDD, a significant contaminant of some of the herbicides. But this has not simplified the risk assessment process, because the toxicologic profile of TCDD is rather complex. In general, there is consensus that most of the toxic effects of TCDD involve interaction with the aryl hydrocarbon receptor (AhR), a protein that binds TCDD and other aromatic hydrocarbons with high affinity. Formation of an active complex between the receptor, ligand (the TCDD molecule), and other protein factors is followed by interaction of the activated complex with specific sites on DNA. This interaction results in DNA changes that alter the expression of genes involved in the regulation of cellular processes. In this manner, TCDD and other AhR ligands modulate target cells and presumably exert toxic effects.

Attempts to establish correlations between the effects of TCDD in experimental systems and in humans have become particularly problematic, because species differences in susceptibility to acute TCDD toxicity have been documented. Humans may actually be more resistant than other species to the toxic effects of this chemical (Dickson and Buzik, 1993). Differences in susceptibility involve a toxico-kinetic component, since elimination rates in humans may be slower than in rodents (Ahlborg and Hanberg, 1992). Toxico-dynamic interactions are also important, because the affinity of TCDD for the AhR is species-specific (Lorenzen and Okey, 1991), and the responses to occupancy of the receptor vary among different cell types and during different developmental stages.

If TCDD is assumed to be primarily responsible for the harmful effects of herbicides, then toxicity would be predicted to be receptor-mediated. Such deductive reasoning, however, has faced considerable challenges, because several inconsistencies in the receptor model have been identified, as discussed in Chapter 3. Of particular significance is the recognition that a variable region is present in the AhR (Dolwick et al., 1993), which may account for the presence of multiple forms of the AhR that dictate both species and cell-specific differences in responsiveness to receptor ligands. Although studies in which transformed human cell lines are employed to study AhR biology minimize the inherent error associated with species extrapolations, caution must be exercised, because the extent to which transformation itself affects toxicity outcomes has yet to be fully defined. It is generally accepted that genetic susceptibility plays a key role in determining the adverse effects of environmental chemicals. In the case of TCDD, the drug-metabolizing enzymes induced in humans are different from those induced in rodents (Neubert, 1992), suggesting that the impact of different genetic backgrounds on AhR function is not yet completely understood. This issue is particularly central to the assessment of biologic plausibility, because polymorphisms of the AhR in humans similar to those in laboratory animals would place some individuals at greater risk of the toxic and carcinogenic effects of TCDD. Ultimately, the major challenge in the assessment of biologic plausibility for the toxicity of herbicides and TCDD is not restricted to the understanding of receptor-mediated events. The dose-response relationships that arise from multiple toxico-kinetic and toxico-dynamic interactions must also be considered. The gene regulation models described to date do not consider the intricacies of the multiprotein interactions between the AhR and other proteins. Thus, future attempts to define the quantitative relationship between receptor occupancy and biological response to TCDD must consider that multiple biochemical changes may influence the overall cellular response.

Epidemiologic Studies

Environmental and/or occupational exposure to herbicides or TCDD have provided data on human responses that can be directly compared to data obtained in experimental studies. Higher-than-background body burdens of dioxin have been documented in many of these groups, and details describing the major findings from these studies are reviewed in Chapters 7-11 of this report. In general, the elevated risks of cancers at various sites reported in epidemiologic studies are consistent with the known biological actions of the agents present in herbicide formulations. Although its full potential has yet to be realized, the application of molecular and cellular measurements to epidemiologic research promises to be useful in facilitating correlations between herbicide exposure and disease occurrence. Such correlations will allow transfer of information to the study, prevention, and control of health risks of herbicide exposure in human populations. This evolution may provide a significant advantage in the assessment of biologic plausibility, because biologically based epidemiologic data allow for more accurate identification and quantification of exposures. For instance, the analytical data available from individuals known to have been exposed to Agent Orange during the Vietnam War provide a valuable resource for the study of TCDD-related disease, with documented TCDD body burdens providing a quantitative bridge between experimental studies and human epidemiology. Taken together, experimental studies and epidemiologic investigations provide complementary perspectives from which to view human health effects of exposure to herbicides. However, it must be recognized that the ultimate test of associations between exposure and disease occurrence will be data obtained from human populations.

To obtain additional information pertinent to the evaluation of potential effects of herbicide exposure of veterans, the committee decided to review studies of other groups potentially exposed to the herbicides contained in Agent Orange, to other herbicides, and to dioxin, the contaminant believed to be the cause of many of the purported adverse effects of Agent Orange. These study populations include industrial and agricultural workers, Vietnamese citizens, and people exposed environmentally as a result of residing near the site of an accident or a toxic-waste dumping area. The committee felt that considering studies of such groups would help in determining whether these compounds *could* be associated with particular health outcomes in veterans and what is the nature of any dose-response relationship, although the committee acknowledged that findings may have only an indirect bearing on the association in veterans themselves. It is also important to note that the categories of association described below relate to the association between exposure to chemicals and health outcomes in human populations, not to the likelihood that any individual's health problem is associated with or caused by the herbicides in question.

The Role of Case Studies and
Other Studies with No Comparison Groups

With the exception of one condition, the committee did not specifically consider case studies or other published studies lacking a control or comparison group. The one exception involved studies of acute and subacute transient peripheral neuropathy. Because peripheral neuropathies can be induced by common medical disorders and environmental exposures, the presence of neuropathy in an herbicide-exposed population cannot necessarily be attributed to the herbicide without consideration of these other potentially causative agents. Nonetheless, peripheral neuropathies do meet the conditions generally accepted as supporting an association in uncontrolled studies— namely, that the health outcome in question is somewhat unusual, and that the outcome becomes apparent soon after the exposure. Furthermore, a severe transient neuropathy may cause the individual to leave a worksite, thus removing that person from the pool of workers available for properly controlled epidemiologic studies. The very transience of these conditions may also contribute to making it difficult to locate patients with active symptoms. Performing a case-control study of neuropathies at a worksite, when cases may be hard to find, could lead to uninterpretable results. Thus, the committee gave substantial weight to case histories from occupational exposure and the descriptive reports following the Seveso accident when evaluating the association between herbicides and acute and subacute peripheral neuropathies.

Publication Bias

The phenomenon known as publication bias is also of concern to the committee. It has been well documented (Begg and Berlin, 1989; Berlin et al., 1989; Dickersin, 1990; Easterbrook et al., 1991; Dickersin et al., 1992) in biomedical research that studies with a statistically significant finding are more likely to be published than studies with nonsignificant results. Thus, evaluations of disease-exposure associations based solely on published literature could be biased in favor of showing a positive association. In general, however, for reports of overall associations with exposure, the committee did not consider the risk of publication bias to be high among studies of herbicide exposure and health risks. The committee took this position because there are numerous published studies showing no positive association; the committee examined a substantial amount of unpublished material; and the committee felt that the publicity surrounding the issue of exposure to herbicides, particularly regarding Vietnam veterans, has been so intense that any studies showing no association would be unlikely to be viewed as unimportant by the investigators. In short, the pressure to publish such "negative" findings would be considerable.

Nevertheless, publication bias of a more specific and subtle form may still have had a bearing on the committee's evaluation of the evidence. In particular, the relationship between timing and duration of exposure and subsequent changes in risk of disease was a major concern. This more subtle bias would arise if decisions to publish *specific* findings relative to timing of exposure were based on the statistical significance of those findings. For example, the NIOSH study (Fingerhut, 1991) of production workers found a more substantial increase in risk among those whose exposure began more than 20 years previously and lasted for more than one year. Many other studies did not publish data relevant to the issues of duration of and time since exposure. In most cases, it is impossible to know whether or not such issues were examined and simply not discussed in a publication solely because no "interesting" associations were found. Even decisions to examine or not examine such relationships may have been based on the investigators' perception that such analyses would or would not lead to any statistically significant findings.

The Role of Judgment

The evaluation of evidence to reach conclusions about statistical associations goes beyond quantitative procedures at several stages: assessing the relevance and validity of individual reports; deciding on the possible influence of error, bias, or confounding on the reported results; integrating the overall evidence, within and across diverse areas of research; and formulating the conclusions themselves. These aspects of the review required thoughtful consideration of alternative approaches at several points. They could not be accomplished by adherence to a narrowly prescribed formula.

Rather, the approach described here evolved throughout the process of review and was determined in important respects by the nature of the evidence, exposures, and health outcomes at issue. Both the quantitative and the qualitative aspects of the process that could be made explicit were important to the overall review. Ultimately, the conclusions about causation that are expressed in this report about causation are based on the committee's collective judgment. The committee endeavored to express its judgments as clearly and precisely as the data allowed.

Integration of New Evidence

As stated above, this first biennial update concentrates on evaluating the evidence published following the completion of work on *VAO*. For each disease, the new evidence is evaluated, and conclusions are based on the totality of the accumulated evidence, not just on the recently published studies. For only four diseases, *transient peripheral neuropathy (acute and subacute peripheral neuropathy), spina bifida, porphyria cutanea tarda,* and *skin cancer,* the committee found new evidence that was sufficiently strong to change the conclusions stated in *VAO.* For all other diseases, evidence appearing since the publication of *VAO* reinforced, or was not considered strong enough to change, the previous conclusions.

SUMMARY OF THE EVIDENCE

Categories of Association

The categories of association used by the committee were those used in *VAO*. Consistent with the charge to the Secretary of Veterans Affairs in P.L. 102-4, the distinctions between the categories are based on "statistical association," not on causality. Thus, standard criteria used in epidemiology for assessing causality (Hill, 1971) do not strictly apply. The distinctions between the categories reflect the committee's judgment that a statistical association would be found in a large, well-designed epidemiologic study of the outcome in question in which exposure to herbicides or dioxin was sufficiently high, well-characterized, and appropriately measured. The categories of association are:

• *Sufficient Evidence of an Association* Evidence is sufficient to conclude that there is a positive association. That is, a positive association has been observed between herbicides and the outcome in studies in which chance, bias, and confounding could be ruled out with reasonable confidence. For example, if several small studies that are free from bias and confounding show an association that is consistent in magnitude and direction, there may be sufficient evidence for an association.

• *Limited/Suggestive Evidence of an Association* Evidence is suggestive of an association between herbicides and the outcome but is limited because chance, bias, and confounding could not be ruled out with confidence. For example, at least one high-quality study shows a positive association but the results of other studies are inconsistent.

• *Inadequate/Insufficient Evidence to Determine Whether an Association Exists* The available studies are of insufficient quality, consistency, or statistical power to permit a conclusion regarding the presence or absence of an association. For example, studies fail to control for confounding, have inadequate exposure assessment, or fail to address latency.

• *Limited/Suggestive Evidence of No Association* There are several adequate studies, cover the full range of levels of exposure that human beings are known to encounter, that are mutually consistent in not showing a positive association between exposure to herbicides and the outcome at any level of exposure. A conclusion of "no association" is inevitably limited to the conditions, level of exposure, and length of observation covered by the available studies. In addition, the possibility of a very small elevation in risk at the levels of exposure studied can never be excluded.

REFERENCES

Ahlborg UG, Hanberg A. 1992. Toxicokinetics of PCDDs and PCDFs of importance to the development of human risk assessment. Toxic Substances Journal 12:197-211.

Begg CB, Berlin JA. 1989. Publication bias and dissemination of clinical research. Journal of the National Cancer Institute 81:107-115.

Berlin JA, Begg CB, Louis TA. 1989. An assessment of publication bias using a sample of published clinical trials. Journal of the American Statistical Association 84:381-392.

Dickersin K. 1990. The existence of publication bias and risk factors for its occurrence. Journal of the American Medical Association 263:1385-1389.

Dickersin K, Min Y-I, Meinert CL. 1992. Factors influencing publication of research results: followup of applications submitted to two institutional review boards. Journal of the American Medical Association 267:374-378.

Dickson LC, Buzik SC. 1993. Health risks of "dioxins": a review of environmental and toxicological considerations. Veterinary and Human Toxicology 35:68-77.

Dolwick KM, Swanson HI, Bradfield CA. 1993. In vitro analysis of Ah receptor domains involved in ligand-activated DNA recognition. Proceedings of the National Academy of Sciences (USA) 90:8566-8570.

Easterbrook PJ, Berlin JA, Gopalan R, Matthews DR. 1991. Publication bias in clinical research. Lancet 337:867-872.

Fingerhut MA, Halperin WE, Marlow DA, Piacitelli LA, Honchar PA, Sweeney MH, Greife AL, Dill PA, Steenland K, Suruda AJ. 1991. Cancer mortality in workers exposed to 2,3,7,8-tetrachlorodibenzo-p-dioxin. New England Journal of Medicine 324:212-218.

Hill, AB. 1971. Principles of Medical Statistics, 9th ed. New York: Oxford University Press.

Huff J. 1993. Chemicals and cancer in humans: first evidence in experimental animals. Environmental Health Perspectives 100:201-210.

Huff J, Lucier G, Tritscher A. 1994. Carcinogenicity of TCDD: experimental, mechanistic, and epidemiologic evidence. Annual Review of Pharmacology and Toxicology 34:343-372.

Lorenzen A, Okey AB. 1991. Detection and characterization of Ah receptor in tissue and cells from human tonsils. Toxicology and Applied Pharmacology 107:203-214.

Neubert D. 1992. Evaluation of toxicity of TCDD in animals as a basis for human risk assessment. Toxic Substances Journal 12:237-276.

5

Exposure Assessment

In this chapter, the committee addresses the question of whether studies published since *VAO* should change how assessments of exposure are used in the evaluation of epidemiologic studies. The committee's perspectives on the exposure assessment issues as presented in *VAO* are summarized, and then a review of recent literature is presented.

EXPOSURE ASSESSMENT IN THE EVALUATION OF EPIDEMIOLOGIC STUDIES

Assessment of individual exposure to herbicides and 2,3,7,8-tetrachloro-dibenzo-*p*-dioxin (TCDD) or other chemical compounds found in the herbicides used in Vietnam is a key element in determining whether specific health outcomes are associated with exposure to these compounds. The committee has found in its review, however, that the definition and quantification of exposure represent the weakest methodologic aspects complicating the interpretation of epidemiologic studies. Chapter 6 in *VAO* describes the criteria used by the committee in assessing the quality and validity of exposure measures. This chapter provides a brief review of that discussion.

When epidemiologists assess the potential health risks of exposure to a toxic chemical, they compare the disease experience of groups of people with different levels of exposure to that substance. Accurate estimation of any risk associated with exposure depends on the ability to identify those who are "exposed" and those who are not. When the concern is with low-level, possibly intermittent exposure to a chemical such as an herbicide, it becomes important to assess not only the presence or absence of exposure, but also to characterize the *degree* of exposure—its *intensity* and *duration*. Exposure assessment contributes to the epidemiologic study process in several ways. First, well-defined contrasts in exposure in the groups being studied increase the validity of individual and group risk assessments. A poorly defined contrast could result, for example, if a group of people assumed to be exposed to a particular agent contained many individuals who were not, in fact, truly exposed. Second, very large groups must be studied in order to identify the small risks associated with low levels of exposure, whereas a relatively small study may be able to detect the effect of heavy or sustained exposure to a toxic substance. In this way, a study's *precision* or statistical power is also linked to the extent of the exposure and the accuracy of its measurement.

The strength of association between an exposure and a disease is only one of the criteria used in evaluating epidemiologic evidence. Another criterion often used in evaluating an association is whether or not there is evidence that as exposure increases, the risk of the disease also increases (Hill, 1971). This dose-response pattern can be detected only if the degree of exposure among different cohorts or subcohorts of the study can be determined. Inaccurate assessment of exposure can obscure the existence of such a trend and thus make it less likely that a true risk will be identified.

Once an exposure-disease association has been established, it is often desirable to consider the implications for some exposed population other than the population in which the study was performed. In making this inference, it is important to have exposure assessments that allow valid comparative assessments of exposure of the different study populations. For example, if an increased risk of a certain disease has been demonstrated in workers occupationally exposed to a herbicide for a long period, what would the risk be for a Vietnam veteran who was exposed only occasionally or for just a short period? The proper scale on which to compare these risks is the scale of quantitative exposure (integrating both level and duration), with risk assessed per unit of exposure. If the exposure levels are unknown or poorly characterized, then extrapolating from one population to another may be difficult.

Exposure assessment is the weakest aspect in most of the epidemiologic studies that the committee has reviewed. Rarely is there precise information on the intensity and duration of individual exposure. Rather, surrogates such as the length of employment and job location in the workplace are measured. In some cases, not even the specific chemicals to which a cohort has been exposed are specified. Many studies use overall membership in a group to assign exposure. Exceptions are studies conducted by Fingerhut et al. (1991) and Saracci et al. (1991), which involve chemical production workers and evaluate subgroups with presumed higher, longer, or better-characterized exposure.

The types of occupational and environmental exposure situations studied, and the likely intensity and duration of the exposures to herbicides and TCDD, are diverse. In principle, this provides an opportunity to compare results between studies in order to determine whether certain diseases are more common in populations likely to have higher exposures. However, because of the complex pattern of exposures to the various herbicides and TCDD in the available epidemiologic studies, the committee was generally not able to differentiate among multiple chemical exposures to determine whether specific health effects were associated with a particular herbicide or TCDD in the mixed exposure setting.

Studies of occupational and environmental exposures to air contaminants often observe that although most exposures occur at lower levels, a few people are exposed to much higher concentrations. Those with the highest exposures are at the highest risk for disease, and their risks are not well represented by the average or median exposure of the group. The importance of the "tail" of the exposure distribution can be illustrated by examining the serum TCDD concentrations among the sample of Ranch Hand ground crews studied by Michalek et al. (1995). Although the geometric mean (approximately the median) serum TCDD concentration for 397 ground crewmen was 26 ppt, a quarter of these men had serum TCDD levels above 150 ppt, and some were above 500 ppt. Note that those with the highest exposures had serum TCDD concentrations 20 times greater than the geometric mean. Thus, the mean or median exposure of Vietnam veterans, either as a whole or of any military occupation group, will not adequately represent the exposure of maximally exposed veterans. In *VAO*, the committee estimated that some unknown, but likely small, fraction of Vietnam veterans may have had phenoxy herbicide exposures comparable in intensity to members of the occupational cohorts (the NIOSH and IARC cohorts, for example). It is not currently possible to identify this heavily exposed fraction of Vietnam veterans (outside the Ranch Hand and Chemical Corps groups), although in *VAO* the committee recommended the testing of exposure reconstruction methods that might have this capability.

ESTIMATES OF EXPOSURE TO HERBICIDES AND TCDD DURING VIETNAM SERVICE

Different approaches have been used in estimating the exposure of Vietnam veterans, including self-reported exposures, records-based exposure estimates, or biomarkers of TCDD exposure. Each approach is limited in its ability to determine precisely the degree of individual exposure. Some studies rely on gross markers such as service in Vietnam—perhaps enhanced by branch of service, military region, military specialty, or exposure to combat—as proxies for exposure to herbicides. Studies of this type include the CDC Vietnam Experience Study and Selected Cancers Study, the Department of Veterans Affairs (DVA) mortality studies, and most veterans studies conducted by states. This approach almost surely dilutes whatever health effects of herbicides exist, because many members of the cohort presumed to be exposed to herbicides may, in reality, not have been. At the other extreme, some studies rely on fine details of military records of troop movements and herbicide spraying, perhaps combined with self-reported retrospective data, for individuals or small units on a daily basis. Examples of this approach include are a study performed by Stellman and Stellman (1986) and the CDC Agent Orange Study (1988). The latter study was proposed but never completed. Although measures of this type may be accurate for many individuals, such fine detail may exceed the accuracy of a record system not designed for this purpose (for example data on troop movements), and the accuracy of the resulting exposure measure cannot be guaranteed for all potential subjects. However, recent application of such a method for estimating exposures of Vietnamese civilians (summarized below) did find evidence supporting the utility of a records-based exposure reconstruction strategy (Verger, 1994).

Serum TCDD measurements may provide valuable information about past herbicide exposure under some conditions. They are best used to detect differences in exposure levels among large groups for epidemiologic studies. However, serum TCDD measurements should not be considered the "gold standard" measure of exposure to herbicides in Vietnam, for several reasons. First, all Americans have some exposure to TCDD from a variety of environmental sources, primarily food. This background exposure varies among individuals depending on their diets and other poorly understood factors. Second, there are variations among individuals in the way that TCDD is metabolized. For example, a person's fat content affects his or her rate of clearance of TCDD (see below for further discussion of TCDD clearance studies). Third, because not all herbicides used in Vietnam contained TCDD, serum TCDD levels may not be good indicators of overall exposure to herbicides. Agent White did not contain TCDD, and the 2,4-D contained in Agent Orange did not contain TCDD. Additionally, the concentration of TCDD in the 2,4,5-T in Agent Orange varied widely over time. A further complication, as noted below, is that exposures to other dioxin congeners contained in some herbicides may not be well-correlated with serum TCDD levels years after exposure, because of differences in their environmental fate after they were sprayed in Vietnam, as well as in their metabolism in the human body. Finally, the committee reported in *VAO* that there was evidence to suggest that exposure to the herbicide 2,4-D (which contains no TCDD) was associated with one cancer, non-Hodgkin's lymphoma (NHL), while exposure to TCDD has no such association.

Despite these concerns, the committee concluded that any group differences in serum TCDD levels probably reflect group differences in exposure to TCDD. Group differences are more meaningful, because in groups the factors leading to differences in serum dioxin measurements unrelated to past dioxin exposure would tend to average out. However, even if there was at one time a difference in TCDD exposure between two groups, it may disappear over time as serum concentrations fade to background levels. Thus, the failure to detect group mean differences does not necessarily indicate that there were not small differences in past exposure.

Current serum TCDD levels in Vietnam veterans, with the exception of measured levels in Ranch Hand veterans, suggest that exposure to TCDD in Vietnam was substantially less, *on average*, than that of occupationally exposed workers or of persons exposed as a result of the industrial explosion in Seveso, Italy. As noted above, this estimation of *average* exposure does not preclude the existence of a heavily exposed subgroup. The CDC's Validation Study found that study subjects could not be distinguished from controls based on serum TCDD levels. The median TCDD levels for Vietnam veterans and non-Vietnam veterans were both 4 ppt. Serum TCDD levels obtained from Ranch Hand veterans in 1987, however, did differ among groups defined by military duties, although the median levels for the Ranch Hand groups were lower than those of several occupational cohorts and Seveso residents. The best-studied of the occupational cohorts (Fingerhut et al., 1991) had serum TCDD measurements performed 23 years (on average) after their occupational exposure, which is not very different from the 15 to 25 years in the Ranch Hand studies. The estimated (back extrapolated) mean maximum serum TCDD level (see below) was approximately 1,400 ppt for the NIOSH cohort, 200 ppt for the Ranch Hands and Chemical Corps veterans, and very low on average for other Vietnam veterans. The Ranch Hand and Chemical Corps veterans appear to be the most highly exposed groups of veterans. The available evidence concerning TCDD exposure shows that, as a group, Vietnam veterans had much lower exposures to TCDD than heavily exposed occupational workers.

Historical data, personal testimony, and other information made available to the committee suggest that there was substantial variability in individual wartime experiences and that opportunities for exposure are also likely to have varied. Approximately 1.5 million U.S. military personnel served in South Vietnam from 1967 through 1969, the period of heaviest herbicide use. According to Air Force operations data, nearly 14 million gallons of herbicide were sprayed over Vietnam during this period. In addition to Ranch Hands, an unknown number of veterans were likely to have received varying degrees of exposure to herbicides. Localized spraying, while conducted on a smaller scale than Ranch Hand spraying, may have resulted in higher degrees of exposure because it was done in close proximity to ground troops. Most military bases had vehicle-mounted and backpack spray units available for use in routine vegetation-control programs conducted around the perimeters of base camps. Approximately 750 personnel who were assigned to the Army Chemical Corps have been followed (Thomas and Kang, 1990). These individuals were responsible for the storage, preparation, and application of chemicals around the perimeters of base camps and, as a group, were likely to have been more highly exposed than most other military personnel. U.S. Army Special Forces camps were often located in enemy territory throughout Vietnam and may have been in the target areas of Ranch Hand missions. Construction of Special Forces camps or fire-support bases often required defoliation, so soldiers in these units may have been exposed to high levels of herbicides. Navy riverine units operating along the rivers and canals of the Mekong Delta reportedly sprayed base perimeters with herbicides (Zumwalt, 1993).

Although the CDC Validation Study (CDC, 1988) found no correlations between a range of possible herbicide exposure measures, including serum TCDD levels, oral and written testimony suggests that substantial numbers of veterans were exposed to Agent Orange and other herbicides. Surveys of Vietnam veterans indicate that 25 to 55 percent believe they were exposed to herbicides (Erickson et al., 1984a,b; Stellman and Stellman, 1986; CDC, 1989). It appears that many veterans other than those involved in Operation Ranch Hand were likely to have been exposed to herbicides during their service in Vietnam.

It is clear that the military use of herbicides in Vietnam was not uniform, either spatially or temporally, and that the movement and behavior of troops also varied. Thus, it cannot be assumed that all troops were equally exposed to herbicides. In the committee's judgment, a sufficiently large range of exposures may exist among Vietnam veterans (including those who served in Ranch Hand and the Chemical Corps) to conduct a valid epidemiologic study for certain health outcomes. The difficulty (from the perspective of epidemiologic studies) is that the available data do not precisely quantify individual exposures for most veterans. None of the measures that the committee has reviewed would be free of nondifferential misclassification bias. The effect of this bias on relative risk estimates would likely be to underestimate true effects of exposure if they existed, possibly to such an extent that these effects could be missed entirely by future studies.

REVIEW OF THE RECENT LITERATURE

Several studies published since the release of *VAO* provided useful information for the refinement of exposure assessment strategies. While none of these studies led the committee to revise its basic view of the role of exposure assessment in the evaluation of the epidemiologic studies, several recent reports warrant brief discussion here. The studies fall into three categories: investigations of the clearance of TCDD from the human body, evaluations of other types (congeners) of dioxins found in humans exposed to herbicides and related chemicals, and descriptions of the development of several different exposure indices for epidemiologic studies.

TCDD Half-Life Investigations

Estimates of the body burden half-life of 2,3,7,8-TCDD have been undertaken in several recent studies. An early pilot study was undertaken in a collaborative effort by the Air Force and the Centers for Disease Control and Prevention (CDC) personnel using data collected on 36 Ranch Hand veterans (Pirkle et al.,

1989). The initial study was expanded to 337 individuals, with serum measurements collected during 1982 and from May 1987 through March 1988 (Wolfe et al., 1994).

The Air Force-CDC study was further extended with an additional five years of follow-up for 213 of the subjects (Michalek et al., 1995). Excluded from study were about 23 percent of the population who had serum TCDD levels below a set level, in order to avoid a biased estimate of decay rate because of serum levels that approach the background level. Using a repeated measures regression analysis, the investigators estimated a mean half-life of 8.7 years, with a 95 percent confidence interval around the mean half-life that ranged from 8.0 to 9.5 years. However, half-life was found to increase with increasing body fat, and the mean half-life does not address individual variability in half-life that would derive from differences in body fat among an exposed population. For example, for a high but plausible percent body fat (35 percent), the predicted mean half-life is about 20 years, while for a low percent body fat (15 percent), the predicted mean half-life is about seven years.

Other recently published studies find similar mean serum TCDD half-life estimates. A study of 27 individuals exposed during the Seveso accident and followed for 15.9 years yielded a half-life estimate of 8.2 years (Needham et al., 1994). A study of 48 German workers in a plant producing herbicides showed a half-life of 10.3 years (Flesch-Janys et al., 1994). In this case, however, the time between the first and last analysis was only 6.3 years. These studies did not investigate possible heterogeneity in half-life due to such variables as body fat.

TCDD Exposure Levels for Selected Epidemiologic Studies

Using an estimate of the mean half-life for TCDD—the committee used 8.7 years (Michalek et al., 1995)—it is possible to back-extrapolate from measurements of serum TCDD made years after exposure to the mean maximum levels that were likely to have occurred for an exposed population at the time they were exposed (see Appendix B for calculations). There are, unfortunately, only a few studies for which this can be done with data in the published literature. Nevertheless, the committee found these data useful in evaluating epidemiologic studies, because they provide some reference with which to rank exposures in these studies. It becomes apparent, for example, that the NIOSH cohort probably had considerably higher levels of exposure to TCDD than the average member of the Ranch Hand cohort. The heavily exposed Zone A cohort in the Seveso population probably had higher mean maximum TCDD exposure than even the NIOSH cohort, but its small size severely limits its usefulness for the evaluation of all but the most common health effects. The committee estimated serum TCDD levels for the Seveso Zones B and R cohorts by assuming a proportional relationship between soil TCDD levels in the zones and the residents' mean serum TCDD levels. The mean serum TCDD levels for residents of Zones B and R were estimated by this method to be roughly 100 times less than in Zone A.

The committee noted several limitations in using these serum TCDD data in the evaluation of studies. First, as noted earlier, there may have been other toxic agents in the herbicides sprayed in Vietnam as well as in the chemicals to which other cohorts were exposed. Second, it is possible that the patterns of exposure (for example, short intense exposures, long-term low-level exposures, periods of no exposure interspersed among periods of heavy exposure) are relevant to disease risk, so that simply knowing mean maximum serum TCDD level at the time of exposure may not be an adequate way to summarize exposure. Third, TCDD and other dioxin congeners persist in the body for long periods, and these periods of "internal exposure" may be important to risk.

The committee noted that quantitative estimates of the magnitude of the risks faced by Vietnam veterans from herbicide exposure can only be made if quantitative data on exposure are available. Thus, there is a need for more measurements of serum TCDD levels in exposed populations, as well as for the development of quantitative measures of exposure to the other herbicide constituents.

Other Dioxin Congeners

In addition to 2,3,7,8-TCDD, other congeners of dioxin and dibenzofuran contaminated the herbicides sprayed in Vietnam as well as the products used and manufactured by the occupational cohorts whose health experience forms the basis for many of the committee's conclusions. Because these may contribute to cancer risk, "dioxin toxic equivalent factors" (Teq factors) have been estimated for the various other congeners of dioxin and dibenzofuran (U.S. EPA, 1989). A Teq factor for each dioxin or furan congener is estimated by comparing its toxicity to that of 2,3,7,8-TCDD, which is arbitrarily assigned a Teq factor of 1.0. Other congeners have lower Teq factors, some as much as 1,000 times lower. In principle, it is possible to measure each congener and calculate a toxic equivalent for the entire mixture, but this is costly. Most studies of dioxin-exposed individuals have related health effects to TCDD levels only and have not considered the other associated dioxins or furans.

The use of 2,3,7,8-TCDD alone as a measure of risk when exposure includes many congeners must be considered cautiously. Different sources of dioxin contamination may have different distributions of congeners. Also, the stability of the different congeners in the environment differs, so that human exposures occurring long after spraying may differ from those at the time of spraying. Finally, the half-lives of the different congeners in the body differ, so that an exposed individual will have different and varying patterns of exposure to each congener over time.

The degree to which these differences may be of importance is seen in some measured distributions of the various congeners in human tissue. While having lower Teq factors, some of the other dioxins or furans may be present in the body at concentrations hundreds of times greater than TCDD. For example, in a study by Verger et al. (1994) of dioxin levels in adipose tissue of Vietnamese civilians, the geometric mean concentration of TCDD was 7.8 ppt, that of 2,3,7,8-dibenzofuran was 1.7 ppt, and those of other congeners of dioxin ranged up to 384 ppt. By explicitly considering Teqs, Schecter et al. (1995) have shown that the total potential toxicity of all dioxins and furans measured in pooled serum samples of 433 southern, 183 central, and 82 northern Vietnamese civilians during 1991 and 1992 was, respectively, 2.4, 3.8, and 7.0 times the potential toxicity of TCDD alone. Other studies provide similar data (Schecter, 1994). Such Teq studies of Vietnam veterans and occupational cohorts would be valuable.

In summary, the magnitude of the effect of other congeners may be large, and it may vary among exposure settings. While it is probably not feasible to conduct a total congener analysis in every study, the use of TCDD measurements alone may represent an oversimplification of the full exposure picture.

Development of Exposure Indices

As noted in *VAO*, the committee emphasized the importance of exposure indices that could account for the full range of exposures, not just for TCDD. Several recent studies are relevant to this effort.

Occupational Cohorts

Two recent publications examined the development of exposure indices for cohorts exposed to herbicides, dioxins, or related compounds during chemical manufacture (Kauppinen et al., 1994; Ott et al., 1993). Both illustrate methods of exposure reconstruction for cohorts with past exposures to chemicals for which no actual exposure monitoring data exist. In both cases, an indirect validation or evaluation of the model was accomplished.

Kauppinen et al. (1994) estimated past exposures to phenoxy herbicides, chlorophenols, and dioxins for workers engaged in the manufacture or spraying of phenoxy herbicides and related compounds. The procedure was carried out for two diseases (soft-tissue sarcoma and non-Hodgkin's lymphoma), using controls chosen from the multicountry IARC cohort (Saracci et al., 1991). A team of three industrial hygienists, blind to case-control status, evaluated the exposure histories of each subject using a standardized procedure. The main steps of the reconstruction procedure were qualitative exposure assessment, determination of the duration of exposure, estimation of the intensity, or level of exposure, calculation of cumulative exposure, and the ranking of the subjects. The procedure was performed separately for more than a dozen agents, including the principal phenoxy herbicides (2,4-D, 2,4,5-T), several chlorophenols, dioxins, and dibenzofurans. This procedure could not be directly validated because almost no quantitative exposure data existed. However, in a separate paper discussed in detail elsewhere in this report, Kogevinas et al. (1995) used the exposure estimates to study the association with soft-tissue sarcoma (STS) and non-Hodgkin's lymphoma (NHL) in nested case-control studies. The authors report considerably stronger associations between estimated exposure and risk of STS than was seen with the simpler exposure classification used in the full cohort study (Saracci et al., 1991). The relationship between estimated exposure and NHL was equivocal, although some evidence of increasing risk with increasing estimated exposure to some agents was observed.

In the second report on exposure reconstruction for an occupational cohort (Ott et al., 1993), workers at a German chemical plant involved in a 1953 industrial accident resulting in TCDD exposure and the subsequent cleanup operations have been followed to study potential health effects (Zober et al., 1990). Of the 254 workers followed, serum TCDD data were available on 138. Ott et al. (1993) have constructed a model to characterize the relationships between current (1988-92) serum TCDD levels and information on the workers' activities during and after the accident for those members with measured serum TCDD levels. The model was then used to estimate TCDD levels for those cohort members without measurements. The investigators also used a simple back-extrapolation procedure to estimate serum TCDD levels for all cohort members during the time of the accident and cleanup.

Using such factors as the time period of exposure (varying from the first few days after the accident to 15 years later), physical location of the worker during exposure, type of work performed, use of protective equipment, and duration of exposure, the authors could explain 65 percent of the variability in the measured serum TCDD levels. The authors found that estimated back-extrapolated serum TCDD levels were higher in those who experienced severe chloracne (geometric mean = 1,008 ppt, n = 56) than in workers with moderate chloracne (geometric mean = 421 ppt, n = 59) and those with no chloracne (geometric mean = 38 ppt, n = 139).

Vietnamese Civilians

Verger et al. (1994) developed an exposure index based on the U.S. military's HERBS tapes of aerial spraying and investigated its association with serum TCDD levels in 27 South Vietnamese civilians. The HERBS tapes contain information regarding the location, content, and amount of herbicides applied in aerial missions from August 1965 through February 1971. The subjects were patients undergoing abdominal surgery in 1989 for whom adipose tissues were readily available. Residential histories were obtained from all. Five had always lived in Ho Chi Minh City and were considered not exposed to Agent Orange; the remainder had varying degrees of exposure in spray areas. The data indicated that 2,3,7,8-TCDD lipid concentrations in 24 samples ranged from 0.3 ppt to 49.6 ppt, with a geometric mean concentration of 7.8 ppt. Geometric mean concentrations of other dioxin congeners ranged from 10 ppt to 384 ppt for octochlorodibenzo-dioxin and from 1.7 ppt to 233 for various furan congeners. Two important results were reported from the analyses of these Vietnamese tissue specimens collected 19 years after the cessation of Operation Ranch Hand. First, there was a moderately strong correlation between lipid concentrations of 2,3,7,8-TCDD and an exposure index based on spraying patterns, after log-transformation of the two variables. Second, strong correlations were found among the serum levels of the different dioxin and furan congeners, but the correlation between congeners other than 2,3,7,8-TCDD and the exposure index were generally weak. The analyses assumed the same degradation half-life in the environment (a range of four to 17 years was considered) and biological half-life (five and seven years were considered) for all congeners. One would expect differences to exist among congeners for each of these two half-lives.

These data, although limited by small numbers, suggest that Agent Orange exposures among South Vietnamese civilians may be estimated by using of an appropriate exposure model and information on residence and spraying patterns during the Vietnam conflict.

Ranch Hand

Michalek and colleagues (1995) developed several indices of herbicide exposure for members of the Ranch Hand cohort and tried to relate these to the levels of serum TCDD measured between 1987 and 1992. Self-administered questionnaires completed by veterans of Operation Ranch Hand were used to develop three indices for herbicide or TCDD exposure: the number of days of skin exposure; the percentage of skin area exposed; and the number of days of skin exposure, times the percentage of skin exposed, times a factor for the concentration of TCDD in the herbicide. A fourth index used no information gathered from the individual subject. It was calculated as the volume of herbicide sprayed during a specific individual's tour of duty, times the concentration of TCDD in herbicides sprayed in that period, divided by the number of crew members at that time in each job specialty.

Each of the four models tested was significantly related to the serum TCDD level, although each explained only between 10 and 27 percent of the variability in serum TCDD. Military job classification (non-Ranch Hand combat troops, Ranch Hand administrators, Ranch Hand flight engineers, and Ranch Hand ground crew), which is separate from the four indices, explained 60 percent of the variance in serum TCDD concentrations. When the questionnaire-derived indices were applied within each job classification, none of the indices added significantly to the variability explained by job alone.

REFERENCES

Centers for Disease Control. 1988. Serum 2,3,7,8-tetrachlorodibenzo-*p*-dioxin levels in U.S. Army Vietnam-era veterans. The Centers for Disease Control Veterans Health Studies [see comments]. Journal of the American Medical Association 260:1249-1254.

Centers for Disease Control. 1989. Health Status of Vietnam Veterans. Vietnam Experience Study. Atlanta: U.S. Department of Health and Human Services. Vols. I-V, Supplements A-C.

Erickson JD, Mulinare J, Mcclain PW. 1984a. Vietnam veterans' risks for fathering babies with birth defects. Journal of the American Medical Association 252:903-912.

Erickson JD, Mulinare J, Mcclain PW, Fitch TG, James LM, McClearn AB, Adams MJ. 1984b. Vietnam Veterans' Risks for Fathering Babies with Birth Defects. Atlanta: U.S. Department of Health and Human Services, Centers for Disease Control.

Fingerhut MA, Halperin WE, Marlow DA, Piacitelli LA, Honchar PA, Sweeney MH, Greife AL, Dill PA, Steenland K, Suruda AJ. 1991. Cancer mortality in workers exposed to 2,3,7,8-tetrachlorodibenzo-*p*-dioxin. New England Journal of Medicine 324:212-218.

Flesch-Janys D, Gurn P, Jung D, Konietzke J, Papke O. 1994. First results of an investigation of the elimination of polychlorinated dibenzo-*p*-dioxins and dibenzofurans (PCDD/F) in occupationally exposed persons. Organohalogen Compounds 21:93-99.

Hill AB. 1971. Principles of Medical Statistics, 9th ed. New York: Oxford University Press

Kauppinen TP, Pannett B, Marlow DA, Kogevinas M. 1994. Retrospective assessment of exposure through modeling in a study on cancer risks among workers exposed to phenoxy herbicides, chlorophenols and dioxins. Scandinavian Journal of Work, Environment, and Health 20:262-271.

Kogevinas M, Kauppinen T, Winkelmann R, Becher H, Bertazzi PA, Bueno de Mesquita HB, Coggon D, Green L, Johnson E, Littorin M, Lynge E, Marlow DA, Mathews JD, Neuberger M, Benn T, Pannett B, Pearce N, Saracci R. 1995. Soft tissue sarcoma and non-Hodgkin's lymphoma in workers exposed to phenoxy herbicides, chlorophenols, and dioxins: two nested case-control studies. Epidemiology 6:396-402.

Michalek JE, Pirkle JL, Caudill SP, Tripathi RC, Patterson G, Needham LL. 1995. Pharmacokinetics of TCDD in veterans of Operation Ranch Hand: 10 year follow-up. Journal of Exposure Analysis and Environmental Epidemiology (in press).

Needham LL, Gerthoux PM, Patterson DG, Brambilla P, Pirkle JL, Tramacere PI, Turner WE, Beretta C, Sampson EJ, Mocarelli P. 1994. Half-life of 2,3,7,8-tetrachlorodibenzo-*p*-dioxin in serum of Seveso adults: interim report. Organohalogen Compounds 21:81-85.

Ott MG, Messerer P, Zober A. 1993. Assessment of past occupational exposure to 2,3,7,8-tetrachlorodibenzo-*p*-dioxin using blood lipid analyses. International Archives of Occupational and Environmental Health 65:1-8.

Pirkle JL, Wolfe WH, Patterson DG, Needham LL, Michalek JE, Miner JC, Peterson MR, Phillips DL. 1989. Estimates of the half-life of 2,3,7,8-tetrachlorodibenzo-*p*-dioxin in Vietnam veterans of Operation Ranch Hand. Journal of Toxicology and Environmental Health 27:165-171.

Saracci R, Kogevinas M, Bertazzi PA, Bueno De Mesquita BH, Coggon D, Green LM, Kauppinen T, L'Abbe KA, Littorin M, Lynge E, Mathews JD, Neuberger M, Osman J, Pearce N, Winkelmann R. 1991. Cancer mortality in workers exposed to chlorophenoxy herbicides and chlorophenols. Lancet 338:1027-1032.

Schecter A. 1994. Exposure Assessment: Measurement of Dioxins and Related Chemicals in Human Tissues. In: Dioxins and Health (ed. A Schecter). New York: Plenum Press. pp. 449-485.

Schecter A, Dai LC, Thuy LT, Quynh HT, Minh DQ, Cau HD, Phiet PH, Nguyen NT, Constable JD, Baughman R. 1995. Agent Orange and the Vietnamese: the persistence of elevated dioxin levels in human tissues. American Journal of Public Health 85:516-522.

Stellman SD, Stellman JM. 1986. Estimation of exposure to Agent Orange and other defoliants among American troops in Vietnam: a methodological approach. American Journal of Industrial Medicine 9:305-321.

Thomas TL, Kang HK. 1990. Mortality and morbidity among Army Chemical Corps Vietnam veterans: a preliminary report. American Journal of Industrial Medicine 18:665-673.

U.S. Environmental Protection Agency. 1989. Interim Procedures for Estimating Risks Associated with Exposures to Mixtures of Chlorinated Dibenzo-*p*-dioxins and Dibenzofurans (CDDs and CDFs) and 1989 Update. Springfield: U.S. Department of Commerce: National Technical Information Service. PB90-145756.

Verger P, Cordier S, Thuy LT, Bard D, Dai LC, Phiet PH, Gonnord MF, Abenhaim L. May 1994. Correlation between dioxin levels in adipose tissue and estimated exposure to Agent Orange in south Vietnamese residents. Environmental Research 65:226-242.

Wolfe WH, Michalek JE, Miner JC, Pirkle JL, Caudill SP, Patterson DG Jr, Needham LL. 1994. Determinants of TCDD half-life in veterans of Operation Ranch Hand. Journal of Toxicology and Environmental Health 41:481-488.

Zober A, Messerer P, Huber P. 1990. Thirty-four-year mortality follow-up of BASF employees exposed to 2,3,7,8-TCDD after the 1953 accident. International Archives of Occupational and Environmental Health 62:139-157.

Zumwalt ER Jr. 1993. Letter to the Institute of Medicine Committee to Review the Health Effects in Vietnam Veterans of Exposure to Herbicides regarding draft version of the IOM chapter on the U.S. military and herbicide program in Vietnam. May 20, 1993.

6

Epidemiologic Studies

In seeking evidence for associations between health outcomes and exposure to herbicides and TCDD, many different kinds of epidemiologic studies must be considered. Each study has varying degrees of strengths and weaknesses and contributes evidence to an association with the health outcomes considered in Chapters 7, 9, 10 and 11. There are three main groups of individuals studied with respect to herbicide exposure: those with occupational, environmental, and military exposures. The historical basis for the groups studied was examined in Chapter 2 of *VAO*. A description of how the articles to be reviewed were selected from the literature can be found in Appendix A of *VAO*.

This chapter summarizes epidemiologic studies and reports reviewed by the committee. Included are studies published after *VAO*, studies that were not reviewed by the committee that wrote *VAO*, and studies that have been updated since to the publication of *VAO*. Tables 6-1, 6-2, and 6-3 present a brief overview of all of the epidemiologic studies reviewed for both *VAO* and this report. The summaries of the study present the study methods used, including, how the study subjects were ascertained; how the data were collected; the inclusion criteria; and how the exposure was determined, including 2,4,5-T (2,4,5-trichlorophenoxy-acetic acid), 2,4-D (2,4-dichlorophenoxyacetic acid), chlorophenols, and the TCDD (2,3,7,8-tetrachlorodibenzo-p-dioxin) contaminant. Additionally, the numbers in the study and comparison populations, when available, are given along with a brief description of the study in Tables 6-1, 6-2, and 6-3. No results are presented here; rather, the chapter provides a methodologic framework for the health outcome chapters that follow. Qualitative critique of the study design, population size, methods of data collection, case and control ascertainment, or quality of exposure assessment has been reserved for the individual health outcome chapters in which the results of these studies are discussed. The text and tables in this chapter are organized in three basic sections—occupational studies, environmental studies, and studies in Vietnam veterans—with subsections included under each heading. The studies focused on exposures to 2,4,5-T (2,4,5-trichlorophenoxyacetic acid), 2,4-D (2,4-dichlorophenoxyacetic acid), chlorophenols, and the TCDD (2,3,7,8-tetrachlorodibenzo-*p*-dioxin) contaminant, 2,4-D, 2,4,5-T, 4-chloro-2-methylphenoxyacetic acid (MCPA), picloram, hexachlorophene, and chlorophenols, including trichlorophenol. In several instances, the investigators did not indicate which specific chemicals study participants were exposed to, or levels of exposure. Where available, details are given with regard to exposure assessment and how exposure was subsequently used in the analysis.

The occupational section includes studies of production workers, agricultural/forestry workers (including herbicide/pesticide applicators), and paper/pulp workers, as well as case-control studies of specific cancers and the association with exposures to herbicides and related compounds in many of these occupations. The environmental section includes studies of populations exposed to excessive herbicides as a result of where they live, such as the residents of Seveso, Italy, Times Beach, Missouri, and the southern portion of Vietnam. The section on Vietnam veterans includes studies conducted in the United States by the Air Force, the Centers for Disease Control and Prevention (CDC), Department of Veterans Affairs (DVA, formerly the Veterans Administration), the American Legion, and the state of Michigan, as well as other groups. Studies of Australian veterans of Vietnam are also presented here.

OCCUPATIONAL STUDIES

Several occupational groups in the United States and elsewhere have been exposed to the types of herbicides used in Vietnam and, more specifically, to TCDD, a contaminant of some herbicides and other products. Occupational groups exposed to these chemicals include farmers, agricultural/forestry workers, herbicide sprayers, workers in chemical production plants, and workers involved in paper/pulp manufacturing. In addition, studies that use job titles as broad surrogates of exposure and studies that rely on disease registry data have been conducted. Exposure measures vary widely in these studies in terms of measurement, quantification, level of detail, confounding by other exposures, and individual versus surrogate or group (ecological) measures.

TABLE 6-1 Epidemiologic Studies—Occupational Exposure

Reference	Study Design	Description	Study Group (N)	Comparison Group (N)[a]
Production Workers				
NIOSH				
New studies				
Egeland et al., 1994	Cohort	Study of total serum testosterone and gonadotropin levels in chemical production workers exposed to dioxin, in same group as Calvert et al. (1991)	248	231
Calvert et al., 1994	Cross-sectional	Study of porphyria cutanea tarda in same group as Calvert et al. (1991)	281	260
Studies reviewed in VAO				
Fingerhut et al., 1991	Cohort	Cancer mortality in male workers from 12 plants producing TCDD-contaminated chemicals (1942-1984) compared to U.S. population	5,172	—
Calvert et al., 1991	Cohort	Study of workers employed at one of two plants manufacturing substances contaminated with TCDD 15 years or more prior to assessment of chronic bronchitis, COPD, ventilatory function, and thorax and lung abnormalities compared to neighborhood controls without exposure to TCDD	281	260
Calvert et al., 1992	Cohort	Assessment of liver and gastrointestinal systems in same group as Calvert et al. (1991)	281	260
Alderfer et al., 1992	Cohort	Assessment of psychological variables to determine depression in same group as Calvert et al. (1991)	281	260
Sweeney et al., 1993	Cohort	Peripheral neuropathy in same group as Calvert et al. (1991)	281	260
Monsanto				
Zack and Suskind, 1980	Cohort	Evaluation of mortality experience among employees with chloracne exposed to TCP process accident in 1949 at Monsanto compared to U.S. male population standard	121	—
Zack and Gaffey, 1983	Cohort	Study of mortality experience of all white male workers (1955-1977) employed at a Monsanto plant through December 31, 1977, compared to mortality of standardized U.S. population rates	884	—
Suskind and Hertzberg, 1984	Cohort	Evaluation of health outcomes (1979) at clinical examination among workers exposed to 2,4,5-T (1948-1969) compared to non-exposed workers at same Monsanto plant	204	163

Reference	Study Design	Description	Exposed	Comparison Population
Moses et al., 1984	Cohort	Study of health outcomes in Monsanto workers (1948-1969) with chloracne reported as a surrogate to 2,4,5-T exposure compared to health outcomes in workers without chloracne as surrogate for no exposure	117	109
Collins et al., 1993	Cohort	Mortality of workers (through 1987) exposed and unexposed to dioxin between March 8, 1949, and November 22, 1949, as indicated by presence of chloracne, compared to local population mortality rates	122 With chloracne 632 Without chloracne	—
Dow				
New studies				
Bloeman et al., 1993	Cohort	Additional years of follow-up of Bond et al. (1988) study cohort through 1986	878	(1) U.S. population (2) 36,804 Unexposed workers
Studies reviewed in *VAO*				
Ott et al., 1980	Cohort	Mortality experience among workers exposed to 2,4,5-T in manufacturing (1950-1971) compared to mortality experience of U.S. white men	204	—
Cook et al., 1980	Cohort	Mortality experience (through 1978) of male workers involved in a chloracne incident (1964) from TCDD exposure compared to mortality experience of U.S. white men	61	—
Bond, 1987	Cohort	Extension of Cook et al. (1980) study, mortality through 1982	322	(1) U.S. white male population (2) 2,026 Employees without chloracne
Bond et al., 1983	Cross-sectional	Study of differences in workers potentially exposed and unexposed to TCDD during chemical production for (1) morbidity and (2) medical examination frequency between 1976 and 1978	(1) 183 (2) 114	(1) 732 (2) 456
Cook et al., 1986	Cohort	Mortality experience (1940-1979) of men manufacturing chlorinated phenols compared to U.S. white men	2,189	—
Ott et al., 1987 Cook et al., 1987	Cohort	Expanded Cook et al. (1986) study an additional three years, through 1982	2,187	—

Continued

TABLE 6-1 *Continued*

Reference	Study Design	Description	Study Group (N)	Comparison Group (N)[a]
Bond et al., 1989b	Cohort	Extension of Ott et al. (1987) study through 1984	2,187	—
Bond et al., 1989a	Cohort	Study of incidence of chloracne among a cohort of workers potentially exposed to TCDD, and association with other risk factors	2,072	Internal comparison
Bond et al., 1988	Cohort	Study of mortality (through 1982) among workers potentially exposed to 2,4-D (1945-1983) compared to U.S. white males and all other male employees not exposed	878	(1) U.S. white male population (2) 36,804 Employees not exposed
Sobel et al., 1987	Case-control	Study of STS among Dow Chemical employees (1940-1979) compared to employees without STS for possible association with several chemical exposures	14	126
Townsend et al., 1982	Cohort	Study of adverse reproductive outcomes among wives of Dow Chemical employees potentially exposed to TCDD (1939-1975) compared to reproductive outcomes among wives whose husbands were not exposed	370	345
Other Chemical Plants **New studies**				
Zober et al., 1994	Cohort	Morbidity experience in the same group as Zober et al. (1990)	158	161
Lynge et al., 1993	Cohort	Cancer incidence in the same group as Lynge (1985), with follow-up extended through 1987	3,390 Men 1,071 Women	—
Kogevinas et al., 1993	Cohort	Cancer incidence and mortality experience of female workers in seven countries potentially exposed to chlorophenoxy herbicides, chlorophenols, and dioxin compared to national death rates and cancer incidence rates	701	—
Kogevinas et al., 1992	Cohort	Study of mortality from STS and malignant lymphomas in an international cohort of production workers and herbicide sprayers (same group as Saracci et al., 1991)	14,439 (13,482 exposed, 416 probably exposed, 541 with unknown exposure)	3,951 Non-exposed employees
Kogevinas et al., 1995	Case-control	Two nested case-control studies of the relationship between STS and NHL and occupational exposures in members of the IARC cohort	STS: 11 cases NHL: 32 cases	5 Controls per case

Studies reviewed in VAO

Study	Type	Description	Number	External controls
Thiess et al., 1982	Cohort	Study of mortality experience among BASF employees potentially exposed to TCDD during November 17, 1953, accident compared to population and other workers not exposed	74	External controls: 180,000 town 1.8 million district 60.5 million Federal Republic of Germany Two groups of 74 each from other cohort studies
Zober et al., 1990	Cohort	Mortality experience of workers exposed to TCDD (1954-1987) at BASF plant compared to population of Federal Republic of Germany	247	—
Manz et al., 1991	Cohort	Mortality experience of workers (1952-1984) at Hamburg plant of Boehringer exposed to TCDD compared to national mortality and workers from another company	1,184 Men 399 Women	(a) Population (b) 3,120 Gas workers
Saracci et al., 1991	Cohort	Study of mortality experience of 20 international cohorts of herbicide sprayers and production workers compared to mortality experience expected for the nation	16,863 Men 1,527 Women	—
Coggon et al., 1986	Cohort	Study of mortality experience (through 1983) among workers manufacturing and spraying MCPA (1947-1975) compared to expected numbers of deaths among men in England and Wales and for rural areas	5,754	—
Coggon et al., 1991	Cohort	Mortality experience among four cohorts of workers potentially exposed (1963-1985) to phenoxy herbicides and chlorophenols compared to national (England and Wales) expected numbers and to the local population where factory is located	1,104 Factory A 271 Factory B 345 Factory C 519 Factory D	—
Jennings et al., 1988	Cohort	Assessment of immunological abnormalities among workers exposed to TCDD during accident manufacturing 2,4,5-T compared to matched controls	18	15
May, 1982, 1983	Cohort	Health outcomes among workers exposed and probably exposed to TCDD following a 1968 accident compared to unexposed workers	41 Exposed 54 Possibly exposed	31

Continued

TABLE 6-1 Continued

Reference	Study Design	Description	Study Group (N)	Comparison Group (N)[a]
Bueno de Mesquita et al., 1993	Cohort	Mortality experience of production workers exposed to phenoxy herbicides and chlorophenols in the Netherlands compared to national rates	2,310	—
Bashirov, 1969	Cross-sectional	Descriptive results of examination of workers involved in production of herbicides and study of workers at examination of cardiovascular and digestive systems compared to unexposed controls	292 (descriptive) 50 (examined)	20 (examined)
Lynge, 1985	Cohort	Study of cancer incidence among Danish workers exposed to phenoxyherbicides compared to expected results from the general population	3,390 Men 1,069 Women	—
Pazderova-Vejlupkova et al., 1981	Descriptive	Study of development of TCDD intoxication among men in Prague (1965-1968)	55	No comparison group
Poland et al., 1971	Cross-sectional	Assessment of PCT, chloracne, hepatotoxicity, and neuropsychiatric symptoms among 2,4-D and 2,4,5-T workers compared to other plant workers	73 Total 20 Administrators 11 Production supervisors 28 Production workers 14 Maintenance workers	Internal comparison
Thomas, 1987	Cohort	Assessment of mortality experience as of January 1, 1981, for white men employed in fragrance and flavors plant with possible exposure to TCDD compared to U.S. white men, and for cancers compared to local men	1,412	—
Agricultural/Forestry Workers **1. COHORT STUDIES** *Agricultural Workers* New studies				
Blair et al., 1993	Cohort	Study of causes of death, including cancer, among farmers in 23 states (1984-1988)	119,648 White men 2,400 White women 11,446 Nonwhite men 2,066 Nonwhite women	—

Reference	Study type	Description		
Dean, 1994	Cohort	Study of mortality from brain and hematopoietic cancers of agricultural workers compared to nonagricultural workers in Ireland (1971-1987)	(population size unclear)	—
Morrison et al., 1994	Cohort	Update of mortality experience in Wigle et al. (1990) cohort, through 1987, with addition of farmers from Alberta and Manitoba.	155,547	—
Semenciw et al., 1993	Cohort	Study of multiple myeloma mortality of male farmers compared to male population of the three prairie provinces of Canada (1971-1987)	155,547	—
Semenciw et al., 1994	Cohort	Study of leukemia mortality in same group as Morrison et al. (1993)	155,547	—
Senthilselvan et al., 1992	Cross-sectional	Study of the association between pesticide exposure and asthma in male farmers	1,939	No comparison group
Studies reviewed in VAO				
Burmeister, 1981	Cohort	Study of mortality of farmers compared to nonfarmers in Iowa (1971-1978)	6,402	13,809
Wigle et al., 1990	Cohort	Mortality experience from NHL of male farmers 35 years or older (1971-1985) in Saskatchewan, Canada, compared to age- and period-specific mortality rates expected for Saskatchewan males	69,513	—
Morrison et al., 1993	Cohort	Mortality experience of male Canadian farmers 45 years or older in Manitoba, Saskatchewan, and Alberta, Canada (1971-1987), compared to Canadian prairie province mortality rates	145,383	—
Morrison et al., 1992	Cohort	Mortality experience of male farmers 35 years or older (1971-1987) compared to Canadian prairie province mortality rates	155,547	—
Ronco et al., 1992	Cohort	Study of cancer incidence (1970-1980) among male and female Danish farm workers 15-74 years old compared to expected numbers of cancers among persons economically active, and study of cancer mortality (November 1981-April 1982) among male and female Italian farmers 18-74 years old compared to persons in other occupational groups	No Ns given	No Ns given
Corrao et al., 1989	Cohort	Study of cancer incidence among male farmers licensed (1970-1974) to use pesticides compared to number of cancers expected among licensed nonusers	642	18,839
Lerda and Rizzi, 1991	Cohort	Study of farmers exposed to 2,4-D as measured in urine compared to men unexposed for differences in sperm volume, death, count, motility, and abnormalities between March and June 1989	32	25

Continued

TABLE 6-1 *Continued*

Reference	Study Design	Description	Study Group (N)	Comparison Group (N)[a]
Hansen et al., 1992	Cohort	Study of cancer incidence among male and female Danish gardeners compared to incidence expected among the general population	4,015 859 Women 3,156 Men	—
Wiklund, 1983	Cohort	Study of cancer incidence (diagnosed 1961-1973) among agricultural workers in Sweden compared to rates expected from the 1960 population census	19,490	—
Wiklund and Holm, 1986	Cohort	STS incidence among agricultural and forestry workers in Sweden compared to the general population of men, 1960 census	354,620	1,725,845
Wiklund et al., 1988a	Cohort	Malignant lymphoma incidence among agricultural and forestry workers in Sweden compared to the general population of men, 1960 census	354,620	1,725,845
Eriksson et al., 1992	Cohort	Study of incidence of NHL, HD, and multiple myeloma (1971-1984) among selected occupational groups in Swedish men and women compared to expected rates of disease in general population	Number in occupational group unknown	—
Forestry Workers				
Green, 1987	Cohort	Suicide experience in a cohort of Canadian forestry workers by number of years in forestry trade as a surrogate for exposure to phenoxy herbicides compared to population	1,222	—
Green, 1991	Cohort	Mortality experience of male forestry workers (1950-1982) in Ontario compared to the expected mortality of the male Ontario population	1,222	—
van Houdt et al., 1983	Cross-sectional	Study of acne and liver dysfunction in a select group of Dutch forestry workers exposed to 2,4,5-T and unexposed	54	54
Herbicide/Pesticide Sprayers **New studies**				
Asp et al., 1994	Cohort	Mortality and cancer morbidity experience of male chlorophenoxy herbicide applicators (same cohort as Riihimaki et al., 1982 and 1983) in Finland (1955-1971), through 1989, compared to general population rates for morbidity and mortality.	1,909	—
Garry et al., 1994	Cross-sectional	Evaluation of health outcomes resulting from exposure to pesticides by male pesticide appliers in Minnesota	719	No comparison group

Studies reviewed in VAO

Reference	Type	Description	Exposed
Axelson and Sundell, 1974	Cohort	Study of mortality and cancer incidence among cohorts of Swedish railroad workers spraying herbicides (>45 days) compared to the expected number of deaths (1957-1972) from Swedish age- and sex-specific rates	348 Total herbicide exposure 207 Phenoxy acids and combinations 152 Amitrole and combinations 28 Other herbicides and combinations	—
Axelson et al., 1980	Cohort	Additional years of follow-up to cohort established in Axelson and Sundell (1974)	348	—
Blair, 1983	Cohort	Mortality experience of white male Florida pesticide applicators compared to U.S. and Florida men	3,827	—
Riihimaki et al., 1982	Cohort	Study of mortality among herbicide applicators exposed to 2,4-D and 2,4,5-T in Finland compared to mortality expected in the population	1,926	—
Riihimaki et al., 1983	Cohort	Cancer morbidity and mortality in cohort (Riihimaki et al., 1982) through 1980	1,926	—
Smith et al., 1981	Cohort	Study of chemical applicators (1973-1979) in New Zealand compared to agricultural contractors for differences in adverse reproductive outcomes	459	422
Smith et al., 1982	Cohort	Study of adverse reproductive outcomes among chemical applicators and agricultural contractors by category of exposure: none; chemicals not 2,4,5-T; and 2,4,5-T	113 Pregnancies (chemicals not 2,4,5-T) 486 Pregnancies (2,4,5-T)	401 Pregnancies (not exposed)
Wiklund, 1987	Cohort	Risk of HD and NHL among Swedish pesticide applicators from date of license through 1982 compared to expected number of cases in the total population	20,245	—
Wiklund et al., 1988b	Cohort	Risk of STS in Wiklund et al. (1987) cohort through 1984	20,245	—
Wiklund et al., 1989a	Cohort	Risk of cancer in Wiklund et al. (1987) cohort through 1982	20,245	—
Wiklund et al., 1989b	Cohort	Risk of STS, HD, and NHL in Wiklund et al. (1987) cohort through 1984	20,245	—
Swaen et al., 1992	Cohort	Cancer mortality experience (through 1987) among Dutch male herbicide applicators licensed before 1980 compared to the total male Dutch population	1,341	—
Bender et al., 1989	Cohort	Cancer mortality of Minnesota highway maintenance workers compared to expected numbers based on white Minnesota men	4,849	—

Continued

TABLE 6-1 *Continued*

Reference	Study Design	Description	Study Group (N)	Comparison Group (N)[a]
Barthel, 1981	Cohort	Study of male agricultural production workers (1948-1972) for incidence of cancer compared to incidence rates expected in the population	1,658	—
2. CASE-CONTROL STUDIES				
New studies				
Persson et al., 1993	Case-control	Study of risk factors potentially associated with HD and NHL in males identified from the Regional Cancer Registry in Sweden	HD: 31 NHL: 93	204
Hardell et al., 1994	Case-control	Study of the association between occupational exposures and parameters related to NHL in white males in Sweden	105	335
Brown et al., 1993	Case-control	Population-based case-control study of multiple myeloma in Iowa men for association with pesticide exposures	173	650
Zahm et al., 1993	Case-control	Study of NHL and exposure to pesticides in white women diagnosed with NHL between July 1, 1983, and June 30, 1986	206	824
Mellemgaard et al., 1994	Case-control	Study of cases of renal-cell carcinoma (20-79 years) in Denmark compared to population-based sample without cancer for identification of occupational risk factors	365	396
McDuffie et al., 1990	Case-control	Study of pesticide exposure in male cases of primary lung cancer in Saskatchewan compared to control subjects matched by age, sex, and location of residence	273	187
Nurminen et al., 1994	Case-control	Study of infants with structural defects born to mothers engaged in agricultural work during the first trimester of pregnancy compared to infants with structural defects born to mothers who did not engage in agricultural work during the first trimester	1,306	1,306
Semchuk, 1993	Case-control	Study of cases of Parkinson's disease (36-90 years) in Canada compared to population-based sample for association with occupational exposure to herbicides and other exposures	75 Men 55 Women	150 Men 110 Women
Studies reviewed in VAO				
Hardeli and Sandstrom, 1979	Case-control	Study of male cases of STS (26-80 years) diagnosed between 1970 and 1977 in northern Sweden compared to population-based sample without cancer for association with occupational exposure to phenoxyacetic acids and chlorophenols	52	206
Eriksson et al., 1979, 1981	Case-control	Study of cases of STS diagnosed between 1974 and 1978 in southern Sweden compared to population-based sample without cancer for association with occupational exposure to phenoxyacetic acids and chlorophenols	110	219

Reference	Study type	Description	Cases	Controls
Hardell and Eriksson, 1988	Case-control	Study of male cases of STS (25-80 years) diagnosed between 1978 and 1983 in northern Sweden compared to two referent groups: (1) population based and (2) with other cancers, for association with occupational exposure to phenoxyacetic acids and chlorophenols	55	330 Population based 190 Other cancers
Wingren et al., 1990	Case-control	Study of male cases of STS (25-80 years) diagnosed between 1975 and 1982 in southeast Sweden compared to two referent groups: (1) population-based sample and (2) with other cancers, for association with phenoxyacetic acids and chlorophenols	71	315 Population based 164 Other cancers
Eriksson et al., 1990	Case-control	Study of male cases of STS (25-80 years) diagnosed between 1978 and 1986 in central Sweden compared to population-based sample without cancer for association with occupational exposure to phenoxyacetic acids and chlorophenols	218	212
Hardell et al., 1980 Hardell et al., 1981	Case-control	Study of malignant lymphomas (HD, NHL, unknown) diagnosed between 1974 and 1978 in men age 25-85 in northern Sweden compared to population-based sample without cancer for association with occupational exposure to phenoxyacetic acids and chlorophenols	60 HD 109 NHL	338
Hardell and Bengtsson, 1983	Case-control	Study of HD diagnosed between 1974 and 1978 in men 25-85 in northern Sweden compared to population-based sample without cancer for association with occupational exposure to phenoxyacetic acid and chlorophenols	60	335
Hardell, 1981	Case-control	Study (1) of cases of STS (Hardell and Sandstrom, 1979) and malignant lymphomas (Hardell et al., 1981) compared to colon cancer cases, and (2) study of colon cancer compared to population-based controls for association with occupational exposure to phenoxyacetic acids and chlorophenols	(1) 221 (2) 154	154 541
Hardell et al., 1982	Case-control	Study of nasal and nasopharyngeal cancers diagnosed between 1970 and 1979 in men 25-85 years residing in northern Sweden compared to controls selected from previous studies (Hardell and Sandstrom, 1979; Hardell et al., 1981) for association with occupational exposure to phenoxyacetic acids and chlorophenols	44 Nasal 27 Nasopharyngeal	541
Hardell et al., 1984	Case-control	Study of primary liver cancer diagnosed between 1974 and 1981 in men 25-80 years residing in northern Sweden compared to population-based controls for association with occupational exposure to phenoxyacetic acids and chlorophenols	98	200
Persson et al., 1989	Case-control	Study of HD and NHL among living men and women in Sweden compared with those without these cancers for association with occupational exposures, including phenoxy herbicides	54 HD 106 NHL	275

Continued

TABLE 6-1 Continued

Reference	Study Design	Description	Study Group (N)	Comparison Group (N)[a]
Olsson and Brandt, 1988	Case-control	Study of NHL (1978-1981) in Swedish men compared to two groups of men without NHL for association with occupational exposures including phenoxy acids	167	50 Same area 80 Other parts of Sweden
Smith et al., 1983	Case-control	Preliminary report of men with STS reported between 1976 and 1980 in New Zealand compared to controls with other cancers for association with phenoxyacetic acid exposure	80	92
Smith et al., 1984	Case-control	Study of STS among New Zealand residents (1976-1980) compared to those without these cancers for association with occupational exposures, including phenoxy herbicides	82	92
Smith and Pearce, 1986	Case-control	Update of Smith et al. (1983) with diagnoses through 1982	51 In updated study 133 When combined with Smith et al., 1983	315 407
Pearce et al., 1985	Case-control	Study of malignant lymphoma and multiple myeloma in men diagnosed between 1977 and 1981 in New Zealand compared to men with other cancers for association with agricultural occupations	734	2,936
Pearce et al., 1986b	Case-control	Study of NHL cases (ICD 202) in men diagnosed between 1977 and 1981 in New Zealand compared to sample with other cancers and population sample, for association with occupational exposure to phenoxy herbicides and chlorophenols	83	168 Other cancers 228 General population
Pearce et al., 1986a	Case-control	Study of male multiple myeloma cases diagnosed between 1971 and 1981 in New Zealand compared to controls for other cancers for potential association with phenoxy herbicides and chlorophenols	76	315
Pearce et al., 1987	Case-control	Expanded study (Pearce et al., 1986b) of NHL to include ICD 200-diagnosed cases and additional controls for association with farming exposures	183	338
Blair and Thomas, 1979	Case-control	Study of leukemia cases in Nebraska (1957-1974) compared to deaths from other causes for association with agricultural practices	1,084	2,168
Blair and White, 1985	Case-control	Study of leukemia cases by cell type in Nebraska (1957-1974) compared to nonleukemia deaths for association with agricultural practices	1,084	2,168
Brown et al., 1990	Case-control	Population-based case-control study of leukemia in Iowa and Minnesota men for association with farming exposures	578	1,245

Reference	Study type	Description	Cases	Controls
Cantor et al., 1992	Case-control	Population-based case-control study of NHL in Iowa and Minnesota men for association with farming exposures	622	1,245
Zahm et al., 1990	Case-control	Study of white men 21 years or older diagnosed with NHL (1983-1986) in Nebraska compared to residents of the same area without NHL, HD, multiple myeloma, and chronic lymphocytic leukemia for association with herbicide use (2,4-D) on farms	201	725
Boffetta et al., 1989	Nested case-control	National study of multiple myeloma compared to other cancer controls for association with exposures including pesticides and herbicides	282	1,128
Burmeister et al., 1982	Case-control	Study of leukemia deaths (1964-1978) in white men 30 years or older in Iowa compared to nonleukemia deaths for association with farming	1,675	3,350
Burmeister et al., 1983	Case-control	Study of multiple myeloma, NHL, and prostate and stomach cancer mortality (1964-1978) in white men 30 years or older compared to mortality from other causes for association with farming practices including herbicide use in Iowa	550 Multiple myeloma 1,101 NHL 4,827 Prostate 1,812 Stomach	1,100 2,202 9,654 3,624
Hoar et al., 1986	Case-control	Study of STS, NHL, and HD in Kansas (1976-1982) compared to controls without cancer for association with 2,4-D, 2,4,5-T, and other herbicides in white men 21 years or older	133 STS 121 HD 170 NHL	948
Cantor, 1982	Case-control	Study of NHL in Wisconsin among men (1968-1976) compared to men dying from other causes for association with farming exposures	774	1,651
Dubrow et al., 1988	Case-control	Death certificate study (1958-1983) of NHL and HD among white male residents of Hancock County, Ohio, compared to a random sample of those dying from other causes for association with farming	61 NHL 15 HD	304
Morris et al., 1986	Case-control	Study of multiple myeloma (1977-1981) in four SEER areas compared to population controls for risk factors associated with the disease, including farm use of herbicides	698	1,683
Carmelli et al., 1981	Case-control	Cases of spontaneous abortions occurring to women (1978-1980) compared to live births for association with father's exposure to 2,4-D	134	311
Woods et al., 1987	Case-control	Study of STS or NHL in men 20-79 years old (1983-1985) in western Washington State compared to a population sample without these cancers for association with occupational exposure to phenoxy herbicides and chlorinated phenols	128 STS 576 NHL	694

Continued

126

TABLE 6-1 *Continued*

Reference	Study Design	Description	Study Group (N)	Comparison Group (N)[a]
Woods and Polissar, 1989	Case-control	Study of NHL from the Woods et al. (1987) study for association with phenoxy herbicides in farm workers	576	694
Alavanja et al., 1988	PMR analysis with nested case-control	Mortality experience of USDA extension agents (1970-1979) evaluated for specific cancer excess; case-control study of specific cancers identified from PMR analysis	1,495	—
Alavanja et al., 1989	PMR analysis with nested case-control	Mortality experience of USDA forest/soil conservationists (1970-1979) evaluated for specific cancer excess; case-control study of specific cancers identified from PMR analysis	1,411	—
Hardell et al., 1987	Case-control	Study of Kaposi's sarcoma in AIDS patients (23-53 years of age) compared to controls for association with TCDD and pesticide exposure in Sweden	50	50
Donna et al., 1984	Case-control	Study of ovarian cancer in women (1974-1980) for association with herbicide use compared to women without ovarian cancer	60	127
Musicco et al., 1988	Case-control	Study of brain gliomas diagnosed between 1983 and 1984 in men and women in Italy compared to (1) patients with nonglioma nervous system tumors and (2) patients with other neurologic diseases, for association with chemical exposures in farming	240	(1) 465 (2) 277
Vineis et al., 1987	Case-control	Study of cases of STS in men and women diagnosed between 1981 and 1983 in northern Italy compared to population sample of controls for association with phenoxy herbicide exposure	37 Men 31 Women	85 Men 73 Women
Balarajan and Acheson, 1984	Case-control	Study of STS (1968-1976) diagnosed in men in England and Wales compared to men with other cancers for association with farming, agriculture, and forestry occupations	1,961	1,961
Smith and Christophers, 1992	Case-control	Study of STS and malignant lymphomas in men diagnosed between 1982 and 1988 in Australia compared to other cancers for association with exposure to phenoxy herbicides and chlorophenols	82	82 Other cancers 82 Population
LaVecchia et al., 1989	Case-control	Study of Italian men and women with HD, NHL, and multiple myeloma (1983-1988) compared to population of Italy for association with occupations and herbicide use	69 HD 153 NHL 110 MM	396
Paper/Pulp Workers				
Robinson et al., 1986	Cohort	Mortality experience through March 1977 of white male workers employed in five paper/pulp mills compared to expected number of deaths among U.S. population	3,572	—

Henneberger et al., 1989	Cohort	Mortality experience through August 1985 of white men employed in Berlin, N.H., paper and pulp industry compared to expected mortality in U.S. white men	883	—
Solet et al., 1989	Cohort	Mortality (1970-1984) among white male United Paperworkers International Union members compared to expected number of deaths in U.S. men	201	—
Jappinen and Pukkala, 1991	Cohort	Cancer incidence (through 1987) among male Finnish pulp and paper workers (1945-1961) compared to rates in the local central hospital district	152	Approx. 135,000
Other Occupational Studies				
Fitzgerald et al., 1989	Cohort	Health outcomes in group exposed to electrical transformer fire in 1981 compared to standardized rates among upstate New York residents	377	—

NOTE: COPD = chronic obstructive pulmonary disease; HD = Hodgkin's disease; IARC = International Agency for Research on Cancer; ICD = International Classification of Diseases; NHL = non-Hodgkin's lymphoma; PMR = proportionate mortality ratio; SEER = surveillance, epidemiology, and end results; STS = soft-tissue sarcoma; and *VAO = Veterans and Agent Orange: Health Effects of Herbicides Used in Vietnam* (Institute of Medicine, 1994).

[a]The dash (—) indicates the comparison group is based on a population (e.g., U.S. white males, country rates), and details are given in the text for specifics of the actual population.

Production Workers

National Institute for Occupational Safety and Health

In 1978, the National Institute for Occupational Safety and Health (NIOSH) began a study to identify all U.S. workers potentially exposed to TCDD between 1942 and 1984 (Fingerhut et al., 1991). In a total of 12 chemical companies, 5,000 workers were identified from personnel and payroll records as having been involved in production or maintenance processes associated with TCDD contamination. Their exposure resulted from working with certain contaminated chamicals, including 2,4,5-trichlorophenol and in which TCDD was a contaminant included 2,4,5-trichlorophenoxyacetic acid, Silvex, Erbon, Ronnel, and hexachlorophene. An additional 172 workers identified previously by their employers as being exposed to TCDD were also included in the study cohort. TCDD was also measured in serum from a sample of 253 workers. The health status of the workers was determined as of December 31, 1987, and death certificates were used to establish numbers of deaths from each cause. Person-years were calculated from the first documented assignment to a process involving TCDD contamination until date of death or December 31, 1987. Vital status was determined for all but 77 members (2 percent) of the cohort. Those with unknown vital status were assumed to be alive. General U.S. population rates were used to calculate the number of expected deaths. The 12 plants involved were large manufacturing sites of major chemical companies. Thus, many of the study subjects probably were exposed to many other chemicals, some of which could be carcinogenic. Data were analyzed for mortality according to duration of exposure to processes involving TCDD contamination (determined from personnel records) and latency; total years of employment at the plant were also considered. A number of studies were later conducted that looked at health outcomes in the exposed worker population.

Prior to this study, NIOSH conducted a cross-sectional study that included a comprehensive medical history, medical examination, and measurement of pulmonary function of workers employed in the manufacture of chemicals with TCDD contamination at chemical plants in Newark, New Jersey (from 1951 through 1969), and in Verona, Missouri (from 1968 through 1969, and from 1970 through 1972) (Sweeney et al., 1989, 1993; Calvert et al., 1991, 1992; Alderfer et al., 1992). The plant in New Jersey manufactured TCP and 2,4,5-T ($N = 490$ eligible); the Missouri plant manufactured TCP, 2,4,5-T, and hexachlorophene ($N = 96$ eligible). TCDD is formed as a contaminant during the production of each of these chemicals. The workers were interviewed to collect information on health status, occupational history, time in Vietnam, time in agriculture, residential history, hospitalizations, medications, demographics, and life-style variables. Health outcomes of interest included peripheral neuropathies, neurobehavioral effects, chloracne, pigmentary changes, skin cancer, hepatic enzyme changes, porphyria, angina, myocardial infarction, ulcers, lipid changes, diabetes, lymphocyte cell types and function, and such adverse reproductive outcomes as fetal loss, reduced fertility, and major malformations (Sweeney et al., 1989). Physical examination included clinical assessment of respiratory function and adverse health outcomes, including chronic bronchitis, chronic obstructive pulmonary disease (COPD), ventilatory function, and thorax and lung abnormalities (Calvert et al., 1991); assessment of hepatic and gastric systems, including determination of laboratory tests associated with liver function, hepatitis, cirrhosis, fatty liver, gastritis, gastrointestinal hemorrhage, and ulcer disease (Calvert et al., 1992); psychological testing to determine the presence of depression (Alderfer et al., 1992); and assessment of peripheral neuropathy through examination, electrophysiologic and quantitative sensory tests, and symptoms (Sweeney et al., 1993). Serum levels of TCDD were determined as indicating exposure and were adjusted for lipids. The matched comparison group consisted of individuals who had no occupational exposure to phenoxy herbicides, who lived in the same communities as the workers, and who were within five years of age and of the same sex and race as the exposed workers. Comparison subjects underwent the same series of medical examinations and interviews as workers exposed to TCDD (Sweeney et al., 1993). A total of 281 workers and 260 unexposed subjects participated in the medical examination; 360 exposed worker interviews and 325 neighborhood interviews were completed. Data on important confounders, including cigarette and alcohol consumption, were collected and adjusted for in the analyses.

The data were further analyzed to evaluate the association between occupational exposure to TCDD and porphyria cutanea tarda (Calvert et al., 1994). Unadjusted odds ratios were calculated to assess the relationship between TCDD exposure and urinary porphyrin and other outcomes of interest.

Total serum testosterone and gonadotropin levels in 248 dioxin-exposed chemical production workers in New Jersey (1951-69) and Missouri (1968-72) were compared with the same parameters in 231 nonexposed individuals from neighborhoods near the plants who participated in a medical evaluation in 1987 (Egeland et al., 1994). The plants in this study are two of the 12 plants in the original NIOSH study at which serum TCDD measurements were performed on workers. A total of 586 workers were identified in these two plants, and 281 (48 percent) participated in the medical examination. Questionnaires on occupational exposures and demographics were administered to study participants by trained interviewers, and serum dioxin, follicle-stimulating hormone, luteinizing hormone, and total serum testosterone were determined by laboratory analyses. The association of each of the hormonal parameters with serum dioxin exposure was analyzed by multiple linear regression analysis.

Dow Chemical Company

Dow Chemical Company undertook a cohort mortality study of workers exposed to 2,4-dichlorophenoxyacetic acid (Bond et al., 1988). The herbicide was manufactured in several Dow plants; in some plants it was the only chemical produced, while other plants also produced 2,4,5-T and other herbicides containing TCDD. It was estimated that 77 percent of the group worked in proximity to 2,4-D manufacturing, and thus had opportunity for exposure to TCDD or H/OCDD. Prior to 1950, levels of 2,4-D ranged from 0.5 to 3.0 mg/m^3. Thereafter, concentrations decreased to 0.2-0.8 mg/m^3, depending on the job classification. After 1978, 2,4-D concentrations were below the detection limit of 0.01 mg/m^3. The cohort consisted of 878 workers from four production areas and was followed from 1945 until employee death, loss to follow-up, or December 31, 1982. Analysis was conducted according to cumulative dose of 2,4-D, as determined from such information as job history lists, industrial hygiene data, and years on the job. Allowance for latent period was made by lagging exposures by an interval of 15 years. Expected numbers were calculated for two comparison groups. The first comparison group consisted of white American males, adjusted for age and calendar year, and the second comparison group consisted of all other male workers at the manufacturing location ($N = 36,804$) who were employed between 1945 and 1982. This comparison was adjusted for age, interval since entry into follow-up, and pay status.

The study was updated with four additional years of follow-up of the cohort of 878 workers, through December 31, 1986 (Bloeman et al., 1993). The method of analysis corresponded closely with that of the first study. Vital status was successfully ascertained for all of the original cohort members through 1986, using company records, the files of Social Security Administration, and the National Death Index.

BASF

In Germany, an accident on November 17, 1953, during the manufacture of trichlorophenol at BASF Aktiengesellschaft, resulted in the exposure to TCDD of some of the workers in the plant. These workers were identified and followed for mortality; other workers who were potentially exposed in the building following the accident were also studied.

Mortality of the employees was evaluated by Zober et al. (1990). Of the 247 employees followed, three study cohorts—a basic cohort and two additional cohorts—were assembled to establish all those exposed during the accident as well as during cleanup operations, for follow-up over 34 years. The potential amount and reliability of exposure information were the defining factors in compiling the cohorts. The basic cohort consisted of those workers who were listed as being exposed during the accident ($N = 69$); of the 69 workers in this group, 66 were included in the cohort of Thiess et al. (1982). The first additional cohort identified by the BASF Occupational Safety and Employee Protection Department consisted of those workers who had been potentially exposed by August 31, 1983, since more people were reporting potential exposures to the company medical department ($N = 84$); the degree of exposure for this group was less clear than the basic cohort. The second additional cohort was assembled (1984 through December 1987) through the "Dioxin Investigation Programme," which informed employees of potential hazards from exposure and identified, through a variety of methods, other employees, investigators, and demolition workers who had potentially been exposed ($N = 94$). Occupational descriptions of jobs held by these employees were investigated, and for those included in the "Dioxin Investigation Programme," medical examinations were conducted. Vital status for the final cohort of 247 persons was established as of December 31, 1987. The cohort mortality was compared with the national mortality rates in the Federal Republic of Germany for different periods of time since the first exposure. Analysis included cancer outcomes for a subcohort of members of the three cohorts described above who experienced chloracne or erythema.

Morbidity follow-up of 151 members of the original cohort, as well as seven additional employees later identified as part of the accident cohort, was continued by Zober and colleagues through 1989 (Zober et al., 1994). Cohort members were assigned to one of three subcohorts based on chloracne status following the accident. Subgroup I consisted of 52 workers with extensive or severe chloracne; Subgroup II consisted of 61 workers with either moderate chloracne or a diagnosis of "erythyema" but no chloracne; and Subgroup III consisted of 45 men without chloracne. Blood lipid TCDD concentrations in the cohort members were also used to assess exposure. Cohort morbidity was compared with a referent group comprised of male employees hired before November 1953. Episodes of acute illness were assessed on the basis of number of illness episodes per time period for each employee; while for chronic illness, an "ever" or "never" basis was used.

International Register of Workers Exposed to Phenoxy Herbicides

A study involving numerous cohorts from different countries was conducted by the International Agency for Research on Cancer (IARC) (Saracci et al., 1991). The cohort of international workers, the "International Register of Workers Exposed to Phenoxy Herbicides and Their Contaminants," included information on mortality and exposures of 18,390 workers—16,863 men and 1,527 women. In an effort to avoid the problems of small studies with insufficient power to detect increased cancer risks, Saracci and colleagues at the IARC created a multinational registry of workers exposed to phenoxy herbicide and chlorophenol (Saracci et al., 1991). The Danish production worker cohort studied by Lynge (1985) is included in this registry, as are the cohorts of Green

(1991), Coggon et al. (1986, 1991), and Bueno de Mesquita et al. (1993). The cohort of Lynge (1985) contributes a very large fraction of all the person-years in the IARC study, and all four of the deaths found in the study were attributed to soft-tissue sarcoma (International Classification of Disease [ICD] 171). The studies are reported in detail in Chapter 8 of *VAO*. Workers are included from 20 cohorts who had ever been involved in herbicide production or spraying, with the exception of the Australian, Canadian, and New Zealand cohorts, which required a minimum employment of one year, six months, and one month, respectively. Follow-up for all cohorts was either through the computerized systems for the particular country or from medical records and cancer registries.

In the study, questionnaires were distributed to workers in factories producing chlorophenoxy herbicides or chlorinated phenols and to workers involved in spraying operations at the plants; job histories were examined if available. The cohort was subdivided according to whether members were exposed and whether they were producers or sprayers. Workers who sprayed chlorophenoxy herbicides or worked in factory departments in contact with these chemicals were considered "exposed" ($N = 13,482$); workers "probably exposed" had no job title but were judged to have been exposed ($N = 416$). Workers with no exposure status information were considered as having "unknown" exposure ($N = 541$), and those who never worked in factory departments with exposure to chlorophenoxy herbicides or who never sprayed these chemicals were considered "nonexposed" ($N = 3,951$). There were 12,492 workers categorized as producers and 5,898 as sprayers. Exposed and probably exposed workers were subclassified according to the chemical they produced or sprayed (9,377 worked with chlorophenoxy herbicides; 408 worked with chlorinated phenols; and 4,133 worked with both) and according to their department (3,034 were in main production; 1,522 in maintenance and cleaning; 1,665 in other departments; and 1,907 were unclassifiable). For the analysis, results are presented for the potential categories of exposure, with the "exposed" category combining production workers and sprayers into one category. Comparison mortality rates were calculated from the World Health Organization Mortality Data Bank, standardized for sex, age, and calendar-year period; mortality coding was done nationally, with a conversion table developed to allow pooling over ICD revisions. Determination of vital status began in 1955 or the date of first exposure thereafter and continued for an average of 17 years. Exposure to TCDD was assumed to be possible for those who worked producing or spraying 2,4,5-TCP and 2,4,5-T (other products). Because certain factories produced no or very little 2,4,5-T, it was possible to differentiate workers by probable TCDD exposure. Exposure was not exclusively focused on TCDD, as in the NIOSH-assembled cohort (Fingerhut et al., 1991), and the workers may have been exposed to multiple chemicals.

In the Netherlands, the National Institute of Public Health and Environmental Protection contributed a cohort to the IARC registry, consisting of workers from two companies that produced several chlorophenoxy herbicides; this cohort was also evaluated apart from the IARC registry for cancer mortality (Bueno de Mesquita et al., 1993). Factory A produced primarily 2,4,5-T; in March 1963, an uncontrolled reaction in the factory resulted in an explosion in which polychlorinated dibenzodioxins (PCDDs), including TCDD, were released. Anyone employed at this factory between 1955 and June 30, 1985, was eligible to be included in the study; workers contracted to clean up after the accident were also included in the cohort. Factory B produced primarily MCPA and MCPP (2-[4-chloro-2-methylphenoxy]propanoic acid), plus smaller amounts of 2,4-D; all persons employed between 1965 and June 30, 1986, were included in the cohort. The total cohort included 2,310 workers, and follow-up was 97 percent complete; analysis was presented for the 2,074 male workers who were exposed and unexposed in the factories. The causes of death were taken from the Netherlands Central Bureau of Statistics. The important steps for phenoxy herbicide exposure, which might occur in a number of different departments, included synthesis of the chemical, formulation of the herbicide, and packaging. Since individual measures of exposure were not available, occupational history, including working in the above departments and exposure to the accident, was used to define exposure. Workers were considered exposed if they worked in departments involving synthesis, finishing, formulation, packing, maintenance/repair, the laboratory, chemical effluent/waste handling, cleaning, shipping/transport, or plant supervision; if they were exposed to the accident; or if they were exposed by proximity to the above departments. Comparisons were made to total and cancer-specific mortality using expected numbers standardized for the Netherlands; exposed and unexposed workers were also compared by selected mortality causes.

In Denmark, cohort study of cancer incidence was conducted among employees of manufacturing facilities that produced phenoxy herbicides, including 2,4-D, 4-chloro-2-methylphenoxyacetic acid (CMPP), 2-[4-chloro-2-methylphenoxy]-propanoic acid (MCPA), and 2-[2,4-dichlorophenoxy]-propanoic acid (2,4-DP) (Lynge, 1985). All workers involved in the manufacture of phenoxy herbicides in Denmark before 1982 were eligible for the exposed study cohort; two factories were the source of identification of 4,461 workers (3,390 men and 1,071 women) who were followed for vital status and cancer incidence through 1982. Vital status was ascertained through the Central Population Register, and cancer incidence was determined through the Danish Cancer Registry. The incidence of cancer in the cohort was compared to the expected incidence in the entire Danish population, by sex, five-year age group, and calendar period. Individual exposure was not indicated; however, department worked in the factory was used as a means of classifying those exposed. Two groups were considered to be potentially exposed to phenoxy herbicides: those in the "phenoxy herbicidal manufacturing and packaging departments"; and those in "manual service functions."

The cohort was followed for cancer incidence for five years, through December 31, 1987 (Lynge, 1993). Workers at each plant were classified according to estimated potential herbicide exposure. Exposure measurement data for the cohort were inferred from data on production. Two types of analyses were performed: the first, with the individual risk periods starting on the first day of employment; and the second, with the inclusion only of persons employed for at least one year and with a ten-year latency period.

In a study covering ten countries, cancer mortality from soft-tissue sarcoma and malignant lymphoma was evaluated in an international cohort of 16,863 male and 1,527 female workers ever employed in the production or spraying of pesticides (Kogevinas et al., 1992). Workers were classified into four exposure categories based on the results of exposure questionnaires and job histories: exposed (N = 13,482), probably exposed (N = 416), unknown exposure (N = 541), or nonexposed (N = 3,951). Workers were further classified as producers (N = 12,492) or sprayers (N = 5,898). There was an average follow-up period of 17 years, and follow-up was successful for 95 percent of the cohort. SMRs were derived for soft-tissue sarcomas and malignant lymphomas using person-years. In many plants and sprayer cohorts, there was exposure to several different chlorophenoxy herbicides or chlorophenols, as well as to various other pesticides, raw materials, intermediates, and processing chemicals. The authors differentiated workers who were and were not probably exposed to TCDD, on the basis of whether 2,4,5-T or 2,4,5-trichlorophenol were manufactured.

A cohort study of cancer incidence and mortality was conducted among 701 women occupationally exposed to chlorophenoxy herbicides, chlorophenols, and dioxins from seven countries (Kogevinas et al., 1993). One hundred and sixty nine of the workers had potential exposure to TCDD during the production of 2,4,5-T or 2,4,5-trichlorophenol. Five hundred and thirty two workers were unlikely to have had TCDD exposure. Female workers on the International Register of Workers who were ever employed in production or spraying of chlorophenoxy herbicides and/or chlorophenols were eligible for the study. Exposure histories were reconstructed using company records, exposure questionnaires and analyses of TCDD and other dioxin congeners in end products, reactor products, and waste streams. Vital status of workers was ascertained either by using computerized national death certificate records or by using active follow-up procedures. The overall follow-up rate was greater than 95 percent and 44 percent of the subjects were followed for ten years or more. Data on cancer incidence were available for 634 workers from Denmark, Finland, New Zealand, and Switzerland. Cancer incidence and mortality among exposed subjects were compared with national death rates and cancer incidence rates.

Two nested case-control studies were undertaken to evaluate the relationship between soft-tissue sarcoma and non-Hodgkin's lymphoma in the Saracci et al. (1991) cohort and occupational exposures, including dioxin (Kogevinas et al., 1995). Eleven cases of soft-tissue sarcoma and 32 cases of non-Hodgkin's lymphoma NHL were identified through examination of death certificates for members of the International Agency for Researchers on Cancer (IARC) cohort. Five controls, matched for age, sex, and country of residence, were assigned to each case. Cases and controls were interviewed by an industrial hygienist to determine occupational exposures, including phenoxy herbicides, chlorophenols, and polychlorinated dibenzodioxins and furans. Actual measurements of past exposure for the study subjects were largely unavailable, but company exposure questionnaires, company reports, and individual job records were used in an attempt to reconstruct past exposure. A relative scale was used to assess level of exposure, and a cumulative exposure score was assigned based on the estimated level of exposure and duration of exposure in years. Logistic regression analysis was performed to estimate risk in each study.

Agricultural Workers

Cohort Studies

The Canadian Farmer Cohort In Canada, the Mortality Study of Canadian Male Farm Operators covering the years 1971-85 was undertaken to investigate the relationship of farm practices, especially herbicide spraying, to the risk of all causes of mortality (Wigle et al., 1990; Morrison et al., 1992, 1993). The cohort was established by linking records from the 1971 Census of Agriculture, the 1971 Census of Population, and the 1971 Central Farm Register, which combined agricultural, population, and personal identifying information on the cohort. A second step linked the 1971 Central Farm Register to the 1981 Central Farm Register as a follow-up of the cohort. A third step linked the cohort to the Mortality Data Base (1971-85) for the mortality experience. The agriculture census included information on number of acres sprayed with herbicides (types not specified) and insecticides, total acreage of land operated, and surrogate measures for pesticide exposure. In order to determine duration of exposure, indices for individual farmers were developed from 1971 and 1981 data; farmers appearing in both censuses on the same farm were considered to have had a continuing exposure for those years. Farmers not appearing in both censuses had more uncertain continual exposure to herbicides. Also, subgroups of farmers who did not employ outside workers were assumed to be more likely to be exposed. No other information on individual exposures was available. The Farm Register, established as a mailing list for agricultural questionnaires, contained all farm operators in the 1971 agriculture census, in addition to agricultural variables and personal identifiers.

In Saskatchewan, Canada, a total of 69,513 men over age 35 were identified using the methods described above. A detailed multivariate analysis of the risk of death from NHL was undertaken (Wigle et al., 1990). The study, with a larger cohort ($N = 155,547$), was updated to further evaluate the risk of death from NHL (Morrison et al., 1994). There were two additional years of follow-up through 1987. Two additional provinces were added—Alberta and Manitoba. Death certificates were obtained for farmers whose underlying cause of death was recorded as NHL. SMRs due to NHL were calculated with the combined Manitoba, Saskatchewan, and Alberta male mortality rates as the reference and were stratified by number of acres sprayed with herbicides.

Another study of the Canadian farmer cohort focused on evaluating mortality from multiple myeloma from 1971 to 1987 (Semenciw et al., 1993). The mortality experience of male Canadian farmers from multiple myeloma was compared to mortality in the general male population of the three prairie provinces of Canada. Death certificates were used to identify subjects whose underlying cause of death was multiple myeloma. SMRs were calculated using age-specific mortality rates and were stratified by number of acres sprayed with herbicides.

The Canadian farmer cohort was also evaluated for leukemia mortality (Semenciw et al., 1994). Census records from 1971 for 155,547 male farmers who were at least 35 years of age at some point during the follow-up period (June 1971 to December 1987) were linked with mortality records through 1987. Subjects with leukemia listed as the cause of death on death certificates were included in the cohort. SMRs were calculated using age-specific mortality rates for males in Manitoba, Saskatchewan, and Alberta.

A cross-sectional study examining the association between pesticide exposure and asthma was conducted in 1982-83 using a cohort of male farmers from Saskatchewan (Senthilselvan et al., 1992). Of 2,375 farmers in 17 municipalities visited at their homes by a volunteer and asked to participate in the study, 1,939 agreed. Participants were administered questionnaires that contained questions on occupational exposures, including exposure to pesticides, and questions on respiratory health and smoking habits taken from the Epidemiology Standardization Questionnaire of the American Thoracic Society. Pulmonary function tests were also performed on the participants. Prevalence odds ratios were used to estimate the association between asthma and factors.

Other Agricultural Workers   A cluster of deaths from brain cancer, leukemia, and Hodgkin's disease among employees of the former Agricultural Institute of the Republic of Ireland provided the impetus for performing a cohort study of mortality from brain, lymphatic, and hematopoietic cancers in Irish agricultural workers (Dean, 1994). Information on deaths from 1971 to 1987 coded as cancer of the brain (ICD 191) or lymphatic or hematopoietic cancer (ICD 200-208) was obtained from the Central Statistics Office of Ireland. Computer analysis was performed to stratify deaths by socioeconomic group, age, and sex using data from the 1971 and 1981 national censuses and from death certificates. Deaths were grouped into two time periods (1971-78 and 1979-87). Cause-specific mortality rates in individuals classified as farmers (using census data) were compared with the rates by sex and age group for all deaths in Ireland for the time periods 1968-77 and 1978-87. Agricultural workers were divided into two groups: farmers, relatives assisting farmers and farm managers; and other agricultural occupations and fishermen.

In the United States, a proportionate mortality study was performed using data on male and female farmers from 23 states (Blair et al., 1993). Mortality data were obtained using death certificates from the years 1984-88. Occupation and industry were coded based on the information listed on the death certificate. Relative risks were estimated by calculating proportionate mortality ratios and proportionate cancer mortality ratios for white men (N = 119,648), white women (N = 2,400), non-white men (N = 11,446), and non-white women (N = 2,066). The deaths among non-farmers from the same states were used to generate expected numbers. There was no individual verification of the death certificate information on farming history, so some misclassification of exposure might have been possible.

Herbicide/Pesticide Applicators In Finland, 1,971 male herbicide applicators who had been exposed for at least two weeks to 2,4-D and 2,4,5-T between 1955 and 1971 were identified from the personnel records of the four main Finnish employers involved with chemical brushwood control (Riihimaki et al., 1982). After excluding 45 individuals who had died before 1971, the final cohort of 1,926 workers was followed from 1972 to 1980 for mortality, by checking the names with the population register of the Social Insurance Institution. Underlying cause of death was determined from death certificates. Expected numbers of deaths were determined by using age- and cause-specific death rates for the nation in 1975. Data on new cancer cases were obtained from the Finnish Cancer Registry. Since data on exposure were collected from personnel records, files did not always contain assignment information, and in some cases, recall of exposures was based on the memory of clerks or foremen. Cancer morbidity and mortality in this cohort were reported separately (Riihimaki et al., 1983).

An 18-year prospective follow-up of cancer morbidity and mortality for 1,909 members of the original cohort was reported in 1994 (Asp et al., 1994). Cancer incidence and mortality was followed through 1989. A questionnaire addressing exposure history and smoking history was mailed to all living cohort members and to the next-of-kin for deceased subjects. The median total duration of exposure was six weeks. SMRs were calculated based on zero, ten, and 15 years of latency since first exposure.

A cross-sectional study of 1,000 pesticide appliers in Minnesota was conducted to evaluate health outcomes associated with pesticide use (Garry et al., 1994). Study participants were selected from a current list of licensed pesticide appliers obtained from the state Department of Agriculture. All persons certified and/or recertified within the past five years were eligible to participate in the study. One thousand pesticide appliers were chosen by random selection and contacted by telephone. Seven hundred and nineteen individuals who chose to participate in the study received a questionnaire in the mail regarding general health, occupation, pesticide use, and use of protective gear. Medical record verification of each diagnosis of cancer was obtained, and death certificates were obtained from state agencies. The study population was divided into groups based on the use of four different groups of pesticides, and intergroup comparisons of health status were performed using chi square analysis. Cholinesterase levels in the study group were also ascertained.

Case-Control Studies

Sweden   Risk factors potentially associated with Hodgkin's Disease (HD) and NHL were evaluated in a recent case-control study (Persson et al., 1993). Cases of HD ($N = 31$) and NHL ($N = 93$) among males at least 20 years of age were ascertained from the Regional Cancer Registry at the University Hospital in Linkoping. Cases were confirmed by histopathologic analysis. Controls ($N = 204$), also males at least 20 years of age, were selected at random from population registers. Study participants were mailed a questionnaire that contained questions about exposure to herbicides and other occupational exposures. For an exposure to be considered relevant, exposure time had to be at least one year, and the exposure must have occurred five to 45 years before the diagnosis of malignant lymphoma. Individuals who reported exposure to herbicides through occupations related to farming or forestry were categorized as being exposed to phenoxy herbicides, due to the prevalence of phenoxy herbicides used in agriculture and forestry in Sweden. Odds ratios were calculated to estimate the risk associated with various occupational exposures.

The relationship between occupational exposure to phenoxyacetic acids and chlorophenols and various parameters related to NHL, including histopathology, stage, and anatomical location, was examined in a case-control study (Hardell et al., 1994). Cases ($N = 105$) were selected from white males between the ages of 25 and 85 with histopathologically confirmed NHL who were admitted between 1974 and 1978 to the Department of Oncology in Umea. Three hundred and fifty five control subjects from an earlier study of malignant lymphoma and chemical exposure were utilized for the current study (Hardell et al., 1981). Controls were matched to cases on the basis of sex, age, residence, and vital status. A questionnaire was administered to participants to ascertain occupational exposures and working history. Control subjects had completed the questionnaire as part of the earlier study. Exposure to chlorophenols or organic solvents was classified as low-grade if the exposure was less than one week continuously or less than one month total; all other exposures were classified as high-grade. Odds ratios stratified by age and vital status were calculated to estimate the risk of NHL associated with various occupations and exposures.

United States   White males in Iowa were the subjects of a population-based case-control study examining the association between pesticide exposure and multiple myeloma (Brown et al., 1993). Cases of multiple myeloma ($N = 173$) were identified through the Iowa Health Registry and included men aged 30 or older diagnosed between 1981 and 1984. White men without lymphatic or hematopoietic cancer were selected as controls ($N = 650$) through random-digit dialing, Medicare records, and state death certificate files. Detailed information regarding general farm activities, the use of a variety of pesticides, and the first and last year each pesticide was used was obtained through a standardized questionnaire administered in person to subjects or relatives of deceased subjects. Odds ratios were calculated for multiple myeloma from agricultural exposures and from individual pesticides. Nonfarmers were used as the referent group for all odds ratio calculations. A case-control study of white women 21 years or older residing in the 66 counties of eastern Nebraska and diagnosed with NHL between July 1, 1983, and June 30, 1986, was conducted (Zahm et al., 1993). Cases ($N = 206$) were identified through the Nebraska Lymphoma Study group and area hospitals. Histological confirmation of NHL was necessary for inclusion in the study cohort. Residents of the same 66 counties were selected as controls ($N = 824$) and matched on a three to one basis to cases of race, sex, vital status, and age. Cases (or next of kin) and controls were interviewed by telephone to determine pesticide exposures. Odds ratios stratified by age were calculated as the measure of association.

Other Case-Control Studies   A case-control study on the association between pesticide use and primary lung cancer was conducted using cases chosen from the Saskatchewan Cancer Foundation, a population based registry (McDuffie et al., 1990). Two hundred and seventy three male cases were matched with 187 male population-based controls, selected from enrollees in the Saskatchewan Hospital Services Plan on the basis of year of birth, sex, and geographic area of residence. Identical questionnaires were administered to cases and controls to ascertain occupational, smoking, and other exposures. Cases and community controls were compared; in addition, cases were divided into farmer and nonfarmer groups. A farmer was defined as a person who had farmed for at least 15 years on more than 80 acres of land. Odds ratios were calculated on the basis of exposure to different classes of pesticides, as well as smoking history.

Cases of renal cell carcinoma ($N = 365$) were identified from the Denmark Cancer Registry and from pathology records and compared to control cases ($N = 396$) selected from the Central Population Register for a study of the association between occupational risk factors and renal cell carcinoma (Mellemgaard et al., 1994). Cases ranged from 20 to 79 years of age and were matched by gender to controls in five-year intervals. There was a 79 percent response rate among cases (365/402) and 79% response rate among controls (396/500). Study subjects were interviewed in person to determine past and present occupation and exposure to occupational risk factors, including herbicides, as well as their medical history, education, medication use, smoking history, and diet. Classification of occupation was done according to the International Standard Classification of Occupation. Socioeconomic status of each subject was determined according to guidelines developed by the Danish National Institute for Social Research. Odds ratios were calculated according to socioeconomic strata, high-risk industries, high-risk occupations, and high-risk agents. Occupational exposures were considered only if the job that resulted in exposure lasted one year or more and if the exposure took place ten years or more before the interview.

In Canada, a population-based study was conducted to evaluate the etiologic importance of various potential risk factors such as occupational herbicide exposure in the development of Parkinson's disease (Semchuk et al., 1993). Living cases without dementia (N = 130) were selected from a population-based case registry of individuals in Calgary with Parkinson's disease and were each matched with two community controls selected by random-digit dialing. Cases and controls were matched by sex and age (± 2.5 years), and institutionalized cases were matched with an additional institutionalized control. Subjects were interviewed to obtain occupational histories, including dates of exposure, and descriptive information on occupational exposures to herbicides and other chemicals. Logistic regression was used to estimate the relative risk for Parkinson's disease associated with each exposure variable.

The relationship between birth defects and maternal agricultural work during pregnancy was the focus of a case-control study in Finland (Nurminen et al., 1994). One thousand three hundred and six infants born with structural malformations between 1976 and 1982 were chosen as cases from the Finnish Register of Congenital Malformations and each was matched with one control infant born in the same maternity welfare district. Mothers of cases and controls were interviewed within two to four months of giving birth to determine their agricultural exposures, including exposure to pesticides, within the first trimester of pregnancy. Exposure questionnaires were reviewed by an industrial hygienist and mothers were classified into one of five categories: nonexistent exposure, slight exposure, moderate short-term exposure, heavy short-term exposure, or moderate or heavy long-term exposure. Odds ratios were calculated for agricultural and for nonagricultural work during the first trimester of pregnancy and birth defects.

ENVIRONMENTAL STUDIES

The occurrence of accidents and industrial disasters has offered opportunities to evaluate the long-term health effects of exposure to dioxin and other potentially hazardous chemicals. One of the largest industrial accidents involving environmental exposures to TCDD occurred in Seveso, Italy in July 1976, as a result of an uncontrolled reaction during trichlorophenol production. A variety of indicators were used to estimate individual exposure; soil contamination by TCDD has been the most extensively used. On the basis of soil sampling, three areas were defined about the release point. They were Zone A, the most heavily contaminated, from which all residents were evacuated within 20 days; Zone B, an area of lesser contamination that children and pregnant women in their first trimester were urged to avoid during daytime; and Zone R, a region with some contamination, in which consumption of local crops was prohibited (Bertazzi et al., 1989a,b).

Seveso

The incidence of neurological disorders following exposure to TCDD was the focus of one study initiated shortly after the Seveso accident (Boeri et al., 1978). Residents from Zone A were invited for neurological examination, and 470 of 723 residents volunteered; invitation was by letter or personal invitation during home screening visits (Filippini et al., 1981). Some residents of Zone R also requested examination, although they were not originally designated for inclusion in the study. However, since examinations of controls were not completed, volunteers from this zone ($N = 152$) were examined for comparison with the Zone A participants. Neurologic testing occurred in March 1977. Although actual individual exposures were unknown, residence in a high- versus low-exposure potential area was considered as the exposure. As a follow-up, residents were invited to return in April 1978 for a second neurological screening, to be compared with results from neurological tests of those in unpolluted areas around Seveso (Filippini et al., 1981). Of the 709 Seveso residents invited, 308 who attended the second screening were eligible for inclusion; subjects were examined clinically, completed a medical history questionnaire, and underwent an electrophysiologic investigation. A nonexposed population of 305 individuals provided referent levels of neurological functioning. Analyses were done by comparing those people with symptoms of neuropathy or indicators of TCDD exposure (chloracne, gamma-glutamyl transpeptidase, glutamic-oxalacetic transaminase, or glutamic-pyruvic transaminase) to those with neither symptoms nor indicators.

A ten-year mortality follow-up of individuals exposed to TCDD following the accident has been reported (Bertazzi et al., 1989b). All persons who resided in any of the 11 towns included in the two health districts that were in the contaminated zones (A, B, and R) were eligible for study follow-up; information collected included demographics, residence at time of and following the accident, and date of first residence for those moving into the area. Classification of exposed residents of the Seveso area was according to Zones A ($N = 556$), B ($N = 3,920$), and R ($N = 26,227$), or outside the contaminated boundaries, based on residence at the time of the accident or at first entry to the area. Study subjects were followed through national records throughout the country as of December 31, 1986; cause of death for those deceased was as certified by the attending physician and reported to the National Statistics Institute of Italy. The reference population was the cohort residing outside the contaminated A, B, and R zones ($N = 167,391$).

Cancer incidence over the same period for this cohort has also been evalu-

TABLE 6-2 Epidemiologic Studies—Environmental Exposure

Reference	Study Design	Description	Study Group (N)	Comparison Group (N)[a]
Seveso				
New studies				
Bertazzi et al., 1993	Cohort	Study of cancer incidence in Seveso residents aged 20-74 years in contaminated zones (A, B, and R) exposed to TCDD on July 10, 1976, compared to neighboring residents in unexposed areas	724 Zone A 4,824 Zone B 31,647 Zone R	181,579
Pesatori et al., 1993	Cohort	Evaluation of cancer incidence in Seveso residents aged 1-19 years in the first postaccident decade compared to age-matched residents of neighboring unexposed areas	Approximately 20,000	167,391
Studies reviewed in *VAO*				
Boeri et al., 1978	Cohort	Evaluation of neurological disorders among Seveso residents exposed to TCDD on July 10, 1976, compared to residents in unexposed areas	470 Zone A	152 Zone R
Filippini et al., 1981	Cohort	Comparison of prevalence of peripheral neuropathy on two screening examinations among Seveso residents compared to residents in unexposed areas	308	305
Barbieri et al., 1988	Cohort	Comparison of prevalence of peripheral nervous system involvement among Seveso residents with chloracne compared to residents in unexposed areas	152	123
Bisanti et al., 1980	Descriptive	Descriptive report of selected health outcomes among residents of Seveso located in zones A, B, and R	730 Zone A 4,737 Zone B 31,800 Zone R	No comparison group
Caramaschi et al., 1981	Cohort	Evaluation of chloracne among children in Seveso compared to children with no chloracne, and association with other health outcomes between chloracne and no-chloracne groups	146	182

Reference	Study type	Description		
Mocarelli et al., 1986	Cross-sectional	Study of laboratory measures of seru and urine in Seveso zone A and B children measured over six years (1977-1982) compared to zone R children	69 Zone A 528 Zone B 874 Zone R	241, Subset of zone R
Assennato et al., 1989a	Cohort	Comparison of dermatologic and laboratory findings in children during periodic exams following accident in Seveso	193 With chloracne	123
Ideo et al., 1982	Cross-sectional	Evaluation of hepatic enzymes in children exposed in Seveso compared to normal values	16 Zone A 51 Zone B	60 Bristo Assizio 26 Cannero
Ideo et al., 1985	Cross-sectional	Evaluation of levels of enzyme activity among residents of Seveso zone B and an uncontaminated community	117 Adults	127 Adults
Bertazzi et al., 1989a, 1989b	Cohort	Comparison of mortality experience (1976-1986) of residents of contaminated zones (A, B, and R) around Seveso to the mortality experience of unexposed residents in neighboring towns	556 Zone A 3,920 Zone B 26,227 Zone R	167,391
Pesatori et al., 1992	Cohort	Cancer incidence (1976-1986) among those in zones A, B, and R around Seveso compared to residents of uncontaminated surrounding areas	Data given in person-years	Data given in person-years
Bertazzi et al., 1992	Cohort	Comparison of mortality of children (1976-1986) exposed during Seveso accident compared to children in uncontaminated areas	306 Zone A 2,727 Zone B 16,604 Zone R	95,339
Assennato et al., 1989b	Cohort	Study of health outcomes in workers assigned to cleanup or referent group following Seveso accident	36	36
Tenchini et al., 1983	Cross-sectional	Cytogenetic analysis of maternal and fetal tissue among Seveso exposed compared to control sample	19	16
Mastroiacovo et al., 1988	Cohort	Comparison of birth defects occurring among zone A, B, and R mothers with live and stillbirths to mothers with births from non-A, -B, or -R residents	26 Zone A 435 Zone B 2,439 Zone R	12,391 (non-A, -B, or -R)

Continued

TABLE 6-2 *Continued*

Reference	Study Design	Description	Study Group (N)	Comparison Group (N)[a]
Times Beach/Quail Run				
Stehr et al., 1986	Cross-sectional	Pilot study of Missouri residents exposed to TCDD in the environment (1971) for health effects, comparing potentially high-exposed to low-exposed residents	68 High exposed	36 Low exposed
Webb et al., 1987	Cross-sectional	Pilot study of Missouri residents exposed to TCDD in the environment (1971) for health effects, comparing potentially high-exposed to low-exposed residents	68 High exposed	36 Low exposed
Evans et al., 1988	Cross-sectional	Comparison of retesting for skin delayed-type hypersensitivity among nonresponders in earlier test (Stehr et al., 1986)	28	15
Hoffman et al., 1986 Stehr-Green et al., 1987	Cohort	Study of the health effects (1971-1984) of residents of Quail Run Mobile Home Park compared to residents in uncontaminated mobile parks	154	155
Stockbauer et al., 1988	Cohort	Study of adverse reproductive outcomes (1972-1982) among mothers potentially exposed to TCDD-contaminated areas of Missouri (1971) compared to births among unexposed mothers	402 Births	804 Births
Vietnam				
New studies				
Cordier et al. 1993	Case-control	Study of cases of hepatocellular carcinoma (1989-1992) in males living in Vietnam compared to other hospitalized patients for association with a range of exposures including herbicides	152	241
Studies reviewed in *VAO*				
Dai et al., 1990	Cohort	Study of infant mortality (1966-1986) in two South Vietnam villages exposed to Agent Orange spraying compared to infant mortality in unsprayed area	5,609	3,306

Phuong et al., 1989b	Cohort	Comparison of reproductive anomalies among births to women (May 1982-June 1982) living in areas heavily sprayed with herbicides in southern Vietnam and women from Ho Chi Minh city	7,327 Births	6,690 Births
Phuong et al., 1989a	Case-control	Study of deformed babies and hydatidiform mole compared to normal births (1982) in Ho Chi Minh City for association with mother's exposure to Agent Orange and TCDD in Vietnam conflict	15 Birth defects 50 Hydatidiform moles	104 134
Constable and Hatch, 1985	Review	Summaries of reproductive outcomes among Vietnamese populations; includes nine unpublished studies		
Other Environmental Studies **New studies**				
Butterfield et al., 1993	Case-control	Study of possible environmental risk factors associated with young-onset Parkinson's disease	63	68
Peper, 1993	Descriptive	Study of environmental exposure to dioxins and furans and potential association with adverse neuropsychological effects in Germany	19	None
Studies reviewed in *VAO*				
Cartwright et al., 1988	Case-control	Study of living cases of NHL (1979-1984) in Yorkshire, England, compared to other hospitalized patients for association with a range of exposures including fertilizers/herbicides	437	724
Gordon and Shy, 1981	Case-control	Study of agricultural chemical exposures and potential association with cleft palate/lip in Iowa and Michigan compared to other live births	187	985
Hanify et al., 1981	Ecological design	Study of adverse birth outcomes occurring 1960-1966 compared to 1972-1977 for association with 2,4,5-T spraying in the later period	9,614 Births	15,000 Births
Jansson and Voog, 1989	Cohort/ case study	Case study of facial cleft (April-August 1987) and study of facial clefts (1975-1987) compared to the rates expected in Swedish county with incinerators	20,595 Births after incineration 6 Case study	71,665 Births before incineration

Continued

TABLE 6-2 *Continued*

Reference	Study Design	Description	Study Group (N)	Comparison Group (N)[a]
Lampi et al., 1992	Nested case-control/cohort	Study of cancer incidence among a community in Finland exposed to water and food contaminated with chlorophenols (1987) compared to other communities; study of several cancers compared to population controls for association with potential risk factors including food and water consumption	56 Colon cancer 40 Bladder cancer 8 STS 7 HD 23 NHL 43 Leukemia	688
Nelson et al., 1979	Ecological	Study of prevalence of oval cleft palates in high-, medium-, and low-2,4,5-T sprayed areas in Arkansas (1948-1974)	—	—
Vineis et al., 1991	Ecological	Presentation of rates (1985-1988) of NHL, HD, and STS in men and women 15-74 years old living in provinces in Italy where phenoxy herbicides are used in weeding rice and defined in two categories	63 HD 253 NHL 49 STS	No control/unexposed
White et al., 1988	Case-control and ecological	Study of chemical exposures in agricultural activity for potential association with birth defects and stillbirths in New Brunswick, Canada, 1973-1979	(a) 392 Defects (b) 298 Stillbirths	(a) 384 Matched date of birth/sex 386 Matched county/date of birth (b) 299 Matched date of birth/sex 302 Matched county/date of birth
Michigan Dept. of Health, 1983	Descriptive	Comparison of Michigan county rates of mortality for STS and connective tissue cancer (1960-1981) compared to state and national rates for potential excess in areas where dioxin may be in the environment	County rates	State and national rates
U.S. EPA, 1979	Ecological	Study of spontaneous abortions occurring during 1972-1977 in herbicide sprayed areas around Alsea, Oregon, compared to spontaneous abortions occurring in unsprayed areas	2,344 Births	(a) 1,666 Control births—unsprayed area (b) 4,120 Births—urban area

NOTE: HD = Hodgkin's disease; NHL = non-Hodgkin's lymphoma; STS = soft-tissue sarcoma; and *VAO = Veterans and Agent Orange: Health Effects of Herbicides Used in Vietnam* (Institute of Medicine, 1994).

[a] The dash (—) indicates the comparison group is based on a population (e.g., U.S. white males, country rates), and details are given in the text for specifics of the actual population.

ated, using rates for the Lombardy region from hospital discharge registration as a comparison (Pesatori et al., 1992).

Reported separately are the results of a ten-year follow-up mortality study (1976-86) of children age one to 19 at the time of the accident (Bertazzi et al., 1992), The study used methods similar to those used for adults described previously. The 19,637 subjects who were exposed (Zones A, B, and R) and a reference group of 95,339 people living in the surrounding districts formed the basis of this study. The follow-up was nearly 99 percent for vital status as of December 31, 1986. Exposure data are reasonably good for the amount of TCDD on the ground in different zones beyond the factory. However, there is no individual quantification of exposures.

The incidence of cancer following exposure to TCDD was the focus of another cohort study on individuals exposed to TCDD following the accident (Bertazzi et al., 1993). The cohort consisted of all subjects aged 20 to 74 years who lived in the study area at the time of the accident. The study included individuals from the three exposure zones around the plant: Zone A (N = 724); Zone B (N = 4,824); Zone R (N = 31,647). The referent population consisted of residents from the noncontaminated area surrounding the exposure zones (N = 181,579). The follow-up period was from January 1, 1977, to December 31, 1986, and ascertainment of vital status was greater than 99 percent. Since a nationwide cancer registry does not exist in Italy, ascertainment of cancer cases was limited to the region of Lombardy where hospital admission and discharge information is routinely recorded. Information on individuals admitted to Lombardy hospitals was electronically linked with the records of study population members to identify any study subjects admitted for treatment of neoplasms. The authors determined the proportion of cancer cases admitted to hospitals outside Lombardy to be negligible. Incidence rates were calculated separately for males and females in five-year time periods (1977-81 and 1982-86) and within five-year age classes.

Cancer incidence in a young population in the Seveso area was also evaluated (Pesatori et al., 1993). The study group consisted of all subjects aged 0 to 19 years during the first post-accident decade (1977 to 1986) and living in Zones A, B, or R on the day of the accident (N = 97,774). Subjects were assigned to one of the exposure areas or to the reference area based on their home address at the time of the accident. Control subjects lived in the nearly uncontaminated reference area (N = 447,085). Case ascertainment was performed through hospital discharge records for hospitals in the Lombardy region. Lombardy hospital records were electronically linked with records of study participants in order to determine the occurrence of neoplasms. Since the main cancer hospitals are located in the Lombardy region, the number of cases admitted to hospitals outside of Lombardy was determined to be negligible. The three contaminated zones were combined into one exposure group for the purpose of calculating relative risk, since the population of exposure Zones A and B were small and the outcomes under study were rare. Ascertainment of vitals status was successful for more than 99 percent of the subjects.

Many of the studies looking at health outcomes and mortality in Seveso residents contain overlapping information and results (Bertazzi et al., 1989a,b; Bertazzi et al., 1992; Pesatori et al., 1992). Since the most recent cancer incidence study by Bertazzi and colleagues (1993) updates much of the information reported in the previous studies on Seveso residents, the committee focused primarily on the results of Bertazzi et al. (1993) when evaluating the effects of TCDD exposure on the Seveso population.

A two-year prospective controlled study was conducted of workers potentially exposed to TCDD during the cleanup of the most highly contaminated areas following the accident (Assennato et al., 1989b). Preemployment examinations were performed from March to June 1980 to select the study groups. Workers who met certain criteria (age and certain health characteristics) were assigned to either the cleanup group or the comparison group. Periodic examinations were conducted every six months. The cleanup group was provided with protective clothing and was subject to safety measures designed to minimize the potential for exposure. At the conclusion of the study, TCDD-related clinical disease (i.e., chloracne, liver disease, peripheral neuropathy, porphyria cutanea tarda) and differences in biochemical outcomes were compared between the two groups.

Vietnam

A case-control investigation of possible risk factors, related to hepatocellular carcinoma, including exposure to Agent Orange, was conducted in Hanoi (Cordier et al., 1993). Cases ($N = 152$) were selected from male patients born before January 1, 1953, with a first diagnosis of hepatocellular carcinoma at one of two hospitals in Hanoi. Most cancer cases had no histological confirmation and were made on clinical or biochemical grounds. Controls ($N = 241$) were chosen from male patients born before January 1, 1953, admitted to the same hospitals for abdominal surgery, for reasons other than neoplasms or liver disease. Cases were matched to controls on the basis of age ($\pm$ five years) and place of residence. Blind interviews using a standard questionnaire were conducted in person with each patient in order to determine potential occupational exposures, medical history, and military service. Subjects were also asked about alcohol consumption and tobacco smoking so that these potential confounding variables could be controlled for in the calculation of odds ratios. Potential exposure to herbicides was assessed based on a history of residence in South Vietnam after 1960 and on a history of contact with sprayings.

Other Environmental Studies

A survey of neuropsychological effects was conducted among 22 residents of an area in Germany contaminated with dioxins and furans in the soil due to pyrolitic processes at a metal reclamation plant (Peper et al., 1993). Study participants were randomly chosen from a larger cohort of 450 individuals who had participated in an earlier cross-sectional study of health effects in residents of the contaminated area (Klett et al., 1991). The mean age of participants was 42 years, and the mean duration of exposure was 21 years. Exposure was defined as having lived in the immediate vicinity of the plant (mean distance 100 meters). Biological monitoring for blood PCDD/PCDF levels was also performed. Subjects were evaluated for general intelligence, memory, and attentional and visual-motor performance. Since there was no control group, comparisons were made within the study group, which was divided into high and low exposure. Age norms of psychological test results were determined to evaluate the results of neuropsychological testing.

The association between young-onset Parkinson's disease and a number of environmental and occupational exposures was evaluated in a case-control study (Butterfield et al., 1993). Cases ($N = 63$) included individuals living in Oregon or Washington who were diagnosed with Parkinson's disease on or before the age of 50. Sixty-eight persons living in the same area who were diagnosed with rheumatoid arthritis between the ages of 29 and 51 served as controls. Persons with rheumatoid arthritis were chosen as controls to control for recall bias, because individuals with a chronic disease are more likely to have spent time thinking about past exposures. Cases and controls were frequency matched for sex, year of birth, and year of diagnosis. Study subjects were asked to respond by mail to a questionnaire containing questions on environmental and occupational exposures, including herbicides. The response rate for cases was 69 percent while 41 percent of controls responded. Multivariate analyses were performed using data from the completed questionnaires to evaluate the association between exposures in the environment and workplace and young-onset Parkinson's disease.

VIETNAM VETERANS

Studies of Vietnam veterans who were potentially exposed to herbicides, including Agent Orange, have been conducted in the United States at the national and state levels, as well as in Australia. Exposure measures in these studies have been done on a variety of levels, and evaluations of health outcomes have been made using a variety of different comparison or control groups. This section is organized primarily by the sponsors of the research, as this format was more conducive to the methodologic presentations of the articles. Within these studies, the exposure measures fall along a crude scale of measurement, from the individual level for the Ranch Hands, as reflected in the serum measurements of the amount of dioxin present, to some of the individual state studies, which examined groups of veterans serving in Vietnam as a surrogate for TCDD exposure.

It should also be noted that comparison groups for the veteran cohort studies vary to include unexposed Vietnam veterans who were stationed in areas essentially not exposed to active herbicide missions and were unlikely to have been in areas sprayed with herbicides; Vietnam-era veterans who were in the service at the time of the conflict but did not serve in Vietnam; non-Vietnam veterans who served in other wars or conflicts, such as the Korean War or World War II; and various U.S. male populations (either state or national).

United States

Ranch Hands

The men responsible for the majority of the aerial spraying of herbicides were volunteers from the Air Force who participated in Operation Ranch Hand. Participants in this operation are referred to as "Ranch Hands." To determine whether there are adverse health effects associated with exposure to herbicides, including Agent Orange, the Air Force made a commitment to the Congress and the White House in 1979 to conduct an epidemiologic study of the Ranch Hands (AFHS, 1982).

A retrospective matched cohort study design was implemented to examine morbidity and mortality, with follow-up scheduled to continue until 2002. The National Personnel Records Center and the U.S. Air Force Human Resources Laboratory records were searched and cross-referenced to completely ascertain all Ranch Hand personnel (AFHS, 1982; Michalek et al., 1990). A total of 1,269 participants were originally identified (AFHS, 1983). A control population of 24,971 C-130 crew members and support personnel assigned to duty in Southeast Asia but not occupationally exposed to herbicides (AFHS, 1983) was selected from the same data sources as used to identify the Ranch Hand population. Controls were matched on age, type of job (using Air Force specialty code), and race (white/not white). The rationale for matching on these variables was to control for the clinical aging process, educational and socioeconomic status, and potential differences by race in development of chronic disease. Since Ranch Hands and controls performed similar combat or combat-related jobs, many potential confounders related to the physical/psychophysiologic effects of combat stress and the Southeast Asia environment were potentially controlled (AFHS, 1982).

Ten matches for each exposed subject formed a control set. For the mortality study, each exposed subject and a random sample of half of the subject's control set is being followed for 20 years, in a 1:5 matched design. The morbidity component of follow-up consists of a 1:1 matched design, using the first control randomized to the mortality ascertainment component of the study. If a control is noncompliant, another control from the matched "pool" will be selected; controls who die will not be replaced.

The baseline exam occurred in 1982, and future exams are scheduled until

2002. Morbidity is ascertained through questionnaire and physical examination, which emphasizes dermatologic, neuropsychiatric, hepatic, immunologic, reproductive, and neoplastic conditions. There were 1,208 Ranch Hands and 1,668 comparison subjects eligible for baseline examination. Initial questionnaire response rates were 97 percent for the exposed cohort and 93 percent for the unexposed; baseline physical exam responses were 87 and 76 percent, respectively (Wolfe et al., 1990). For the 1987 examination and questionnaire (Wolfe et al., 1990), 84 percent of the Ranch Hands (N = 955) and 75 percent of the comparison subjects (N = 1,299) were fully compliant. Mortality outcome was obtained and reviewed by using U.S. Air Force Military Personnel Center records, the VA's Death Beneficiary Identification and Record Location System (BIRLS), and the Internal Revenue Service's (IRS) database of active Social Security numbers. Death certificates were obtained from the appropriate health departments (Michalek et al., 1990). Eighty-four percent of the 1,148 eligible Ranch Hands (N = 952), 76 percent of the original comparison group (N = 912), and 65 percent of the 567 replacement comparisons (N = 369) invited to the 1992 follow-up chose to participate in the examination and questionnaire (AFHS, 1995). The methods used to assess mortality and morbidity were identical to the methods described previously for the 1982 and 1987 examinations.

The Ranch Hands were divided into three categories on the basis of their potential exposures:

1. Low potential. This group included pilots, copilots, and navigators. Exposure was primarily through preflight checks and during actual dissemination of the spray.

2. Moderate potential. This group included crew chiefs, aircraft mechanics, and support personnel. Exposure was possible by contact during dedrumming and aircraft loading operations, on-site repair of aircraft, and spray equipment.

3. High potential. This group included spray console operators and flight engineers.

Results have been published for the baseline morbidity (AFHS, 1984a) and baseline mortality studies (AFHS, 1983); first (1984b), second (1987), and third (1992) follow-up examinations (AFHS, 1987, 1990, 1995); and reproductive outcomes study (AFHS, 1992). Mortality updates have been published for 1984-86, 1989, and 1991 (AFHS, 1984b, 1985, 1986, 1989, 1991a). Serum dioxin levels were measured in 1982 (36 Ranch Hands) (Pirkle et al., 1989), 1987 (866 Ranch Hands) (AFHS, 1991b), and 1992 (455 Ranch Hands) (AFHS, 1995). The serum dioxin analysis of the 1987 follow-up examinations was published in 1991 (AFHS, 1991b). Continued follow-up and results will be forthcoming.

The relationship between paternal serum dioxin and reproductive outcomes was updated in a 1995 study (Wolfe et al., 1995). These data are a reanalysis of reproductive outcome information that was previously published (AFHS, 1992).

Subjects consisted of children and conceptions of male veterans of Operation Ranch Hand while the comparison cohort was comprised of children and conceptions of Air Force veterans who served in Southeast Asia during the same time but were not involved with spraying pesticides. Parents were asked to provide full access to their children's medical records through the age of 18. Paternal serum dioxin levels were also ascertained. Children and conceptions were stratified into four comparison groups based on paternal serum dioxin, and relative risks were calculated to evaluate the association between serum dioxin levels and offspring birth defects.

The 1989 serum dioxin analysis (Pirkle et al., 1989) was updated in 1994 and expanded to include 337 individuals (Wolfe et al., 1994) and was further extended with five years of follow-up for 213 of the subjects involved in the previous study (Michalek et al., 1996). Details of the updates are discussed in Chapter 5.

Department of Veterans Affairs

The Department of Veterans Affairs conducted a study of mortality among women Vietnam veterans (Thomas et al., 1991). The study cohort consisted of women who served in Vietnam at any time between 1964 and 1972. They were identified from the service branches by various means: Army women were identified from morning report records of 91 Army hospital and administrative support units that were likely to have had female personnel; Air Force women were identified from a computerized personnel file maintained by the Air Force Human Resources Laboratory; Navy women were identified through a review of all personnel on the muster rolls of the four Navy facilities in Vietnam; and Marine Corps women were identified from listings of all women in the Corps who were assigned to Vietnam.

Women who had never served in Vietnam were selected in a manner similar to that for the Vietnam cohort to serve as a comparison group. For the Army, Environmental Support Group (ESG) identified 90 units with female personnel stationed in the United States between 1964 and 1972; the other service branches selected women at random from their automated personnel files. These women were frequency matched to the Vietnam veterans by rank and military occupation. All personnel records for the potential study subjects were obtained from the National Personnel Records Center and the Army Reserve Personnel Center; 89 percent of the records were available for abstracting. Initially, 4,644 of the Vietnam cohort and 6,575 of the comparison cohort met the eligibility criteria. Vital status on December 31, 1987, was determined for study subjects using the DVA Beneficiary Records and records from the Social Security Administration, the IRS, National Death Index, and the military. An official certificate of death was obtained for deceased subjects. Personnel who died during active military duty before March 28, 1973, were excluded from the analyses.

The final study cohorts consisted of 4,582 women Vietnam veterans and

5,324 women who had served in the U.S. military but not in Vietnam or the Pacific theater. Person-years for risk of dying were calculated for each subject starting with either the date she left military service or March 28, 1973. Analyses were adjusted for rank, military occupation (nurse or non-nurse), duration of military service, age at entry, and race. The mortality experiences in the cohort of women serving in Vietnam and the non-Vietnam cohort were each compared to the mortality experience of U.S. women, adjusted for race, age, and calendar year. No information on any individual exposures, particularly to herbicides, was available.

This study was updated in 1995 to include follow-up through December 31, 1991 (Dalager et al., 1995). The updated mortality study included 4,586 female veterans who served in Vietnam between July 4, 1965, and March 28, 1973, and 5,325 female controls who had served outside Vietnam between 1964 and 1972. The study excluded as controls 1,213 female veterans who had not served in Vietnam but had served elsewhere in the Pacific theater, because their exposures were deemed too similar to those experienced by women in Vietnam. Data from the Social Security Administration, the IRS, the National Death Index, military records, and DVA beneficiary records were used to determine vital status of all study subjects. Identical statistical methods to those used in the first study were used to approximate risk for persons in the updated study.

A case-control study that examined the relationship between testicular cancer and surrogate measures of exposure to Agent Orange was conducted by the DVA in 1994 (Bullman et al., 1994). Cases ($N = 97$) and controls ($N = 311$) were selected from male Vietnam veterans who participated in an Agent Orange Registry examination between March 1982 and January 1991. While 127 veterans were identified from the computerized registry as currently having testicular cancer (ICD-9 code 186), 21 cases were excluded from the study due to data entry errors or unknown date of diagnosis. Surrogate measures of exposure to Agent Orange were chosen on the basis of assumptions about the association between certain aspects of military service in South Vietnam and documented uses and methods of applications of Agent Orange. Military records were used to obtain information on surrogate measures of exposure for each study participant, including branch of service, combat or noncombat military occupation specialty code (MOS), geographic area in which the individual served in Vietnam, and location of study subject's unit in relation to a sprayed area. Crude odds ratios were calculated to estimate the risk of testicular cancer associated with each surrogate measure. Odds ratios were not adjusted to account for confounding variables.

State Studies

Michigan   A proportionate mortality study examining causes of death among veterans on the Michigan Department of Management and Budget's Vietnam-era Bonus List was conducted (Visintainer et al., 1995). Veterans were classified as

TABLE 6-3 Epidemiologic Studies—Vietnam Veterans

Reference	Study Design	Description	Study Group (N)	Comparison Group (N)[a]
Ranch Hands				
New studies				
Wolfe et al., 1995	Cohort	Paternal serum dioxin levels and reproductive outcomes of Ranch Hand veterans compared with Air Force veterans from Southeast Asia who did not participate in herbicide spraying missions	932	1,202
AFHS, 1995	Cohort	Mortality updates of Ranch Hands tasked with herbicide spraying operations during the Vietnam conflict compared with Air Force C-130 air and ground crew veterans in Southeast Asia who did not participate in herbicide spraying missions	1,261 (original cohort)	19,101 (original cohort)
Studies reviewed in VAO				
AFHS, 1983, 1984b, 1985, 1986, 1989, 1991a	Cohort	Mortality updates of Ranch Hands tasked with herbicide spraying operations during the Vietnam conflict compared with Air Force C-130 air and ground crew veterans in Southeast Asia who did not participate in herbicide spraying missions	1,261 (original cohort)	19,101 (original cohort)
AFHS, 1984, 1987, 1990, 1991b, 1995	Cohort	Baseline morbidity and follow-up exam results of the Air Force Health Study	1,208 (baseline)	1,668 (baseline)
AFHS, 1992	Cohort	Reproductive outcomes of participants in the Air Force Health Study	791	942
Michalek et al., 1990	Cohort	Mortality of Ranch Hands compared with Air Force C-130 air and ground crew veterans in Southeast Asia	1,261	19,101
Wolfe et al., 1990	Cohort	Health status of Ranch Hands at second followup compared with Air Force C-130 air and ground crew veterans in Southeast Asia	995	1,299

Centers for Disease Control

Reference	Study type	Description		
Erickson et al., 1984a,b	Case-control	CDC birth defects study of children born in the Atlanta area between 1968 and 1980, comparing fathers' Vietnam experience and potential Agent Orange exposure between birth defects cases and normal controls	7,133	4,246
CDC, 1989	Cohort	Vietnam Experience Study—random sample of U.S. Army enlisted men 1965-1971	2,490	1,972
CDC, 1988a	Cohort	Vietnam Experience Study—random sample of U.S. Army enlisted men 1965-1971: psychosocial outcomes	2,490	1,972
CDC, 1988b	Cohort	Vietnam Experience Study: physical health outcomes	2,490	1,972
CDC, 1988c	Cohort	Vietnam Experience Study: reproductive outcomes	12,788 Children	11,910 Children
CDC, 1987; Boyle et al., 1987	Cohort	Vietnam Experience Study: mortality	9,324	8,989
O'Brien et al., 1991	Cohort	Interview report and mortality for NHL based on Vietnam Experience Study	8,170	7,564
Decoufle et al., 1992	Cohort	Association between self-reported health outcomes and perception of exposure to herbicides based on Vietnam Experience Study	7,924	7,364
CDC, 1990a	Case-control	Selected Cancers Study—population-based case-control study of all men born between 1921 and 1953; cases diagnosed area covered by eight cancer registries and controls selected by random-digit dialing	1,157 NHL 342 STS 310 HD 48 Nasal carcinoma 80 Nasopharyngeal carcinoma 130 Primary liver cancer	1,776
CDC, 1990b	Case-control	Selected Cancers Study—population-based case-control study of all men born between 1921 and 1953; cases diagnosed area covered by eight cancer registries and controls selected by random-digit dialing: NHL	1,157	1,776
CDC, 1990c	Case-control	Selected Cancers Study: soft-tissue sarcomas	342	1,776

Continued

TABLE 6-3 Continued

Reference	Study Design	Description	Study Group (N)	Comparison Group (N)[a]
CDC, 1990d	Case-control	Selected Cancers Study: HD, nasal cancer, nasopharyngeal cancer, and primary liver cancer	310 HD 48 Nasal carcinoma 80 Nasopharyngeal carcinoma 130 Primary liver cancer	1,776
Department of Veterans Affairs				
New studies				
Dalager et al., 1995	Cohort	Update of Thomas et al. (1991) through December 31, 1995	4,586	5,325
Bullman et al., 1994	Case-control	Study of the association between testicular cancer and surrogate measures of exposure to Agent Orange in male Vietnam veterans	97	311
Studies reviewed in VAO				
Burt et al., 1987; Breslin et al., 1988	Cohort	Mortality experience (1965-1982) of Army and Marine Corps Vietnam veterans compared to Vietnam-era veterans who did not serve in Southeast Asia standardized by age and race; nested case-control study of NHL	24,235	26,685
Bullman et al., 1990	Cohort	Mortality experience of Army I Corps Vietnam veterans compared to Army Vietnam-era veterans	6,668 Deaths	27,917 Deaths
Watanabe et al., 1991	Cohort	Mortality experience (1965-1984) of Army and Marine Corps Vietnam veterans compared to: (1) branch-specific (Army and Marine) Vietnam-era veterans, (2) all Vietnam-era veterans combined, (3) and the U.S. male population	24,145 Army 5,501 Marines	(1) 27,145 Army 4,505 Marines (2) 32,422 Combined Vietnam era (3) U.S. male population
Thomas and Kang, 1990	Cohort	Morbidity and mortality experience (1968-1987) of Army Chemical Corps Vietnam veterans compared to U.S. men	894	—
Thomas et al., 1991	Cohort	Mortality experience (1973-1987) among women Vietnam veterans compared to women non-Vietnam veterans and for each cohort compared to U.S. women	4,582	5,324

Reference	Design	Description		
Kang et al., 1986	Case-control	STS cases (1969-1983) in Vietnam-era veterans for association with branch of Vietnam service as a surrogate for Agent Orange exposure	234	13,496
Kang et al., 1987	Case-control	STS cases (1975-1980) diagnosed at the Armed Forces Institute of Pathology compared to controls identified from patient logs of referring pathologists or their departments for association with Vietnam service and likelihood of Agent Orange exposure	217	599
Dalager et al., 1991	Case-control	Cases of NHL diagnosed between 1969 and 1985 among Vietnam-era veterans compared to cases of other malignancies among Vietnam-era veterans for association with Vietnam service	201	358
True et al. 1988	Cross-sectional	PTSD and Vietnam combat experience evaluated among Vietnam-era veterans	775	1,012
Bullman et al., 1991	Case-control	PTSD cases in Vietnam veterans compared to Vietnam veterans without PTSD for association with traumatic combat experience	374	373
Farberow et al., 1990	Case-control	Psychological profiles and military factors associated with suicide and motor vehicle accident (MVA) fatalities in Los Angeles County Vietnam-era veterans (1977-1982)	22 Vietnam suicides 19 Vietnam-era suicides	21 Vietnam MVAs 20 Vietnam-era MVAs
Eisen et al., 1991	Cohort	Health effects of male monozygotic twins serving in the armed forces during Vietnam era (1965-1975)	2,260	2,260
American Legion				
Snow et al., 1988	Cohort	Assessment of PTSD in association with traumatic combat experience among American Legionnaires serving in Southeast Asia (1961-1975)	2,858	Study group subdivided for internal comparison
Stellman et al., 1988b	Cohort	Assessment of physical health and reproductive outcomes among American Legionnaires who served in Southeast Asia (1961-1975) for association with combat and herbicide exposure	2,858	3,933
Stellman et al., 1988c	Cohort	Assessment of social and behavioral outcomes among American Legionnaires who served in Southeast Asia (1961-1975) for association with combat and herbicide exposure	2,858	3,933

Continued

TABLE 6-3 *Continued*

Reference	Study Design	Description	Study Group (N)	Comparison Group (N)[a]
State Studies				
New studies				
Visintainer et al., 1995	Cohort	Mortality experience (1965-1971) among male Michigan Vietnam veterans compared to non-Vietnam veterans from Michigan	3,364 Deaths	5,229 Deaths
Studies reviewed in VAO				
Rellahan, 1985	Cohort	Study of health outcomes in Vietnam-era (1962-1972) veterans residing in Hawaii associated with Vietnam experience	232	186
Wendt, 1985	Descriptive	Descriptive findings of health effects and potential exposure to Agent Orange among Iowa veterans who served in Southeast Asia	10,846	None
Kogan and Clapp, 1985, 1988	Cohort	Mortality experience (1972-1983) among white male Massachusetts Vietnam veterans compared to non-Vietnam veterans and to all other nonveteran white males in Massachusetts	840 Deaths	2,515 Deaths in Vietnam-era veterans
Clapp et al., 1991	Case-control	Selected cancers identified (1982-1988) among Massachusetts Vietnam veterans compared to Massachusetts Vietnam-era veterans with cancers of other sites	214	727
Levy, 1988	Cross-sectional	Study of PTSD in chloracne as indicator of exposure to TCDD and control Vietnam veterans in Massachusetts	6	25
Fiedler and Gochfeld, 1992; Kahn et al., 1992a,b,c	Cohort	New Jersey study of outcomes in select group of herbicide-exposed Army, Marine, and Navy Vietnam veterans compared to veterans self-reported as unexposed	10 Pointman I 55 Pointman II	17 Pointman I 15 Pointman II
Pollei et al., 1986	Cohort	Study of chest radiographs of New Mexico Agent Orange Registry Vietnam veterans compared to control Air Force servicemen radiographs for pulmonary and cardiovascular pathology	422	105
Lawrence et al., 1985	Cohort	Mortality experience of New York State (1) Vietnam-era veterans compared to nonveterans and (2) Vietnam veterans compared to Vietnam-era veterans	(1) 4,558 (2) 555	17,936 941

Study	Type	Description	Number	Comparison/Controls
Greenwald et al., 1984	Case-control	Cases of STS in New York State compared to controls without cancer for Vietnam service and herbicide exposure including Agent Orange, dioxin, or 2,4,5-T	281	281 Live controls 130 Deceased controls
Goun and Kuller, 1986	Case-control	Cases of STS, NHL, and selected rare cancers compared to controls without cancer for Vietnam experience in Pennsylvania men (1968-1983)	349	349 Deaths
Anderson et al., 1986a	Cohort	Mortality experience of Wisconsin veterans compared to nonveterans (Phase 1); mortality experience of Wisconsin Vietnam veterans and Vietnam-era veterans compared to nonveterans and other veterans (Phase 2)	110,815 White male veteran deaths 2,494 White male Vietnam-era veteran deaths 923 White male Vietnam veteran deaths	342,654 White male nonveteran deaths 109,225 White male other veteran deaths
Anderson et al., 1986b	Cohort	Mortality experience of Wisconsin Vietnam-era veterans and Vietnam veterans compared to U.S. men, Wisconsin men, Wisconsin nonveterans, and Wisconsin other veterans	122,238 Vietnam-era veterans 43,398 Vietnam veterans	—
Holmes et al., 1986	Cohort	Mortality experience (1968-1983) of West Virginia veterans, Vietnam veterans, Vietnam-era veterans compared to nonveterans, and Vietnam veterans compared to Vietnam-era veterans	615 Vietnam veterans 610 Vietnam-era veterans	—
Newell, 1984	Cross-sectional	Preliminary (1) cytogenetic, (2) sperm, and (3) immune response tests in Texas Vietnam veterans compared to controls	(1) 30 (2) 32 (3) 66	30 32 66
Deprez et al., 1991	Descriptive	Study of Maine Vietnam veterans compared to atomic test veterans and general population for health status and reproductive outcomes	249	113 Atomic test veterans

Other U.S. Veteran Studies

Study	Type	Description	Number	Comparison/Controls
Aschengrau and Monson, 1989	Case-control	Association between husband's military service and women having spontaneous abortion at 27 weeks compared to women delivering at 37 weeks	201	1,119
Aschengrau and Monson, 1990	Case-control	Study of cases with late adverse pregnancy outcomes compared to normal control births for association with paternal Vietnam service (1977-1980)	857 Congenital anomalies 61 Stillbirths 48 Neonatal deaths	998

Continued

TABLE 6-3 Continued

Reference	Study Design	Description	Study Group (N)	Comparison Group (N)[a]
Goldberg et al., 1990	Cohort	Study of male twin pairs who served in Vietnam era (1965-1975) for association between Vietnam service and PTSD	2,092	2,092
Tarone et al., 1991	Case-control	Study of cases between January 1976 and June 1981 with testicular cancer (18-42 years old) compared to hospital controls for association with Vietnam service	137	130
Australian Studies				
Donovan et al., 1983, 1984	Case-control	Australian study of cases of congenital anomalies in children born between 1969 and 1979 compared to infants born without anomalies for association with paternal Vietnam service	8,517	8,517
Fett et al., 1987a	Cohort	Australian study of mortality experience of Vietnam veterans compared to Vietnam-era veterans through 1981	19,205	25,677
Fett et al., 1987b	Cohort	Australian study of cause-specific mortality experience of Vietnam veterans compared to Vietnam-era veterans through 1981	19,205	25,677
Forcier et al., 1987	Cohort	Australian study of mortality in Vietnam veterans by job classification, location, and time of service	19,205	Internal comparison
Field and Kerr, 1988	Cohort	Tasmanian study of Vietnam veterans compared to neighborhood controls for adverse reproductive and childhood health outcomes	357	281

NOTE: HD = Hodgkin's disease; NHL = non-Hodgkin's lymphoma; PTSD = posttraumatic stress disorder; STS = soft-tissue sarcoma; and VAO = Veterans and Agent Orange: Health Effects of Herbicides Used in Vietnam (Institute of Medicine, 1994).

[a] The dash (—) indicates the comparison group is based on a population (e.g., U.S. white males, country rates), with details given in the text for specifics of the actual population.

having served in Vietnam (N = 151,377) or having served during the Vietnam era but outside the country (N = 225,651). The bonus list was compiled from those veterans or their survivors who knew about the state of Michigan's bonus offer and who chose to apply for it; thus it is unknown whether this list is representative of Michigan Vietnam-era veterans. Determination of vital status was accomplished by matching the list database with the state's Department of Public Health death certificate database covering the years 1974 to 1989. Proportional mortality ratios (PMRs) were calculated, since demographic data were available only for the deceased veterans, and were generated as age, race (black or non-black), and period-specific rates. Among deceased veterans who matched the death certificate database, 3,701 deaths (2.4 percent) were among veterans who served in Vietnam, and 6,026 deaths (2.7 percent) were among veterans who did not serve in Vietnam. Veterans were selected for analysis who were 18 to 29 years old during the period 1965 to 1971; this included 3,364 Vietnam veterans and 5229 veterans who served elsewhere.

REFERENCES

Air Force Health Study. 1982. An Epidemiologic Investigation of Health Effects in Air Force Personnel Following Exposure to Herbicides: Study Protocol, Initial Report. Brooks AFB, TX: USAF School of Aerospace Medicine. SAM-TR-82-44.

Air Force Health Study. 1983. An Epidemiologic Investigation of Health Effects in Air Force Personnel Following Exposure to Herbicides: Baseline Mortality Study Results. Brooks AFB, TX: USAF School of Aerospace Medicine. NTIS AD-A130 793.

Air Force Health Study. 1984a. An Epidemiologic Investigation of Health Effects in Air Force Personnel Following Exposure to Herbicides: Baseline Morbidity Study Results. Brooks AFB, TX: USAF School of Aerospace Medicine. NTIS AD-A138 340.

Air Force Health Study. 1984b. An Epidemiologic Investigation of Health Effects in Air Force Personnel Following Exposure to Herbicides. Mortality Update: 1984. Brooks AFB, TX: USAF School of Aerospace Medicine.

Air Force Health Study. 1985. An Epidemiologic Investigation of Health Effects in Air Force Personnel Following Exposure to Herbicides. Mortality Update: 1985. Brooks AFB, TX: USAF School of Aerospace Medicine.

Air Force Health Study. 1986. An Epidemiologic Investigation of Health Effects in Air Force Personnel Following Exposure to Herbicides. Mortality Update: 1986. Brooks AFB, TX: USAF School of Aerospace Medicine. USAFSAM-TR-86-43.

Air Force Health Study. 1987. An Epidemiologic Investigation of Health Effects in Air Force Personnel Following Exposure to Herbicides. First Followup Examination Results. 2 vols. Brooks AFB, TX: USAF School of Aerospace Medicine. USAFSAM-TR-87-27.

Air Force Health Study. 1989. An Epidemiologic Investigation of Health Effects in Air Force Personnel Following Exposure to Herbicides. Mortality Update: 1989. Brooks AFB, TX: USAF School of Aerospace Medicine. USAFSAM-TR-89-9.

Air Force Health Study. 1990. An Epidemiologic Investigation of Health Effects in Air Force Personnel Following Exposure to Herbicides. 2 vols. Brooks AFB, TX: USAF School of Aerospace Medicine. USAFSAM-TR-90-2.

Air Force Health Study. 1991a. An Epidemiologic Investigation of Health Effects in Air Force Personnel Following Exposure to Herbicides. Mortality Update: 1992. Brooks AFB, TX: Armstrong Laboratory. AL-TR-1991-0132.

Air Force Health Study. 1991b. An Epidemiologic Investigation of Health Effects in Air Force Personnel Following Exposure to Herbicides. Serum Dioxin Analysis of 1987 Examination Results. 9 vols. Brooks AFB, TX: USAF School of Aerospace Medicine.

Air Force Health Study. 1992. An Epidemiologic Investigation of Health Effects in Air Force Personnel Following Exposure to Herbicides. Reproductive Outcomes. Brooks AFB, TX: Armstrong Laboratory. AL-TR-1992-0090.

Air Force Health Study. 1995. An Epidemiologic Investigation of Health Effects in Air Force Personnel Following Exposure to Herbicides. 1992 Followup Examination Results. 10 vols. Brooks AFB, TX: Epidemiologic Research Division. Armstrong Laboratory.

Alavanja MC, Blair A, Merkle S, Teske J, Eaton B. 1988. Mortality among agricultural extension agents. American Journal of Industrial Medicine 14:167-176.

Alavanja MC, Merkle S, Teske J, Eaton B, Reed B. 1989. Mortality among forest and soil conservationists. Archives of Environmental Health 44:94-101.

Alderfer R, Sweeney M, Fingerhut M, Hornung R, Wille K, Fidler A. 1992. Measures of depressed mood in workers exposed to 2,3,7,8-tetrachlorodibenzo-p-dioxin (TCDD). Chemosphere 25/1-2:247-250.

Anderson HA, Hanrahan LP, Jensen M, Laurin D, Yick W-Y, Wiegman P. 1986a. Wisconsin Vietnam Veteran Mortality Study: Proportionate Mortality Study Results. State of Wisconsin, Department of Health and Social Sciences.

Anderson HA, Hanrahan LP, Jensen M, Laurin D, Yick W-Y, Wiegman P. 1986b. Wisconsin Vietnam Veteran Mortality Study: Final Report. State of Wisconsin, Department of Health and Social Sciences.

Aschengrau A, Monson RR. 1989. Paternal military service in Vietnam and risk of spontaneous abortion. Journal of Occupational Medicine 31:618-623.

Aschengrau A, Monson RR. 1990. Paternal military service in Vietnam and the risk of late adverse pregnancy outcomes. American Journal of Public Health 80:1218-1224.

Asp S, Riihimaki V, Hernberg S, Pukkala E. 1994. Mortality and cancer morbidity of Finnish chlorophenoxy herbicide applicators: an 18-year prospective follow-up. American Journal of Industrial Medicine 26:243-253.

Assennato G, Cervino D, Emmett EA, Longo G, Merlo F. 1989a. Follow-up of subjects who developed chloracne following TCDD exposure at Seveso. American Journal of Industrial Medicine 16:119-125.

Assennato G, Cannatelli P, Emmett E, Ghezzi I, Merlo F. 1989b. Medical monitoring of dioxin clean-up workers. American Industrial Hygiene Association Journal 50:586-592.

Axelson O, Sundell L. 1974. Herbicide exposure, mortality and tumor incidence. An epidemiological investigation on Swedish railroad workers. Scandinavian Journal of Work, Environment, and Health 11:21-28.

Axelson O, Sundell L, Andersson K, Edling C, Hogstedt C, Kling H. 1980. Herbicide exposure and tumor mortality: an updated epidemiologic investigation on Swedish railroad workers. Scandinavian Journal of Work, Environment, and Health 6:73-79.

Balarajan R, Acheson ED. 1984. Soft tissue sarcomas in agriculture and forestry workers. Journal of Epidemiology and Community Health 38:113-116.

Barbieri S, Pirovano C, Scarlato G, Tarchini P, Zappa A, Maranzana M. 1988. Long-term effects of 2,3,7,8-tetrachlorodibenzo-p-dioxin on the peripheral nervous system. Clinical and neurophysiological controlled study on subjects with chloracne from the Seveso area. Neuroepidemiology 7:29-37.

Barthel E. 1981. Increased risk of lung cancer in pesticide-exposed male agricultural workers. Journal of Toxicology and Environmental Health 8:1027-1040.

Bashirov AA. 1969. The health of workers involved in the production of amine and butyl 2,4-D herbicides. Vrachebnoye Delo 10:92-95.

Bender AP, Parker DL, Johnson RA, Scharber WK, Williams AN, Marbury MC, Mandel JS. 1989. Minnesota highway maintenance worker study: cancer mortality. American Journal of Industrial Medicine 15:545-556.

Bertazzi A, Pesatori AC, Consonni D, Tironi A, Landi MT, Zocchetti C. 1993. Cancer incidence in a population accidentally exposed to 2,3,7,8-tetrachlorodibenzo-*para*-dioxin [see comments]. Epidemiology 4:398-406.

Bertazzi PA, Zocchetti C, Pesatori AC, Guercilena S, Sanarico M, Radice L. 1989a. Mortality in an area contaminated by TCDD following an industrial incident. Medicina Del Lavoro 80:316-329.

Bertazzi PA, Zocchetti C, Pesatori AC, Guercilena S, Sanarico M, Radice L. 1989b. Ten-year mortality study of the population involved in the Seveso incident in 1976. American Journal of Epidemiology 129:1187-1200.

Bertazzi PA, Zocchetti C, Pesatori AC, Guercilena S, Consonni D, Tironi A, Landi MT. 1992. Mortality of a young population after accidental exposure to 2,3,7,8-tetrachlorodibenzo-*p*-dioxin. International Journal of Epidemiology 21:118-123.

Bisanti L, Bonetti F, Caramaschi F, Del Corno G, Favaretti C, Giambelluca SE, Marni E, Montesarchio E, PuccinelliV, Remotti G, Volpato C, Zambrelli E, Fara GM. 1980. Experiences from the accident of Seveso. Acta Morphologica Acadamiae Scientarum Hungaricae 28:139-157.

Blair A. 1983. Lung cancer and other causes of death among licensed pesticide applicators. Journal of the National Cancer Institute 71:31-37.

Blair A, Thomas TL. 1979. Leukemia among Nebraska farmers: a death certificate study. American Journal of Epidemiology 110:264-273.

Blair A, White DW. 1985. Leukemia cell types and agricultural practices in Nebraska. Archives of Environmental Health 40:211-214.

Blair A, Mustafa D, Heineman EF. 1993. Cancer and other causes of death among male and female farmers from twenty-three states. American Journal of Industrial Medicine 23:729-742.

Bloemen LJ, Mandel JS, Bond GG, Pollock AF, Vitek RP, Cook RR. 1993. An update of mortality among chemical workers potentially exposed to the herbicide 2,4-dichlorophenoxyacetic acid and its derivatives. Journal of Occupational Medicine 35:1208-1212.

Boeri R, Bordo B, Crenna P, Filippini G, Massetto M, Zecchini A. 1978. Preliminary results of a neurological investigation of the population exposed to TCDD in the Seveso region. Rivista di Patologia Nervosa e Mentale 99:111-128.

Boffetta P, Stellman SD, Garfinkel L. 1989. A case-control study of multiple myeloma nested in the American Cancer Society Prospective Study. International Journal of Cancer 43:554-559.

Bond GG, Ott MG, Brenner FE, Cook RR. 1983. Medical and morbidity surveillance findings among employees potentially exposed to TCDD. British Journal of Industrial Medicine 40:318-324.

Bond GG. 1987. Evaluation of mortality patterns among chemical workers with chloracne. Chemosphere 16:2117-2121.

Bond GG, Wetterstroem NH, Roush GJ, McLaren EA, Lipps TE, Cook RR. 1988. Cause specific mortality among employees engaged in the manufacture, formulation, or packaging of 2,4-dichlorophenoxyacetic acid and related salts. British Journal of Industrial Medicine 45:98-105.

Bond GG, McLaren EA, Brenner FE, Cook RR. 1989a. Incidence of chloracne among chemical workers potentially exposed to chlorinated dioxins. Journal of Occupational Medicine 31:771-774.

Bond GG, McLaren EA, Lipps TE, Cook RR. 1989b. Update of mortality among chemical workers with potential exposure to the higher chlorinated dioxins. Journal of Occupational Medicine 31:121-123.

Boyle C, DeCoucle P, Delaney RJ, DeStefano F, Flock ML, Hunter MI, Joesoef MR, Karon JM, Kirk ML, Laude PM, McGee DL, Moyer LA, Pollock DA, Rhodes P, Scully MJ, Worth RM.. 1987. Postservice mortality among Vietnam veterans. Atlanta: Centers for Disease Control. CEH 86-0076

Breslin P, Kang H, Lee Y, Burt V, Shepard BM. 1988. Proportionate mortality study of U.S. Army and U.S. Marine Corps Veterans of the Vietnam War. Journal of Occupational Medicine 30:412-419.

Brown LM, Blair A, Gibson R, Everett GD, Cantor KP, Schuman LM, Burmeister LF, Van Lier SF, Dick F. 1990. Pesticide exposures and other agricultural risk factors for leukemia among men in Iowa and Minnesota. Cancer Research 50:6585-6591.

Brown LM, Burmeister LF, Everett GD, Blair A. 1993. Pesticide exposures and multiple myeloma in Iowa men. Cancer Causes Control 4:153-156.

Bueno de Mesquita HB, Doornbos G, Van der Kuip DA, Kogevinas M, Winkelmann R. 1993. Occupational exposure to phenoxy herbicides and chlorophenols and cancer mortality in the Netherlands. American Journal of Industrial Medicine 23(2):289-300.

Bullman TA, Kang HK, Watanabe KK. 1990. Proportionate mortality among U.S. Army Vietnam veterans who served in military region I. American Journal of Epidemiology 132:670-674.

Bullman TA, Kang H, Thomas TL. 1991. Posttraumatic stress disorder among Vietnam veterans on the Agent Orange Registry: a case-control analysis. Annals of Epidemiology 1:505-512.

Bullman TA, Watanabe KK, Kang HK. 1994. Risk of testicular cancer associated with surrogate measures of Agent Orange exposure among Vietnam veterans on the Agent Orange Registry. Annals of Epidemiology 4:11-16.

Burmeister LF. 1981. Cancer mortality in Iowa farmers. 1971-1978. Journal of the National Cancer Institute 66:461-464.

Burmeister LF, Van Lier SF, Isacson P. 1982. Leukemia and farm practices in Iowa. American Journal of Epidemiology 115:720-728.

Burmeister LF, Everett GD, Van Lier SF, Isacson P. 1983. Selected cancer mortality and farm practices in Iowa. American Journal of Epidemiology 118:72-77.

Burt VL, Breslin PP, Kang HK, Lee Y. 1987. Non-Hodgkin's lymphoma in Vietnam veterans. Washington: Department oi Medicine and Surgery, Veterans Administration.

Butterfield PG, Valanis BG, Spencer PS, Lindeman CA, Nutt JG. 1993. Environmental antecedents of young-onset Parkinson's disease. Neurology 43:1150-1158.

Calvert GM, Sweeney MH, Morris JA, Fingerhut MA, Hornung RW, Halperin WE. 1991. Evaluation of chronic bronchitis, chronic obstructive pulmonary disease, and ventilatory function among workers exposed to 2,3,7,8-tetrachlorodibenzo-p-dioxin. American Review of Respiratory Disease 144:1302-1306.

Calvert GM, Hornung RV, Sweeney MH, Fingerhut MA, Halperin WE. 1992. Hepatic and gastrointestinal effects in an occupational cohort exposed to 2,3,7,8-tetrachlorodibenzo-$para$-dioxin. Journal of the American Medical Association 267:2209-2214.

Calvert GM, Sweeney MH, Fingerhut MA, Hornung RW, Halperin WE. 1994. Evaluation of porphyria cutanea tarda in U.S. workers exposed to 2,3,7,8-tetrachlorodibenzo-p-dioxin. American Journal of Industrial Medicine 25:559-571.

Cantor KP. 1982. Farming and mortality from non-Hodgkin's lymphoma: a case-control study. International Journal of Cancer 29:239-247.

Cantor KP, Blair A, Everett G, Gibson R, Burmeister LF, Brown M, Schuman L, Dick FR. 1992. Pesticides and other agricultural risk factors for non-Hodgkin's lymphoma among men in Iowa and Minnesota. Cancer Research 52:2447-2455.

Caramaschi F, Del Corno G, Favaretti C, Gianbelluca SE, Montesarchi E, Gara GM. 1981. Chloracne following environmental contamination by TCDD in Seveso, Italy. International Journal of Epidemiology 10:135-143.

Carmelli D, Hofherr L, Tomsic J, Morgan RW. 1981. A case-control study of the relationship between exposure to 2,4-D and spontaneous abortions in humans. SRI International: Report for the National Forest Products Association and the U.S. Dept. of Agriculture—Forest Service. August 14, 1981.

Cartwright RA, McKinney PA, O'Brien C, Richards IDG, Roberts B, Lauder I, Darwin CM, Bernard SM, Bird CC. 1988. Non-Hodgkin's lymphoma: case-control epidemiological study in Yorkshire. Leukemia Research 12:81-88.

Centers for Disease Control. 1987. Postservice mortality among Vietnam veterans. Journal of the American Medical Association 257:790-795.

Centers for Disease Control. 1988a. Health status of Vietnam veterans. I. Psychosocial characteristics. Journal of the American Medical Association 259:2701-2707.

Centers for Disease Control. 1988b. Health status of Vietnam veterans. II. Physical health. Journal of the American Medical Association 259:2708-2714.

Centers for Disease Control. 1988c. Health status of Vietnam veterans. III. Reproductive outcomes and child health. Journal of the American Medical Association 259:2715-2717.

Centers for Disease Control. 1989. Health status of Vietnam veterans. Vietnam Experience Study. Atlanta: U.S. Department of Health and Human Services. Vols. I-V, Supplements A-C. .

Centers for Disease Control. 1990a. The association of selected cancers with service in the US military in Vietnam. I. Non-Hodgkin's lymphoma. The Selected Cancers Cooperative Study Group [see comments]. Archives of Internal Medicine 150:2473-2483.

Centers for Disease Control. 1990b. The association of selected cancers with service in the US military in Vietnam. II. Soft-tissue and other sarcomas. The Selected Cancers Cooperative Study Group [see comments]. Archives of Internal Medicine 150:2485-2492.

Centers for Disease Control. 1990c. The association of selected cancers with service in the US military in Vietnam. III. Hodgkin's disease, nasal cancer, nasopharyngeal cancer, and primary liver cancer. The Selected Cancers Cooperative Study Group [see comments]. Archives of Internal Medicine 150:2495-2505.

Centers for Disease Control. 1990d. The Association of Selected Cancers with Service in the U.S. Military in Vietnam: Final Report. Atlanta: U.S. Department of Health and Human Services.

Clapp RW, Cupples LA, Colton T, Ozonoff DM. 1991. Cancer surveillance of veterans in Massachusetts, 1982-1988. International Journal of Epidemiology 20:7-12.

Coggon D, Pannett B, Winter PD, Acheson ED, Bonsall J. 1986. Mortality of workers exposed to 2 methyl-4 chlorophenoxyacetic acid. Scandinavian Journal of Work, Environment, and Health 12:448-454.

Coggon D, Pannett B, Winter P. 1991. Mortality and incidence of cancer at four factories making phenoxy herbicides. British Journal of Industrial Medicine 48:173-178.

Collins JJ, Strauss ME, Levinskas GJ, Conner PR. 1993. The mortality experience of workers exposed to 2,3,7,8-tetrachlorodibenzo-*p*-dioxin in a trichlorophenol process accident [see comments]. Epidemiology 4:7-13.

Constable JD, Hatch MC. 1985. Reproductive effects of herbicide exposure in Vietnam: recent studies by the Vietnamese and others. Teratogenesis, Carcinogenesis, and Mutagenesis 5:231-250.

Cook RR, Townsend JC, Ott MG, Silverstein LG. 1980. Mortality experience of employees exposed to 2,3,7,8-tetrachlorodibenzo-*p*-dioxin (TCDD). Journal of Occupational Medicine 22:530-532.

Cook RR, Bond GG, Olson RA. 1986. Evaluation of the mortality experience of workers exposed to the chlorinated dioxins. Chemosphere 15:1769-1776.

Cook RR, Bond GG, Olson RA, Ott MG. 1987. Update of the mortality experience of workers exposed to chlorinated dioxins. Chemosphere 16:2111-2116.

Cordier S, Le TB, Verger P, Bard D, Le CD, Larouze B, Dazza MC, Hoang TQ, Abenhaim L. 1993. Viral infections and chemical exposures as risk factors for hepatocellular carcinoma in Vietnam. International Journal of Cancer 55:196-201.

Corrao G, Caller M, Carle F, Russo R, Bosia S, Piccioni P. 1989. Cancer risk in a cohort of licensed pesticide users. Scandinavian Journal of Work, Environment, and Health 15:203-209.

Dai LC, Chuong NTN, Le HT, Thuy TT, Van NTT, Le HC, Chi HTK, Le BT. 1990. A comparison of infant mortality rates between two Vietnamese villages sprayed by defoliants in wartime and one unsprayed village. Chemosphere 20:1005-1012.

Dalager NA, Kang HK, Burt VL, Weatherbee L. 1991. Non-Hodgkin's lymphoma among Vietnam veterans. Journal of Occupational Medicine 33:774-779.

Dalager NA, Kang HK, Thomas TL. 1995. Cancer mortality patterns among women who served in the military: the Vietnam experience. Journal of Occupational and Environmental Medicine 37:298-305.

Dean G. 1994. Deaths from primary brain cancers, lymphatic and haematopoietic cancers in agricultural workers in the Republic of Ireland. Journal of Epidemiology and Community Health 48:364-368.

Decoufle P, Holmgreen P, Boyle CA, Stroup NE. 1992. Self-reported health status of Vietnam veterans in relation to perceived exposure to herbicides and combat. American Journal of Epidemiology 135:312-323.

Deprez RD, Carvette ME, Agger MS. 1991. The health and medical status of Maine veterans: a report to the Bureau of Veterans Services Commission of Vietnam and atomic veterans. May 13, 1991.

Donna A, Betta P-G, Robutti F, Crosignani P, Berrino F, Bellingeri D. 1984. Ovarina mesothelial tumors and herbicides: a case-control study. Carcinogenesis 5:941-942.

Donovan JW, Adena MA, Rose G, Battistutta D. 1983. Case-Control Study of Congenital Anomalies and Vietnam Service (Birth Defects Study): Report to the Minister for Veterans Affairs. Canberra: Australian Government Publishing Service.

Donovan JW, MacLennan R, Adena M. 1984. Vietnam service and the risk of congenital anomalies: a case-control study. Medical Journal of Australia 140:394-397.

Dubrow R, Paulson JO, Indian RW. 1988. Farming and malignant lymphoma in Hancock County, Ohio. British Journal of Industrial Medicine 45:25-28.

Egeland GM, Sweeney MH, Fingerhut MA, Wille KK, Schnorr TM, Halperin WE. 1994. Total serum testosterone and gonadotropins in workers exposed to dioxin. American Journal of Epidemiology 139:272-281.

Eisen S, Goldberg J, True WR, Henderson WG. 1991. A co-twin control study of the effects of the Vietnam War on the self-reported physical health of veterans. American Journal of Epidemiology 134:49-58.

Erickson JD, Mulinare J, Mcclain PW, Fitch TG, James LM, McClearn AB, Adams MJ. 1984a. Vietnam Veterans' Risks for Fathering Babies with Birth Defects. Atlanta: U.S. Department of Health and Human Services, Centers for Disease Control.

Erickson JD, Mulinare J, Mcclain PW. 1984b. Vietnam veterans' risks for fathering babies with birth defects. Journal of the American Medical Association 252:903-912.

Eriksson M, Hardell L, Berg NO, Moller T, Axelson O. 1979. Case-control study on malignant mesenchymal tumor of the soft tissue and exposure to chemical substances. Lakartidningen 76:3872-3875.

Eriksson M, Hardell L, Berg NO, Moller T, Axelson O. 1981. Soft-tissue sarcomas and exposure to chemical substances: a case-referent study. British Journal of Industrial Medicine 38:27-33.

Eriksson M, Hardell L, Adami HO. 1990. Exposure to dioxins as a risk factor for soft tissue sarcoma: a population-based case-control study [see comments]. Journal of the National Cancer Institute 82:486-490.

Eriksson E, Hardell L, Malker H, Weiner J. 1992. Malignant lymphoproliferative diseases in occupations with potential exposure to phenoxyacetic acids or dioxins: a register-based study. American Journal of Industrial Medicine 22:305-312.

Evans RG, Webb KB, Knutsen AP, Roodman ST, Roberts DW, Bagby JR, Garrett WA Jr, Andrews JS Jr. 1988. A medical follow-up of the health effects of long-term exposure to 2,3,7,8-tetrachlorodibenzo-p-dioxin. Archives of Environmental Health 43:273-278.

Farberow NL, Kang H, Bullman T. 1990. Combat experience and postservice psychosocial status as predictors for suicide in Vietnam veterans. The Journal of Nervous and Mental Disease 178:32-37.

Fett MJ, Adena MA, Cobbin DM, Dunn M. 1987a. Mortality among Australian conscripts of the Vietnam conflict era. I. Death from all causes. American Journal of Epidemiology 126:869-877.

Fett MJ, Nairn JR, Cobbin DM, Adena MA. 1987b. Mortality among Australian conscripts of the Vietnam conflict era. II Causes of death. American Journal of Epidemiology 125:878-884.

Fiedler N, Gochfeld M. 1992. Neurobehavioral Correlates of Herbicide Exposure in Vietnam Veterans. New Jersey Agent Orange Commission, Pointman Project.

Field B, Kerr C. 1988. Reproductive behavior and consistent patterns of abnormality in offspring of Vietnam veterans. Journal of Medical Genetics 25:819-826.

Filippini G, Bordo B, Crenna P, Massetto N, Musicco M, Boeri R. 1981. Relationship between clinical and electrophysiological findings and indicators of heavy exposure to 2,3,7,8-tetrachlorodibenzo-p-dioxin. Scandinavian Journal of Work, Environment, and Health 7:257-262.

Fingerhut MA, Halperin WE, Marlow DA, Piacitelli LA, Honchar PA, Sweeney MH, Greife AL, Dill PA, Steenland K, Suruda AJ. 1991. Cancer mortality in workers exposed to 2,3,7,8-tetrachlorodibenzo-p-dioxin. New England Journal of Medicine 324:212-218.

Fitzgerald EF, Weinstein AL, Youngblood LG, Standfast SJ, Melius JM. 1989. Health effects three years after potential exposure to the toxic contaminants of an electrical transformer fire. Archives of Environmental Health 44:214-221.

Forcier L, Hudson HM, Cobbin DM, Jones MP, Adena MA, Fett MJ. 1987. Mortality of Australian veterans of the Vietnam conflict and the period and location of their Vietnam service. Military Medicine 152:9-15.

Garry VF, Kelly JT, Sprafka JM, Edwards S, Griffith J. 1994. Survey of health and use characterization of pesticide appliers in Minnesota. Archives of Environmental Health 49:337-343.

Goldberg J, Ture WR, Eisen SA, Henderson WG. 1990. A twin study of the effects of the Vietnam war on posttraumatic stress disorder. Journal of the American Medical Association 263:1227-1232.

Gordon JE, Shy CM. 1981. Agricultural chemical use and congenital cleft lip and/or palate. Archives of Environmental Health 36:213-221.

Goun BD, Kuller LH. 1986. Final Report: A Case-Control Mortality Study on the Association of Soft Tissue Sarcomas, Non-Hodgkin's Lymphomas, and Other Selected Cancers and Vietnam Military Service in Pennsylvania Males. Pittsburgh: University of Pittsburgh.

Green LM. 1987. Suicide and exposure to phenoxy acid herbicides. Scandinavian Journal of Work, Environment, and Health 13:460.

Green LM. 1991. A cohort mortality study of forestry workers exposed to phenoxy acid herbicides. British Journal of Industrial Medicine 48:234-238.

Greenwald P, Kovasznay B, Collins DN, Therriault G. 1984. Sarcomas of soft tissues after Vietnam service. Journal of the National Cancer Institute 73:1107-1109.

Hanify JA, Metcalf P, Nobbs CL, Worsley KJ. 1981. Aerial spraying of 2,4,5-T and human birth malformations: an epidemiological investigation. Science 212:349-351.

Hansen ES, Hasle H, Lander F. 1992. A cohort study on cancer incidence among Danish gardeners. American Journal of Industrial Medicine 21:651-660.

Hardell L. 1981. Relation of soft-tissue sarcoma, malignant lymphoma and colon cancer to phenoxy acids, chlorophenols and other agents. Scandinavian Journal of Work, Environment, and Health 7:119-130.

Hardell L, Bengtsson NO. 1983. Epidemiological study of socioeconomic factors and clinical findings in Hodgkin's disease, and reanlaysis of previous data regarding chemical exposure. British Journal of Cancer 48:217-225.

Hardell L, Eriksson M. 1988. The association between soft tissue sarcomas and exposure to phenoxyacetic acids: a new case-referent study. Cancer 62:652-656.

Hardell L, Sandstrom A. 1979. Case-control study: soft-tissue sarcomas and exposure to phenoxyacetic acids or chlorophenols. British Journal of Cancer 39:711-717.

Hardell L, Eriksson M, Degerman A. 1994. Exposure to phenoxyacetic acids, chlorophenols, or organic solvents in relation to histopathology, stage, and anatomical localization of non-Hodgkin's lymphoma. Cancer Research 54:2386-2389.

Hardell L, Eriksson M, Lenner P. 1980. Malignant lymphoma and exposure to chemical substances, especially organic solvents, chlorophenols and phenoxy acids. Lakartidningen 77:208-210.

Hardell L, Eriksson M, Lenner P, Lundgren E. 1981. Malignant lymphoma and exposure to chemicals, especially organic solvents, chlorophenols and phenoxy acids: a case-control study. British Journal of Cancer 43:169-176.

Hardell L, Johansson B, Axelson O. 1982. Epidemiological study of nasal and nasopharyngeal cancer and their relation to phenoxy acid or chlorophenol exposure. American Journal of Industrial Medicine 3:247-257.

Hardell L, Bengtsson NO, Jonsson U, Eriksson S, Larsson LG. 1984. Aetiological aspects on primary liver cancer with special regard to alcohol, organic solvents and acute intermittent porphyria—an epidemiological investigation. British Journal of Cancer 50:389-397.

Hardell L, Moss A, Osmond D, Volberding P. 1987. Exposure to hair dyes and polychlorinated dibenzo-*p*-dioxins in AIDS patients with Kaposi sarcoma: an epidemiological investigation. Cancer Detection and Prevention Supplement 1:567-570.

Henneberger PK, Ferris BG Jr, Monson RR. 1989. Mortality among pulp and paper workers in Berlin, New Hampshire. British Journal of Industrial Medicine 46:658-664.

Hoar SK, Blair A, Holmes FF, Boysen CD, Robel RJ, Hoover R, Fraumeni JF. 1986. Agricultural herbicide use and risk of lymphoma and soft-tissue sarcoma. Journal of the American Medical Association 256:1141-1147.

Hoffman RE, Stehr-Green PA, Webb KB, Evams. RG, Knutsen AP, Schramm WF, Staake JL, Gibson BB, Steinberg KK. 1986. Health effects of long-term exposure to 2,3,7,8-tetrachlorodibenzo-*p*-dioxin. Journal of the American Medical Association 255:2031-2038.

Holmes AP, Bailey C, Baron RC, Bosenac E, Brough J, Conroy C, Haddy L. 1986. West Virginia Department of Health Vietnam-era Veterans Mortality Study, Preliminary Report. Charleston: West Virginia Department of Health.

Ideo G, Bellati G, Bellobuono A, Mocarelli P, Marocchi A, Brambilla P. 1982. Increased urinary D-glucaric acid excretion by children living in an area polluted with tetrachlorodibenzo-*para*-dioxin (TCDD). Clinica Chimica Acta 120:273-283.

Ideo G, Bellati G, Bellobuono A, Bissanti L. 1985. Urinary d-glucaric acid excretion in the Seveso area, polluted by tetrachlorodibenzo-*p*-dioxin (TCDD): five years of experience. Environmental Health Perspectives 60:151-157.

Jansson B, Voog L. 1989. Dioxin from Swedish municipal incinerators and the occurrence of cleft lip and palate malformations. International Journal of Environmental Studies 34:99-104.

Jappinen P, Pukkala E. 1991. Cancer incidence among pulp and paper workers exposed to organic chlorinated compounds formed during chlorine pulp bleaching. Scandinavian Journal of Work, Environment, and Health 17:356-359.

Jennings AM, Wild G, Ward JD, Ward AM. 1988. Immunological abnormalities 17 years after accidental exposure to 2,3,7,8-tetrachlorodibenzo-*p*-dioxin. British Journal of Industrial Medicine 45:701-704.

Kahn PC, Gochfeld M, Lewis WW. 1992a. Dibenzodioxin and dibenzofuran congener levels in four groups of Vietnam veterans who did not handle Agent Orange. New Jersey: New Jersey Agent Orange Commission.

Kahn PC, Gochfeld M, Lewis WW. 1992b. Immune Status and Herbicide Exposure in the New Jersey Pointman I Project. New Jersey: New Jersey Agent Orange Commission.

Kahn PC, Gochfeld M, Lewis WW. 1992c. Semen Analysis in Vietnam Veterans with Respect to Presumed Herbicide Exposure. New Jersey: New Jersey Agent Orange Commission.

Kang HK, Weatherbee L, Breslin PP, Lee Y, Shepard, BM. 1986. Soft tissue sarcomas and military service in Vietnam: a case comparison group analysis of hospital patients. Journal of Occupational Medicine 28:1215-1218.

Kang HK, Enzinger FM, Breslin P, Feil M, Lee Y, Shepard B, Enziger FM. 1987. Soft tissue sarcoma and military service in Vietnam: a case-control study [published erratum appears in J Natl Cancer Inst 1987;79(5):1173]. Journal of the National Cancer Institute 79:693-699.

Klett M, Peper M, Sennewald E, Heller WD. 1991. [Evaluation of the toxicity of particle-bound dioxins and furans in the environment of a metal plant] Bewertung der Toxizitat partikelgebundener Dioxine und Furane im Umfeld einer Metallhutte. Off Gesundheitswes 53:581-586.

Kogan MD, Clapp RW. 1985. Mortality among Vietnam Veterans in Massachusetts, 1972-1983. Massachusetts Office of Commissioner of Veterans Services. January 18, 1985.

Kogan MD, Clapp RW. 1988. Soft tissue sarcoma mortality among Vietnam veterans in Massachusetts, 1972 to 1983. International Journal of Epidemiology 17:39-43.

Kogevinas M, Saracci R, Bertazzi PA, Bueno De Mesquita BH, Coggon D, Green LM, Kauppinen T, Littorin M, Lynge E, Mathews JD, Neuberger M, Osman J, Pearce N, Winkelmann R. 1992. Cancer mortality from soft-tissue sarcoma and malignant lymphomas in an international cohort of workers exposed to chlorophenoxy herbicides and chlorophenols. Chemosphere 25:1071-1076.

Kogevinas M, Saracci R, Winkelmann R, Johnson ES, Bertazzi PA, Bueno de Mesquita BH, Kauppinen T, Littorin M, Lynge E, Neuberger M. 1993. Cancer incidence and mortality in women occupationally exposed to chlorophenoxy herbicides, chlorophenols, and dioxins. Cancer Causes Control 4:547-553.

Kogevinas M, Kauppinen T, Winkelmann R, Becher H, Bertazzi PA, Bas B, Coggon D, Green L, Johnson E, Littorin M, Lynge E, Marlow DA, Mathews JD, Neuberger M, Benn T, Pannett B, Pearce N, Saracci R. 1995. Soft tissue sarcoma and non-Hodgkin's lymphoma in workers exposed to phenoxy herbicides, chlorophenols and dioxins: two nested case-control studies. Epidemiology 6:396-402.

Lampi P, Hakulinen T, Luostarinen T, Pukkala E, Teppo L. 1992. Cancer incidence following chlorophenol exposure in a community in southern Finland. Archives of Environmental Health 47:167-175.

LaVecchia C, Negri E, D'Avanzo B, Franceschi S. 1989. Occupation and lymphoid neoplasms. British Journal of Cancer 60:385-388.

Lawrence CE, Reilly AA, Quickenton P, Greenwald P, Page WF, Kuntz AJ. 1985. Mortality patterns of New York State Vietnam veterans. American Journal of Public Health 75:277-279.

Lerda D, Rizzi R. 1991. Study of reproductive function in persons occupationally exposed to 2,4-dichlorophenoxyacetic acid (2,4-D). Mutation Research 262:47-50.

Levy CJ. 1988. Agent Orange exposure and posttraumatic stress disorder. Journal of Nervous and Mental Disorders 176:242-245.

Lynge E. 1985. A follow-up study of cancer incidence among workers in manufacture of phenoxy herbicides in Denmark. British Journal of Cancer 52:259-270.

Lynge E. 1993. Cancer in phenoxy herbicide manufacturing workers in Denmark, 1947-87—an update. Cancer Causes and Control 4:261-272.

Manz A, Berger J, Dwyer JH, Flesch-Janys D, Nagel S, Waltsgott H. 1991. Cancer mortality among workers in chemical plant contaminated with dioxin. Lancet 338:959-964.

Mastroiacovo P, Spagnolo A, Marni E, Meazza L, Bertollini R, Segni G, Borgna-Pignatti C. 1988. Birth defects in the Seveso area after TCDD contamination [published erratum appears in JAMA 1988;260(6):792]. Journal of the American Medical Association 259:1668-1672.

May G. 1982. Tetrachlorodibenzo-*p*-dioxin: a survey of subjects ten years after exposure. British Journal of Industrial Medicine 39:128-135.

May G. 1983. TCDD: A study of subjects 10 and 14 years after exposure. Chemosphere 12:771-778.

McDuffie HH, Klaassen DJ, Dosman JA. 1990. Is pesticide use related to the risk of primary lung cancer in Saskatchewan? Journal of Occupational Medicine 32:996-1002.

Mellemgaard A, Engholm G, McLaughlin JK, Olsen JH. 1994. Occupational risk factors for renal-cell carcinoma in Denmark. Scandinavian Journal of Work, Environment, and Health 20:160-165.

Michalek JE, Wolfe WH, Miner JC. 1990. Health status of Air Force veterans occupationally exposed to herbicides in Vietnam. II. Mortality. Journal of the American Medical Association 264:1832-1836.

Michalek JE, Pirkle JL, Caudill SP, Tripathi RC, Patterson G, Needham LL. 1996. Pharmacokinetics of TCDD in veterans of operation Ranch Hand: 10 year follow-up. Journal of Exposure Analysis and Environmental Epidemiology 47:102-112

Michigan Department of Public Health. 1983. Evaluation of Soft and Connective Tissue Cancer Mortality Rates for Midland and Other Selected Michigan Counties. Michigan Department of Public Health.

Mocarelli P, Marocchi A, Brambilla P, Gerthoux P, Young DS, Mantel N. 1986. Clinical laboratory manifestations of exposure to dioxin in children: a six-year study of the effects of an environmental disaster near Seveso, Italy. Journal of the American Medical Association 256:2687-2695.

Morris PD, Koepsell TD, Daling JR, Taylor JW, Lyon JL, Swanson GM, Child M, Weiss NS. 1986. Toxic substance exposure and multiple myeloma: a case-control study. Journal of the National Cancer Institute 76:987-994.

Morrison HI, Semenciw RM, Morison D, Magwood S, Mao Y. 1992. Brain cancer and farming in western Canada. Neuroepidemiology 11:267-276.

Morrison H, Savitz D, Semenciw R, Hulka B, Mao Y, Morison D, Wigle D. 1993. Farming and prostate cancer mortality. American Journal of Epidemiology 137:270-280.

Morrison HI, Semenciw RM, Wilkins K, Mao Y, Wigle DT. 1994. Non-Hodgkin's lymphoma and agricultural practices in the prairie provinces of Canada. Scandinavian Journal of Work, Environment, and Health 20:42-47.

Moses M, Lilis R, Crow KD, Thornton J, Fischbein A, Anderson HA, Selikoff IJ. 1984. Health status of workers with past exposure to 2,3,7,8-tetrachlorodibenzo-*p*-dioxin in the manufacture of 2,4,5-trichlorophenoxyacetic acid: comparison of findings with and without chloracne. American Journal of Industrial Medicine 5:161-182.

Musicco M, Sant M, Molinari S, Filippini G, Gatta G, Berrino F. 1988. A case-control study of brain gliomas and occupational exposure to chemical carcinogens: the risks to farmers. American Journal of Epidemiology 128:778-785.

Nelson CJ, Holson JF, Green HG, Gaylor DW. 1979. Retrospective study of the relationship between agricultural use of 2,4,5-T and cleft palate occurrence in Arkansas. Teratology 19:377-383.

Newell GR. 1984. Development and preliminary results of pilot clinical studies. Report of Agent Orange Advisory Committee to the Texas Department of Health, March 1984.

Nurminen T, Rantala K, Kurppa K, Holmberg PC. 1994. Agricultural work during pregnancy and selected structural malformations in Finland. Epidemiology 1:23-30.

O'Brien TR, Decoufle P, Boyle CA. 1991. Non-Hodgkin's lymphoma in a cohort of Vietnam veterans. American Journal of Public Health 81:758-760.

Olsson H, Brandt L. 1988. Risk of non-Hodgkin's lymphoma among men occupationally exposed to organic solvents. Scandinavian Journal of Work, Environment, and Health 14:246-251.

Ott MG, Holder BB, Olson RD. 1980. A mortality analysis of employees engaged in the manufacture of 2,4,5-trichlorophenoxyacetic acid. Journal of Occupational Medicine 22:47-50.

Ott MG, Olson RA, Cook RR, Bond GG. 1987. Cohort mortality study of chemical workers with potential exposure to the higher chlorinated dioxins. Journal of Occupational Medicine 29:422-429.

Pazderova-Vejlupkova J, Lukas E, Nemcova M, Pickova J, Jirasek L. 1981. The development and prognosis of chronic intoxication by tetrachlorodibenzo-*p*-dioxin in men. Archives of Environmental Health 36:5-11.

Pearce NE, Smith AH, Fisher DO. 1985. Malignant lymphoma and multiple myeloma linked with agricultural occupations in a New Zealand cancer registry-based study. American Journal of Epidemiology 121:225-237.

Pearce NE, Smith AH, Howard JK, Sheppard RA, Giles HJ, Teague CA. 1986a. Case-control study of multiple myeloma and farming. British Journal of Cancer 54:493-500.

Pearce NE, Smith AH, Howard JK, Sheppard RA, Giles HJ, Teague CA. 1986b. Non-Hodgkin's lymphoma and exposure to phenoxy herbicides, chlorophenols, fencing work, and meat works employment: a case-control study. British Journal of Industrial Medicine 43:75-83.

Pearce NE, Sheppard RA, Smith AH, Teague CA. 1987. Non-Hodgkin's lymphoma and farming: an expanded case-control study. International Journal of Cancer 39:155-161.

Peper M, Klett M, Frentzel-Beyme R, Heller WD. 1993. Neuropsychological effects of chronic exposure to environmental dioxins and furans. Environmental Research 60:124-135.

Persson B, Dahlander A-M, Fredriksson M, Brage HN, Ohlson C-G, Axelson O. 1989. Malignant lymphomas and occupational exposures. British Journal of Industrial Medicine 46:516-520.

Persson B, Fredriksson M, Olsen K, Boeryd B, Axelson O. 1993. Some occupational exposures as risk factors for malignant lymphomas. Cancer 72:1773-1778.

Pesatori AC, Consonni D, Tironi A, Landi MT, Zocchetti C, Bertazzi PA. 1992. Cancer morbidity in the Seveso area, 1976-1986. Chemosphere 25:209-212.

Pesatori AC, Consonni D, Tironi A, Zocchetti C, Fini A, Bertazzi PA. 1993. Cancer in a young population in a dioxin-contaminated area. International Journal of Epidemiology 22:1010-1013.

Phuong NTN, Thuy TT, Phuong PK. 1989a. An estimate of differences among women giving birth to deformed babies and among those with hydatidiform mole seen at the ob-gyn hospital of Ho Chi Minh City in the south of Vietnam. Chemosphere 18:801-803.

Phuong NTN, Thuy TT, Phuong PK. 1989b. An estimate of reproductive abnormalities in women inhabiting herbicide sprayed and non-herbicide sprayed areas in the south of Vietnam, 1952-1981. Chemosphere 18:843-846.

Pirkle JL Wolfe WH, Patterson DG, Needham LL, Michalek JE, Miner JC, Peterson MR, Phillips DL. 1989. Estimates of the half-life of 2,3,7,8-tetrachlorodibenzo-*p*-dioxin in Vietnam veterans of operation ranch hand. Journal of Toxicology and Environmental Health 27:165-171.

Poland AP, Smith D, Metter G, Possick P. 1971. A health survey of workers in a 2,4,-D and 2,4,5-T plant. Archives of Environmental Health 22:316-327.

Pollei S, Mettler FA Jr, Kelsey CA, Walters MR, White RE. 1986. Follow-up chest radiographs in Vietnam veterans: are they useful? Radiology 161:101-102.

Rellahan W. 1985. Aspects of the Health of Hawaii's Vietnam-era Veterans. Honolulu: Hawaii State Department of Health, Research and Statistics Office.

Riihimaki V, Asp S, Hernberg S. 1982. Mortality of 2,4-dichlorophenoxyacetic acid and 2,4,5-trichlorophenoxyacetic acid herbicide applicators in Finland: first report of an ongoing prospective cohort study. Scandinavian Journal of Work, Environment, and Health 8:37-42.

Riihimaki V, Asp S, Pukkala E, Hernberg S. 1983. Mortality and cancer morbidity among chlorinated phenoxyacid applicators in Finland. Chemosphere 12:779-784.

Robinson CF, Waxweiler RJ, Fowler DP. 1986. Mortality among production workers in pulp and paper mills. Scandinavian Journal of Work, Environment, and Health 12:552-560.

Ronco G, Costa G, Lynge E. 1992. Cancer risk among Danish and Italian farmers. British Journal of Industrial Medicine 49:220-225.

Saracci R, Kogevinas M, Bertazzi PA, Bueno De Mesquita BH, Coggon D, Green LM, Kauppinen T, L'Abbe KA, Littorin M, Lynge E, Mathews JD, Neuberger M, Osman J, Pearce N, Winkelmann R. 1991. Cancer mortality in workers exposed to chlorophenoxy herbicides and chlorophenols. Lancet 338:1027-1032.

Semchuk KM, Love EJ, Lee RG. 1993. Parkinson's disease: a test of the multifactorial etiologic hypothesis. Neurology 43:1173-1180.

Semenciw RM, Morrison HI, Riedel D, Wilkins K, Ritter L, Mao Y. 1993. Multiple myeloma mortality and agricultural practices in the prairie provinces of Canada. Journal of Occupational Medicine 35:557-561.

Semenciw RM, Morrison HI, Morison D, Mao Y. 1994. Leukemia mortality and farming in the prairie provinces of Canada. Canadian Journal of Public Health 85:208-211.

Senthilselvan A, Mcduffie HH, Dosman JA. 1992. Association of asthma with use of pesticides: results of a cross-sectional survey of farmers. American Review of Respiratory Disease 146:884-887.

Smith AH, Pearce NE. 1986. Update on soft tissue sarcoma and phenoxy herbicides in New Zealand. Chemosphere 15:1795-1798.

Smith AH, Matheson DP, Fisher DO, Chapman CJ. 1981. Preliminary report of reproductive outcomes among pesticide applicators using 2,4,5-T. New Zealand Medical Journal 93:177-179.

Smith AH, Fisher DO, Pearce N, Chapman CJ. 1982. Congenital defects and miscarriages among New Zealand 2,4,5-T sprayers. Archives of Environmental Health 37:197-200.

Smith AH, Fisher DO, Giles HJ, Pearce N. 1983. The New Zealand soft tissue sarcoma case-control study: interview findings concerning phenoxyacetic acid exposure. Chemosphere 12:565-571.

Smith AH, Pearce NE, Fisher DO, Giles HJ, Teague CA, Howard JK. 1984. Soft tissue sarcoma and exposure to phenoxyherbicides and chlorophenols in New Zealand. Journal of the National Cancer Institute 73:1111-1117.

Smith JG, Christophers AJ. 1992. Phenoxy herbicides and chlorophenols: a case control study on soft tissue sarcoma and malignant lymphoma. British Journal of Cancer 65:442-448.

Snow BR, Stellman JM, Stellman SD, Sommer JF. 1988. Post-traumatic stress disorder among American Legionnaires in relation to combat experience in Vietnam: associated and contributing factors. Environmental Research 47:175-192.

Sobel W, Bond GG, Skowronski BJ, Brownson PJ, Cook RR. 1987. A soft tissue sarcoma case control study in a large multi-chemical manufacturing facility. Chemosphere 16:2095-2099.

Solet D, Zoloth SR, Sullivan C, Jewett J, Michaels DM. 1989. Patterns of mortality in pulp and paper workers. Journal of Occupational Medicine 31:627-630.

Stehr PA, Stein G, Webb K, Schramm W, Gedney WB, Donnell HD, Ayres S, Falk H, Sampson E, Smith SJ. 1986. A pilot epidemiologic study of possible health effects associated with 2,3,7,8-tetrachlorodibenzo-*p*-dioxin contaminations in Missouri. Archives of Environmental Health 41:16-22.

Stehr-Green P, Hoffman R, Webb K, Evans RG, Knutsen A, Schramm W, Staake J, Gibson B, Steinberg K. 1987. Health effects of long-term exposure to 2,3,7,8-tetrachlorodibenzo-*p*-dioxin. Chemosphere 16:2089-2094.

Stellman SD, Stellman J.M., Sommer JF Jr. 1988a. Combat and herbicide exposures in Vietnam among a sample of American Legionnaires. Environmental Research 47:112-128.

Stellman JM, Stellman SD, Sommer JF Jr. 1988b. Social and behavioral consequences of the Vietnam experience among American Legionnaires. Environmental Research 47:129-149.

Stellman SD, Stellman JM, Sommer JF Jr. 1988c. Health and reproductive outcomes among American Legionnaires in relation to combat and herbicide exposure in Vietnam. Environmental Research 47:150-174.

Stockbauer JW, Hoffman RE, Schramm WF, Edmonds LD. 1988. Reproductive outcomes of mothers with potential exposure to 2,3,7,8-tetrachlorodibenzo-*p*-dioxin. American Journal of Epidemiology 128:410-419.

Suskind RR, Hertzberg VS. 1984. Human health effects of 2,4,5-T and its toxic contaminants. Journal of the American Medical Association 251:2372-2380.

Swaen GMH, van Vliet C, Slangen JJM, Sturmans F. 1992. Cancer mortality among licensed herbicide applicators. Scandinavian Journal of Work, Environment, and Health 18:201-204.

Sweeney MH, Fingerhut MA, Connally LB, Halperin WE, Moody PL, Marlow DA. 1989. Progress of the NIOSH cross-sectional study of workers occupationally exposed to chemicals contaminated with 2,3,7,8-TCDD. Chemosphere 19:973-977.

Sweeney MH, Fingerhut MA, Arezzo JC, Hornung RW, Connally LB. 1993. Peripheral neuropathy after occupational exposure to 2,3,7,8-tetrachlorodibenzo-*p*-dioxin (TCDD). American Journal of Industrial Medicine 23:845-858.

Tarone RE, Hayes HM, Hoover RN, Rosenthal JF, Brown LM, Pottern LM, Javadpour N, O'Connoll KJ, Stutzman RE. 1991. Service in Vietnam and risk of testicular cancer. Journal of the National Cancer Institute 83:1497-1499.

Tenchini ML, Crimaudo C, Pacchetti G, Mottura A, Agosti S, De Carli L. 1983. A comparative cytogenetic study on cases of induced abortions in TCDD-exposed and nonexposed women. Environmental Mutagenesis 5:73-85.

Thiess AM, Frentzel-Beyme R, Link R. 1982. Mortality study of persons exposed to dioxin in a trichlorophenol-process accident that occurred in the BASF Ag on November 17, 1953. American Journal of Industrial Medicine 3:179-189.

Thomas TL. 1987. Mortality among flavour and fragrance chemical plant workers in the United States. British Journal of Industrial Medicine 44:733-737.

Thomas TL, Kang HK. 1990. Mortality and morbidity among Army Chemical Corps Vietnam veterans: a preliminary report. American Journal of Industrial Medicine 18:665-673.

Thomas TL, Kang H, Dalager N. 1991. Mortality among women Vietnam veterans, 1973-1987. American Journal of Epidemiology 134:973-980.

Townsend JC, Bodner KM, Van Peenen PFD, Olson RD, Cook RR. 1982. Survey of reproductive events of wives of employees exposed to chlorinated dioxins. American Journal of Epidemiology 115:695-713.

True WR, Goldberg J, Eisen SA. 1988. Stress symptomatology among Vietnam veterans. Analysis of the Veterans Administration Survey of Veterans II. American Journal of Epidemiology 128:85-92.

U.S. EPA Epidemiologic Studies Program Human Effects Monitoring Branch. 1979. Report of Assessment of a Field Investigation of Six-Year Spontaneous Abortion Rates in Three Oregon Areas in Relation to Forest 2,4,5-T Spray Practice.

Van Houdt JJ, Fransman LG, Strik JJ. 1983. Epidemiological case control study in personnel exposed to 2,4,5-T. Chemosphere 12:575.

Vineis P, Terracini B, Ciccone G, Cignetti A, Colombo E, Donna A, Maffi L, Pisa R, Ricci P, Zanini E, Comba P. 1987. Phenoxy herbicides and soft-tissue sarcomas in female rice weeders: a population-based case-referent study. Scandinavian Journal of Work, Environment, and Health 13:9-17.

Vineis P, Faggiano F, Tedeschi M, Ciccone G. 1991. Incidence rates of lymphomas and soft-tissue sarcomas and environmental measurements of phenoxy herbicides. Journal of the National Cancer Institute 83:362-363.

Visintainer PF, Barone M, McGee H, Peterson EL. 1995. Proportionate mortality study of Vietnam-era veterans of Michigan. Journal of Occupational and Environmental Medicine 37/4.

Watanabe KK, Kang HK, Thomas TL. 1991. Mortality among Vietnam veterans: with methodological considerations. Journal of Occupational Medicine 33:780-785.

Webb K, Evans RG, Stehr P, Ayres SM. 1987. Pilot study on health effects of environmental 2,3,7,8-TCDD in Missouri. American Journal of Industrial Medicine 11:685-691.

Wendt AS. 1985. Iowa Agent Orange survey of Vietnam veterans. Iowa State Department of Health: April 15, 1985.

White FMM, Cohen FG, Sherman G, McCurdy R. 1988. Chemicals, birth defects and stillbirths in New Brunswick: associations with agricultural activity. Canadian Medical Association Journal 138:117-124.

Wigle DT, Semenciw RB, Wilkins K, Riedel D, Ritter L, Morrison HI, Mao Y. 1990. Mortality study of Canadian male farm operators: non-Hodgkin's lymphoma mortality and agricultural practices in Saskatchewan. Journal of the National Cancer Institute 82:575-582.

Wiklund K. 1983. Swedish agricultural workers: a group with a decreased risk of cancer. Cancer 51:566-568.

Wiklund K Holm LE. 1986. Soft tissue sarcoma risk in Swedish agricultural and forestry workers. Journal of the National Cancer Institute 76:229-234.

Wiklund K. 1987. Risk of malignant lymphoma in Swedish pesticide appliers. British Journal of Cancer 56:505-508.

Wiklund K, Lindefors BM, Holm LE. 1988a. Risk of malignant lymphoma in Swedish agricultural and forestry workers. British Journal of Industrial Medicine 45:19-24.

Wiklund K, Dich J, Holm LE. 1988b. Soft tissue sarcoma risk in Swedish licensed pesticide applicators. Journal of Occupational Medicine 30:801-804.

Wiklund K, Dich J, Holm L-E, Eklund G. 1989a. Risk of cancer in pesticide applicators in Swedish agriculture. British Journal of Industrial Medicine 46:809-814.

Wiklund K, Dich J, Holm LE. 1989b. Risk of soft tissue sarcoma, Hodgkin's disease and non-Hodgkin's lymphoma among Swedish licensed pesticide applicators. Chemosphere 18:395-400.

Wingren G, Fredrikson M, Brage HN, Nordenskjold B, Axelson O. 1990. Soft tissue sarcoma and occupational exposures. Cancer 66:806-811.

Wolfe WH, Michalek JE, Miner JC, Rahe A, Silva J, Thomas WF, Grubbs WD, Lustik MB, Karrison TG, Roegner RH, Williams DE. 1990. Health status of Air Force veterans occupationally exposed to herbicides in Vietnam. I. Physical health. Journal of the American Medical Association 264:1824-1831.

Wolfe WH, Michalek JE, Miner JC, Pirkle JL, Caudill SP, Patterson DG Jr, Needham LL. 1994. Determinants of TCDD half-life in veterans of Operation Ranch Hand. Journal of Toxicology and Environmental Health 41:481-488.

Wolfe WH, Michalek JE, Miner JC, Rahe AJ, Moore CA, Needham LL, Patterson D.G. 1995. Paternal serum dioxin and reproductive outcomes among veterans of Operation Ranch Hand. Epidemiology 6:17-22.

Woods JS, Polissar L, Severson RK, Heuser LS, Kulander BG. 1987. Soft tissue sarcoma and non-Hodgkin's lymphoma in relation to phenoxy herbicide and chlorinated phenol exposure in western Washington. Journal of the National Cancer Institute 78:899-910.

Woods JS, Polissar L. 1989. Non-Hodgkin's lymphoma among phenoxy herbicide-exposed farm workers in western Washington state. Chemosphere 18:401-406.

Zack JA, Gaffey WR. 1983. A mortality study of workers employed at the Monsanto company plant in Nitro, West Virginia. Environmental Science Research 26:575-591.

Zack JA, Suskind RR. 1980. The mortality experience of workers exposed to tetrachlorodibenzo-*p*-dioxin in a trichlorophenol process accident. Journal of Occupational Medicine 22:11-14.

Zahm SH, Weisenburger DD, Babbitt PA, Saal RC, Vaught JB, Cantor KP, Blair A. 1990. A case-control study of non-Hodgkin's lymphoma and the herbicide 2,4-dichlorophenoxyacetic acid (2,4-D) in eastern Nebraska. Epidemiology 1:349-356.

Zahm SH, Weisenburger DD, Saal RC, Vaught JB, Babbitt PA, Blair A. 1993. The role of agricultural pesticide use in the development of non-Hodgkin's lymphoma in women. Archives of Environmental Health 48:353-358.

Zober A, Messerer P, Huber P. 1990. Thirty-four-year mortality follow-up of BASF employees exposed to 2,3,7,8-TCDD after the 1953 accident. International Archives of Occupational and Environmental Health 62:139-157.

Zober A, Ott MG, Messerer P. 1994. Morbidity follow-up study of BASF employees exposed to 2,3,7,8-tetrachlorodibenzo-*p*-dioxin (TCDD) after a 1953 chemical reactor incident. Occupational and Environmental Medicine 51:479-486.

7

Cancer

INTRODUCTION

Cancer is the second leading cause of death in the United States. At present, more than 30 percent of Americans will develop a malignancy at some time in their lives, and approximately half of them will die from it (Seidman et al., 1985).

Many types of cancers are thought to be related to herbicides and/or 2,3,7,8-tetrachlorodibenzo-p-dioxin (TCDD), but the evidence for the association is uneven. Following this introduction about cancer and its epidemiology, the committee summarizes and reaches conclusions about the strength of the evidence in epidemiologic studies regarding associations between exposure to herbicides and TCDD and each type of cancer under consideration in this report. The cancer types are discussed in the order in which they are listed in the International Classification of Diseases (U.S. DHHS, 1991). A section at the end of this chapter summarizes the cancer types for which the strength of the epidemiologic evidence is similar.

In assessing a possible relation between herbicide exposure and risk of cancer, a key issue is the level of exposure of those included in a study. As noted in Chapter 5, for many studies data on exposure are not well measured or defined. Some studies develop an index to approximate a scale of degrees of exposure; some studies use a surrogate measure of exposure, such as veterans' service in Vietnam. The effect of this inadequate exposure measurement is a dilution of the statistical measure of the magnitude of the association. Further, the time from first exposure to cancer development may span decades and in some studies may have been insufficient to rule out a relation. Issues relevant to the time from exposure and the risk of cancer development are discussed in more detail in Chapter 8.

For most types of cancer, a brief summary of the scientific evidence described in *VAO* is presented, followed by an update of the recent scientific literature. There are six cancer sites for which a complete discussion of the evidence is presented, including all the studies cited in *VAO*. These include: three types of cancer of special interest to the Department of Veterans Affairs (hepatobiliary, nasopharyngeal, and prostate cancer); two other types that were classified in the category of limited/suggestive evidence of an association in *VAO* (respiratory cancer and multiple myeloma); and, because of its public health importance, breast cancer.

Plausibility Data

Cancers of a variety of types have been identified in studies of animals exposed to TCDD, as described in detail in Chapter 3. These include liver, lung, and skin tumors in rats and mice. TCDD is not considered a genotoxic carcinogen. However, in multistage models of carcinogenesis, TCDD may act both as a tumor promoter and a tumor initiator. TCDD mediates carcinogenesis through a variety of biochemical effects that are dependent on the presence of a cellular receptor protein referred to as the Ah receptor. This receptor has been identified in both laboratory animals and humans and appears to play a role in regulating cell proliferation and differentiation. The multiple site specificity of TCDD is likely to reflect its multiple mechanisms of action.

In contrast to the experimental data supporting the carcinogenic activity of TCDD, the data regarding the herbicides used in Vietnam are considerably weaker. Only 2,4-D (2,4-dichlorophenoxyacetic acid) has produced positive results in an animal bioassay, and these results are of controversial validity. The herbicides have not been adequately tested, however, so conclusions regarding their carcinogenicity in animals must be drawn with caution.

Given these data, which establish biological plausibility study for cancer in general but not for all specific sites, the committee chose not to summarize biologic plausibility for each cancer reviewed in this chapter. Toxicological data are provided only for a small number of cancer types that have specific, relevant experimental data.

Expected Number of Cancer Cases Among Vietnam Veterans in the Absence of Any Increase in Risk Due to Herbicide Exposure

To provide some background for the consideration of cancer risks in Vietnam veterans, and to evaluate the possibilities for future epidemiologic studies of cancer in this group, the committee estimated the number of cancer cases that could be expected to occur in Vietnam veterans in the absence of any increase in risk due specifically to herbicide exposure, as described in *VAO*. The figures presented for each cancer should be interpreted as providing only approximate estimates, not precise predictions for the Vietnam veteran cohort.

Given the large uncertainties that remain about the magnitude of potential risk from exposure to herbicides in the occupational, environmental, and veterans studies that have been reviewed, inadequate control for important confounders in these studies, and the lack of information needed to extrapolate from the level of exposure in the studies to that of individual Vietnam veterans, the committee cannot quantify the degree of risk likely to have been experienced by Vietnam veterans because of their exposure to herbicides in Vietnam.

GASTROINTESTINAL TRACT TUMORS

Background

As a group, this category includes some of the major cancers in the United States and the world. The committee reviewed the data on colon cancer (ICD-9 153.0-153.9), rectal cancer (ICD-9 154.0-154.1), stomach cancer (ICD-9 151.0-151.9), and pancreatic cancer (ICD-9 157.0-157.9). According to the American Cancer Society, approximately 185,000 new cases of cancers of these types were diagnosed in the United States in 1995, and some 97,000 persons died of these cancers (ACS, 1995). These cases are divided approximately equally between men and women. According to the committee's calculations, assuming that those of veterans have the same cancer rates as the general U.S. population, 1,110 cases of these cancers were expected among male Vietnam veterans and 2.3 among female veterans in 1995. For the year 2000, the expected numbers are 2,184 cases in male veterans and 4.3 in female veterans.

Summary of *VAO*

Numerous studies were considered in *VAO* that examined one or more gastrointestinal tract cancers, and no consistent associations were found. These included studies of chemical production workers in the United States and other countries (Lynge, 1985; Coggon et al., 1986; Thomas, 1987; Bond et al., 1988; Zober et al., 1990; Fingerhut et al., 1991; Manz et al., 1991; Saracci et al., 1991), agricultural workers (Burmeister, 1981; Hardell, 1981; Burmeister et al., 1983; Wiklund, 1983; Hoar et al., 1986; Alavanja et al., 1988, 1989; Wigle et al., 1990; Hansen et al., 1992; Ronco et al., 1992), pesticide applicators (Axelson et al., 1980; Blair et al., 1983; Swaen et al., 1992), paper and pulp workers (Robinson et al., 1986; Henneberger et al., 1989; Solet et al., 1989), the population of Seveso, Italy (Bertazzi et al., 1989a,b; Pesatori et al., 1992), others subjected to environmental exposure (Lampi et al., 1992), and Vietnam veterans (Kogan and Clapp,

1985; Lawrence et al., 1985; Anderson et al., 1986a,b; Boyle et al., 1987; Breslin et al., 1988; CDC, 1988).

VAO observed that the epidemiologic studies examining stomach cancer, pancreatic cancer, rectal cancer, and colon cancer found relative risks were evenly distributed around 1.0. Only the rare study found a statistically significant elevated relative risk. In the heavily exposed production workers in the National Institute for Occupational Safety and Health study, Fingerhut (1991) found elevated, but not statistically significant, standardized mortality ratios (SMRs) in the subcohort with one or more years of exposure and at least 20 years since first exposure (SMR = 1.4 for stomach cancer, and 1.8 for small intestine and colon combined, based on four and 13 deaths, respectively). The small numbers and lack of statistical significance make interpreting these isolated elevations difficult, especially in light of several other studies showing nonsignificant associations in the opposite direction (i.e., relative risks below 1.0). For example, Alavanja (1988) found a relative risk of stomach cancer of 0.7 (95 percent CI 0.4-1.4) for U.S. Department of Agriculture extension agents, based on ten observed cancers.

Update of the Scientific Literature

Occupational Studies

The committee was able to identify only a small number of studies relating to gastrointestinal (GI) cancers that had been published following the release of *VAO*.

A study of a random sample of 1,000 people licensed by the state of Minnesota to perform agricultural pest control examined cancer prevalence in the southern half of the state, which contains the major agricultural areas (Garry et al., 1994). Only 719 people responded to the survey. The study examined prevalent cancers, thus missing any incident cases who died prior to the conduct of the study. Because of small numbers, only overall GI cancer prevalence was examined; the study did not consider site-specific data for GI cancers. No relative risks were calculated because of the small numbers and the lack of availability of population-based prevalence figures for comparison.

Bloemen et al. (1993) provided four additional years of follow-up data for a cohort of 878 chemical workers exposed to 2,4-D at several Dow company plants. This study was previously analyzed by Bond et al. (1988). In this follow-up, only overall digestive system cancers were examined; no site-specific data were provided. The comparisons with both external and internal reference groups showed modest and nonsignificant reductions in the risks of digestive cancer in the exposed workers.

As a subgroup of the International Agency for Research on Cancer (IARC) cohort, a cohort of workers was identified who manufactured chlorophenoxy herbicides in two factories in the Netherlands (Bueno de Mesquita et al., 1993). Cancer-specific mortality rates were compared between workers exposed to herbicides and two comparison groups: unexposed employees and the general population of the Netherlands. No significant increases were observed in the relative risks for the four GI cancer sites.

The mortality experience was evaluated for 754 white male workers with potential exposure to TCDD and 4-aminobiphenyl at a Monsanto Company plant (Collins et al., 1993). This study was an expansion of an earlier study of part of this cohort, a group of 122 workers who had developed chloracne as a result of an accidental release of TCDD (Zack and Suskind, 1980). Reduced risks (nonsignificant) were observed for stomach and colon cancer.

A cohort study of cancer incidence and mortality was conducted among 701 women in the IARC cohort who were occupationally exposed to chlorophenoxy herbicides, chlorophenols, and dioxins (Kogevinas et al., 1993). Cancer incidence and mortality among the exposed employees were compared with national rates. No significant increase was observed in the risk of stomach cancer.

In the United States, a proportionate cancer mortality ratio (PCMR) study was performed for farmers in 23 states, using occupational information from death certificates (Blair et al., 1993). Because of the large population size in this study, the confidence intervals are relatively narrow. Based on 657 deaths from stomach cancer in white male farmers, the PCMR was 1.0 (CI 1.0-1.1). Based on 23 deaths from stomach cancer in nonwhite female farmers, the PCMR was slightly elevated, at 1.9 (CI 1.2-2.8). The numbers of deaths from stomach cancer were small and nonsignificant for the other two racial and gender groups studied: nonwhite males and white females. Based on 2,291 deaths from colon cancer in white males, the PCMR was 1.0 (CI 0.9-1.0); the numbers of deaths were small and nonsignificant for the other three racial and gender groups. Based on 367 deaths from rectal cancer in white male farmers, the PCMR was 1.0 (CI 0.9-1.1). The numbers of deaths from rectal cancer were small and nonsignificant for the other three racial and gender groups. Based on 1,133 deaths from pancreatic cancer among white male farmers, the PCMR was slightly elevated, at 1.1 (CI 1.1-1.2); the numbers of deaths were small and nonsignificant for the other three racial and gender groups.

In Finland, a cohort of 1,909 men was assembled in 1972 from personnel records of the four main employers involved in "chemical brushwood control" (Asp et al., 1994). This study represents further follow-up of two earlier studies discussed in *VAO* (Riihimaki et al., 1982, 1983). It found relative risks close to or less than 1.0 for all four GI sites, regardless of whether or not a latency period of either ten or 15 years was considered.

Environmental Studies

In a follow-up of the cohort of people potentially exposed to TCDD in the industrial accident in Seveso, Italy, the subjects were analyzed by gender (Bertazzi et al., 1993). No elevated relative risks for any of the GI cancers was found, although there was a slight (but not statistically significant) elevation in the risk of rectal cancer in both males and females in Zone B (the second most contaminated area) based on a total of five cases (three males and two females).

Vietnam Veterans Studies

A proportionate mortality study of Vietnam veterans examined the proportion of deaths occurring due to various causes among veterans who had served in Vietnam compared with veterans who had served during the same era but had not been in Vietnam (Visintainer et al., 1995). The study reported deaths from overall gastrointestinal cancer and from pancreatic cancer, but did not report other specific GI sites. No explanation of the failure to report site-specific data, other than pancreas, was provided. Separate estimates of the PMR were calculated for blacks and nonblacks, but it was not clear that distinction was based on any a priori hypotheses as to differential effects of exposure in the different races. The study was not analyzed by the recommended method of treating the data as though they were from a case-control study, with deaths from the cause of interest serving as "cases" and deaths from other causes serving as "controls." Because of an unusual method of identification, it is unknown whether all eligible veterans were identified. The sample was restricted to men who would have been age 18 to 29 during the Vietnam war. Significantly elevated relative risks for all GI cancers and for pancreatic cancer were found in blacks only. Neither risk was elevated in the overall sample. We cannot rule out the possibility that these elevated risks occurred by chance, given the apparent lack of a priori justification for the separate analyses by race, the lack of confirmation of the results in the overall sample, and the weaknesses of the proportionate mortality design (discussed in *VAO*).

A retrospective cohort mortality study was performed among women Vietnam veterans, compared with women veterans who served elsewhere and with women in the general U.S. population (Dalager et al., 1995). This is an extension of a previous study (Thomas et al., 1991). No increased risk was observed for colon cancer. There was a nonsignificant excess risk of death among Vietnam women veterans relative to non-Vietnam veterans (RR = 2.8, CI 0.8-10.2). This excess was confined to Vietnam veteran nurses, who had a statistically significant adjusted RR of 5.7 (95 percent CI 1.2 to 27.0).

Summary

With only rare exceptions, studies on gastrointestinal cancers and herbicide exposure found relative risks close to 1.0, providing no evidence of any increase in risk. Importantly, no evidence of increased risk was observed even with longer latency periods. One recent analysis of a subgroup defined by race found a significant elevation in risk for pancreatic cancer, but it was not clear that this subgroup was defined in advance with any biological explanation for the separate analyses. Two other recent studies found a significant elevation of pancreatic cancer in women Vietnam veterans who were nurses, and in white female farmers.

Conclusions

There is limited/suggestive evidence of <u>no</u> association between exposure to the herbicides (2,4-D, 2,4,5-T and its contaminant, TCDD; cacodylic acid; and picloram) and gastrointestinal cancers (stomach, pancreatic, rectal, and colon cancers). The evidence regarding association is drawn from occupational and other studies in which subjects were exposed to a variety of herbicide and herbicides components.

HEPATOBILIARY CANCERS

Background

According to the American Cancer Society, approximately 18,500 new cases of hepatobiliary cancer (ICD-9 155.0-155.2) were diagnosed in the United States in 1995, and some 14,200 persons died of cancer of the liver and the biliary passages (ACS, 1995). Similar numbers of cases are seen in men and women. According to the committee's calculations, assuming that veterans have the same cancer rate as those in the general U.S. population, 70 cases of cancers of the liver and the biliary passages were expected among male Vietnam veterans and 0.1 among female veterans in 1995. For the year 2000, the expected numbers are 151 cases in male veterans and 0.1 cases in female veterans.

Because this type of cancer is of special interest to the Department of Veterans Affairs (DVA), this discussion integrates the studies reviewed in *VAO* with those published more recently.

In the United States, liver cancers account for about 1.4 percent of new cancer cases and 2.4 percent of cancer deaths. Misclassification of metastatic cancers as primary liver cancer can, however, lead to over-reporting of deaths due to liver cancer (Percy et al., 1990). In developing countries, especially sub-Saharan Africa and Southeast Asia, liver cancers are common and are among the leading causes of death.

About 90 percent of primary liver cancers are hepatocellular carcinomas; tumors of the intrahepatic bile ducts (cholangiocarcinomas) represent approximately 7 percent of malignant tumors of the liver (Mayer and Garnick, 1986). Each form is a separate histological appearance of differentiated cells derived from a common progenitor in the early embryo derived from the foregut epithelium. As such, both forms have many of the same characteristics and can be rationally grouped together for epidemiologic studies. Other liver malignancies, such as angiosarcomas, are extremely rare.

The plausibility of an association of TCDD with liver malignancy follows from the finding of increased risk of liver and biliary cancer among individuals exposed to similar compounds that also act through the Ah receptor that appears to play a role in regulating cell proliferation and differentiation. Kuratsune et al. (1986) found a substantial increase of liver cancer deaths among Yusho patients exposed to dibenzofurans. Nine deaths from liver cancer were observed among males and two among females. The expected numbers of deaths, based on rates of the Fukuoka and Nagasaki prefectures, were 2.3 and 0.8, respectively. A review by Nicholson (1987) of all data on the mortality of industrial workers involved in the manufacture of capacitors who were exposed to PCBs showed seven deaths to have occurred from cancer of the liver, biliary passages, and gallbladder, compared with 2.54 deaths expected. Thus, there is evidence that very high exposures to other compounds that interact with the Ah receptor increase hepatobiliary cancer risk.

Epidemiologists have established hepatitis B virus (HBV) infection as a major risk factor for primary liver cancer (Beasley, 1984). HBV is endemic in the regions where liver cancer is most common, but is also becoming increasingly widespread in Western countries. Recent evidence also links primary liver cancer to the hepatitis C virus (Yu et al., 1990). Alcohol consumption, with or without cirrhosis, appears to be a principal risk factor for liver cancer in Western countries (Yeh et al., 1989). Cancer of the intrahepatic bile duct has been attributed to liver flukes (*Clonorchis* and *Opisthorchis*), which are ingested by humans through uncooked fish and then reside primarily in the intrahepatic bile duct, where they cause chronic damage (Belamaric, 1973). Hepatic angiosarcomas have been associated with exposure to arsenicals, thorotrast, and vinyl chloride (Greenwald and Greenwald, 1983).

Epidemiologic Studies

Occupational Studies

The mortality experience was evaluated for 754 employees who worked at a Monsanto plant with potential exposure to TCDD and 4-aminobiphenyl (Collins et al., 1993). This cohort included 122 employees who developed chloracne as a result of the accident in 1949. This study is an expansion of the study by Zack and Suskind (1980). Two cases of hepatobiliary cancer were observed, which yielded an SMR of 1.4 (CI 0.2-5.2), compared to the general U.S. population.

Production Workers   In a study of production workers at 12 U.S. plants that produced chemicals contaminated with TCDD, six deaths were observed due to cancer of the liver and biliary tract, and the SMR was 1.2 (CI 0.4-2.5) (Fingerhut et al., 1991). When the exposure was limited to those workers who had more than 20 years of latency, only one death was observed due to liver cancer, somewhat lower than expected (1.7), giving an SMR of 0.6 (CI 0.0-3.3).

In another combined cohort of workers exposed to herbicides, Saracci et al. (1991) identified four deaths due to liver cancer among those who were exposed, giving an SMR of 0.4 (CI 0.1-1.1). These reduced rates of liver cancer may reflect the contribution of the "healthy worker effect" to the onset of this cancer; chance or differences in lifestyles may also explain the results.

In a study of workers from Denmark involved in the manufacture of phenoxy herbicides, Lynge (1985) observed three cases of liver cancer among men and none in women. Given that the expected number of cases was 3.1, the relative risk of liver cancer among men was 0.96, showing no elevation.

Agricultural/Forestry Workers   A study of farmers in Denmark and Italy by Ronco et al. (1992) observed no evidence of increased liver cancer in the cohort from Denmark; the group from Italy was too small to be informative. Among self-employed Danish men, 23 were diagnosed with liver cancer, giving a relative risk estimate of 0.4, compared to that of the Danish population. Among Danish men classified as farm employees, nine liver cancers were observed, giving a relative risk estimate of 0.8. Among self-employed women and employees, no cases of liver cancer were observed, but among those women classified as family workers (i.e., those who were actively involved in the work of the farm owned by their husbands), five cases of liver cancer were observed, giving an estimated relative risk of 0.5. In a study of agricultural workers by Wiklund (1983), 103 cases of liver cancer were observed. This was significantly lower than the expected number (306), giving an incidence ratio of 0.3 (99 percent CI 0.3-0.4).

In a study in Finland, 1,909 male herbicide applicators were followed prospectively for 18 years (Asp et al., 1994). This is an update of a previous study (Riihimaki, 1982, 1983). SMRs and standardized incidence ratios (SIRs) were calculated, based on zero, ten, and 15 years latency since first exposure. Assuming zero latency, there were two deaths from hepatobiliary cancer (SMR = 0.6, CI 0.1-2.2) and three cases of hepatobiliary cancer diagnosed (SIR = 0.9, CI 0.2-2.6).

In the United States, a PCMR study was performed for farmers in 23 states, using occupational information from death certificates (Blair et al., 1993). Based on 326 deaths from liver cancer in white male farmers, the PCMR was 1.0 (CI 0.9-1.1). The numbers were small and nonsignificant for the other racial and gender groups studied: nonwhite males and white and nonwhite females.

In a case-control study in Sweden, Hardell et al. (1984) observed a positive relationship between exposure to phenoxy or dichlorophenoxy herbicides and risk of liver cancer. Based on 102 cases, these authors observed an odds ratio (OR) of 1.8 (CI 0.9-4.0).

Paper/Pulp Workers In a study of mortality among pulp and paper workers, Solet et al. (1989) observed two deaths due to liver cancer; only one was expected. Based on this small number of cases, the confidence interval was broad, ranging from 0.2 to 7.3 (PMR = 2.0).

Environmental Studies

Follow-up of the population involved in the Seveso incident (Bertazzi et al., 1989b) showed that during ten years, only three deaths among males due to liver cancer—no more than expected occurred in the population of Zone B. Among those in Zone R, only seven deaths due to liver cancer were recorded, giving a mortality ratio of 0.4 (CI 0.2-0.8). Additional liver cancer incidence data show similar results (Pesatori et al., 1992).

Bertazzi et al. (1993) provides information on combined liver and biliary tract cancer diagnosed among Seveso residents and thus supplements the data on liver cancer alone. In Zone A, where exposure was heaviest, one hepatobiliary cancer occurred; 0.7 cases were expected. In the second most contaminated area, zone B, a nonsignificant increase in the risk of hepatobiliary cancer was observed in both men and women. In Zone R, the least contaminated area, a nonsignificant decrease in the risk of hepatobiliary cancer was also observed in both men and women.

Data from U.S. populations living in contaminated areas do not add any useful information. The residents of the Quail Run trailer park in Times Beach, Missouri, the site of a major realease of TCDD-contaminated oil were free from diagnosed liver cancer, whereas 1.5 cases were expected (Hoffman et al., 1986; Stehr-Green et al., 1987).

A case-control study by Cordier et al. (1993) described the hepatocellular carcinoma risk among 152 North Vietnamese cases and 241 controls, in relation to viral infections and chemical exposures. The dominant risk factor was found to be positive for hepatitis B surface antigen, which carried an odds ratio of 62 (95 percent CI 30-128). Use of organochlorine pesticides did not indicate any statistically significant trend, but military service in South Vietnam did. Those who served for more than ten years in South Vietnam ($N = 11$) had an OR for hepatocellular carcinoma of 8.8 (CI 1.9-41). However, direct contact with aerial sprayings showed only a slight, nonsignificantly increased OR of 1.3. The value of this study is limited because most cancer cases were made on clinical or biochemical grounds and were not confirmed histologically.

Vietnam Veterans Studies

Studies of liver cancer among veterans are hampered by small study size. For example, in the study of Wisconsin Vietnam veterans (Anderson et al., 1986a,b), no men were observed to have died from liver cancer. In the mortality component of the Centers for Disease Control and Prevention's (CDC) Vietnam Experience Study (Boyle et al., 1987) only one death from liver cancer was observed among Vietnam veterans. In a larger mortality study among U.S. Army and Marine Corps Vietnam veterans, Breslin et al. (1988) identified 34 liver cancer deaths among the Army veterans; the PMR was 1.0 (CI 0.8-1.4). The data from the Marines are consistent with this result though there were fewer deaths among Marines. Based on six deaths from cancer of the liver or bile ducts, the PMR was 1.2 (CI 0.5-2.8).

The CDC's Selected Cancers Study (CDC, 1990) included a pathologic review of studies to confirm the diagnosis of 130 men with primary liver cancer. Only 6 percent ($N = 8$) of the men with primary liver cancer served in Vietnam, compared to 7.5 percent of the control subjects. After adjusting for design and a range of established risk factors, the relative risk was 1.2 (CI 0.5-2.7). Of the eight Vietnam veterans with primary liver cancer, four were in the Navy and three were in the Army. (For one, the proxy respondent did not know the branch of service.) The risk for Vietnam veterans was slightly lower than for men who served elsewhere in the military.

Summary

There are relatively few occupational, environmental, or veterans studies of liver cancer (Table 7-1), and most of these are small in size and have not controlled for lifestyle-related risk factors. One of the largest studies (Hardell et al., 1984) indicates an increased risk for liver cancer and exposure to herbicides, but another study of Swedish agricultural workers (Wiklund, 1983) estimates a relative risk that is significantly less than 1.0. The estimated relative risks from other studies are both positive and negative. In summary, given the methodological difficulties associated with most of the few existing studies, the evidence regarding liver cancer is inadequate or insufficient to determine whether an association with herbicides exists.

Conclusions

There is inadequate or insufficient evidence to determine whether an association exists between exposure to the herbicides (2,4-D, 2,4,5-T and its contaminant, TCDD; cacodylic acid; and picloram) and hepatobiliary cancer. The evidence regarding association is drawn from occupational and other studies in which subjects were exposed to a variety of herbicides and herbicide components.

TABLE 7-1   Selected Epidemiologic Studies—Hepatobiliary Cancer

Reference	Study Population	Exposed Cases[a]	Estimated Risk (95% CI)[a]
Occupational			
Cohort studies			
Bond et al., 1988	Dow 2,4-D production workers		1.2
Fingerhut et al., 1991	NIOSH cohort	6	1.2 (0.4-2.5)
	20 years latency	1	0.6 (0.0-3.3)
Lynge, 1985	Danish production workers	3	1.0
Saracci et al., 1991	IARC cohort	4	0.4 (0.1-1.1)
Wiklund, 1983	Swedish agricultural workers	103	0.3 (0.3-0.4)[b]
Ronco et al., 1992	Danish and Italian farm workers		
	Danish male self-employed farmers	23	0.4
	Employees of Danish farmers	9	0.8
	Female family workers	5	0.5
Solet et al., 1989	Paper and pulp workers	2	2.0 (0.2-7.3)
Asp et al., 1994	Finnish herbicide applicators	2	0.6 (0.1-2.2)
Collins et al., 1993	Expansion of Zack and Suskind, 1980	2	1.4 (0.2-5.2)
Blair et al., 1993	U.S. farmers in 23 states	326	1.0 (0.9-1.1)
Case-control studies			
Hardell et al., 1984	Male residents of northern Sweden	102	1.8 (0.9-4.0)
Environmental			
Pesatori et al., 1992	Seveso male residents—zone A and B	4	1.5 (0.5-4.0)
	Female residents—zone A and B	1	1.2 (0.2-9.1)
Stehr et al., 1986	Missouri residents	0	—
Hoffman et al., 1986	Residents of Quail Run Mobile Home Park	0	—
Bertazzi et al., 1993	Seveso male residents—Zone B	5	1.8 (0.7-4.4)
	Female residents—Zone B	5	3.3 (1.3-8.1)
	Seveso male residents—Zone R	11	0.5 (0.3-1.0)
	Female residents—Zone R	12	0.9 (0.5-1.7)
Cordier et al., 1993	Military service in South Vietnam for ≥ 10 years after 1960	11	8.8 (1.9-41.0)

TABLE 7-1 Continued

Reference	Study Population	Exposed Cases[a]	Estimated Risk (95% CI)[a]
Vietnam veterans			
Cohort studies			
Breslin et al., 1988	Army Vietnam veterans	34	1.0 (0.8-1.4)
	Marine Vietnam veterans	6	1.2 (0.5-2.8)
Anderson et al., 1986a,b	Wisconsin Vietnam veterans	0	—
Case-control studies			
CDC, 1990	U.S. men born between 1921 and 1953	8	1.2 (0.5-2.7)

[a]Given when available.
[b]99% CI.

NASAL/NASOPHARYNGEAL CANCER

Background

Nasal and nasopharyngeal cancers (ICD-9 147.0-147.9, 160.0-160.9) can develop from any of the cell types present in any of these organs. The epithelium of the nasal and nasopharyngeal cavities is partly squamous, partly columnar and ciliated pseudostratified columnar. Precise distribution is variable. Also, there are serous and mucous glands and lymphoid aggregates in close association with the epithelium. Several types of adenomas may develop in the nasal cavity ("nasal polyps" papillomas). Squamous-cell carcinomas may develop in dysplastic epithelium at any surface site and are the most common type. They tend to spread locally, eroding into adjacent structures (orbit, cranial cavity, oral cavity), and may metastasize to cervical lymph nodes. Malignant mesenchymal tumors, especially rhabdomyosarcomas, are relatively frequent in this region and are derived from underlying connective tissues. Nasopharyngeal cancers occur in three histological variants: keratinizing squamous-cell, nonkeratinizing squamous-cell, and undifferentiated. Also, sarcomas and lymphomas (both Hodgkin's and non-Hodgkin's) are frequently seen in this region.

Because this type of cancer is of special interest to the DVA, this discussion integrates the studies reviewed in *VAO* with those published more recently.

Surgery, radiation, and chemotherapy are used individually or in combination to treat these neoplasms. Because of the proximity of vital anatomic structures, success of treatment is limited unless the tumor is diagnosed early in the evolution of the tumor cells.

Associations have been found between nasal cancers and occupational exposure to nickel (Doll et al., 1977) and to chromates (Higginson and Muir, 1973). Exposure to wood dust is also a risk factor for nasal cancer (Andersen et al., 1977); smoking (Elwood, 1981) or exposure to formaldehyde (Luce et al., 1993) may increase the risk associated with wood dust. There is also evidence that workers involved in processing leather have an increased risk for nasal cancers (Luce et al., 1993). A study in Shanghai, China, demonstrated an association between chronic nasal diseases and consumption of salt-preserved foods (Zheng et al., 1992b).

Although nasopharyngeal cancers are relatively uncommon, higher incidence is seen in southern China and Southeast Asia. Even among Chinese living in the United States, their cancer rates are higher than for whites or blacks (Burt et al., 1992). Dietary factors, including consumption of salt-preserved foods containing nitrosamines, appear to contribute to increased risk (Ablashi, 1978). A study in Shanghai of occupational risk factors found excess risks for workers in a variety of settings, including textile weaving, baking, and metal smelting, forging, and grinding (Zheng et al., 1992a). Nasopharyngeal cancer has also been associated with the Epstein-Barr virus, but the role of the virus is not yet clear (Henle and Henle, 1981). A genetic risk has been suggested as well (Gajwani et al., 1980).

Incidence of nasopharyngeal cancer in the United States is highest among the Chinese population and lowest among whites (Burt et al., 1992). Rates are generally twice as high in men as in women. Incidence remained stable between 1973 and 1986, but survival appears to have improved (Burt et al., 1992). Age, sex, and histologic type of the tumor each independently influence survival.

Epidemiological Studies

Occupational Studies

The study by Saracci et al. (1991) of production workers and sprayers showed a relative risk of 2.9 (CI 0.6-8.5) for these cancers, based on three cases. In addition, the study of chemical workers involved in the production of MCPA (Coggon et al., 1986) showed an elevated risk of 4.9 (CI 1.0-14.4), based on the same three specific cases. A case-control study by Hardell et al. (1982) found an odds ratio of 2.1 (CI 0.9-4.7) for those exposed to phenoxy acids, based on eight exposed cases.

Other studies showing inconclusive results included studies of agricultural workers (Wiklund, 1983; Ronco et al., 1992) and of paper and pulp workers (Robinson et al., 1986).

Asp et al. (1994), in an 18-year follow-up of 1,909 Finnish herbicide applicators, presented few data and combined cancers of the nasopharynx and larynx into a single category. In this broad category of cancer, four incident cases were observed, giving a relative risk of 1.1 (CI 0.3-2.7). Only one case died, yielding a mortality RR of 0.5 (CI 0.01-2.9).

Environmental Studies

Bertazzi et al. (1993) reported on cancer of the nose and nasal cavity based on follow-up of the Seveso population. There were no cases in Zones A and B, the more contaminated areas. In Zone R, the least contaminated area, two cases were observed among women, giving a relative risk of 2.6 (CI 0.5-13.3), and no cases were observed among men, though 1.5 were expected.

Vietnam Veterans Studies

In the CDC Selected Cancers Study of Vietnam veterans (CDC, 1990), there were 48 cases of nasal cancer and 80 cases of nasopharyngeal cancer, with two and three of the subjects, respectively, having served in Vietnam. No significant associations for Vietnam service and these cancers were found. Results for nasal and nasopharyngeal cancer are summarized in Table 7-2.

Summary

The scientific evidence on the association between herbicide exposure and nasopharyngeal cancer continues to be too sparse to make a definitive statement.

Conclusions

There is inadequate or insufficient evidence to determine whether an association exists between exposure to the herbicides (2,4-D, 2,4,5-T and its contaminant, TCDD; cacodylic acid; and picloram) and nasal/nasopharyngeal cancer. The evidence regarding association is drawn from occupational and other studies in which subjects were exposed to a variety of herbicides and herbicide components.

RESPIRATORY CANCERS

Background

Carcinomas of the lung and bronchus (ICD-9 162.2-162.9) are now the leading causes of cancer death in the United States. According to the American Cancer Society, approximately 169,900 new cases were diagnosed in the United States in 1995, and some 157,400 persons died from respiratory cancers (ACS, 1995). Substantially more men (96,000) than women (73,900) were diagnosed

TABLE 7-2 Selected Epidemiologic Studies—Nasal/Nasopharyngeal Cancer

Reference	Study Population	Exposed Cases[a]	Estimated Risk (95% CI)[a]
Occupational			
Cohort studies			
Coggon et al., 1986	British MCPA production workers	3	4.9 (1.0-14.4)
Saracci et al., 1991	IARC cohort	3	2.9 (0.6-8.5)
Wiklund, 1983	Swedish agricultural workers	64	0.8 (0.6-1.2)
Robinson et al., 1986	Paper and pulp workers	0	—
Asp et al., 1994	Finnish herbicide applicators	1	0.5 (0.01-2.9)
Case-control studies			
Hardell et al., 1982	Residents of northern Sweden		
	Phenoxy acid exposure	8	2.1 (0.9-4.7)
	Chlorophenol exposure	9	6.7 (2.8-16.2)
Environment			
Bertazzi et al., 1993	Residents in Seveso (Zone R)	2	2.6(0.5-13.3)
Vietnam veterans			
CDC, 1990	U.S. men born between 1921 and 1953		
	Vietnam veterans	2	0.7 (0.1-3.0)

[a]Given when available.

with these cancers. According to the committee's calculations, assuming that veterans have the same cancer rates as those of the general U.S. population, 1,266 cases of cancer of the lung and bronchus were expected to be diagnosed among male Vietnam veterans and 2.3 among female veterans in 1995. For the year 2000, the expected numbers are 2,860 cases in male veterans and 4.6 in female veterans. The committee's calculations indicate that 166 cases of cancer of the larynx (ICD-9 161.0-161.9) were expected to be diagnosed among male Vietnam veterans and 0.1 among female veterans in 1995. For the year 2000, the expected numbers are 364 cases in male veterans and 0.3 in female veterans.

Because *VAO* classified respiratory cancers in the category of limited/suggestive evidence of an association with exposure to herbicides, this discussion integrates the studies reviewed in that report with those published more recently.

The incidence and mortality rates for lung cancers have increased markedly during the past half century, reflecting the earlier patterns of smoking among the

U.S. population. Decreases in recent years in the prevalence of smoking among men are now leading to small reductions in the incidence of lung cancer and will eventually result in reductions in mortality. Incidence and mortality rates for lung cancer in women began increasing more recently than those for men. In 1987, lung cancer deaths among women exceeded deaths from breast cancer for the first time (ACS, 1992). For men and women, the incidence of lung cancer increases rapidly beginning at about age 40.

The principal types of lung neoplasms are identified collectively as broncho-genic carcinoma or carcinoma of the lung. The lung is also a common site for the development of a metastatic cancer. It is therefore necessary to have histological examination of the lung tissue to avoid the misclassification of some other type of cancer as primary lung cancer. Squamous-cell carcinoma accounts for 50 to 70 percent of lung tumors, adenocarcinoma for 10 to 25 percent, small-cell (oat-cell) carcinomas for about 5 percent, and large-cell carcinomas for about 5 percent (McGee et al., 1992). Often a neoplasm may be made up of mixtures of these cell types. These different types of lung tumors are often combined in epidemiologic studies for several reasons: (1) there are frequently mixed patterns of a variety of different cell types; (2) there is abundant evidence that these tumors arise from a common stem cell that differentiates along one or more of these pathways; and (3) they often arise in a similar location near the hilum of the lung in the first- or second-order bronchi.

Cigarette smoking is the major risk factor for lung cancer, and is estimated by the American Cancer Society (1992) to be responsible for about 87 percent of lung cancer deaths in the United States. The risk increases with length of time and number of cigarettes smoked (U.S. DHHS, 1987). Tobacco smoke may include both tumor initiators and promoters. Other important risk factors include exposure to radon, arsenic, asbestos, chromium, nickel, and aromatic hydrocar-bons. Asbestos and radon interact with cigarette smoking, increasing the risk of lung cancer beyond that predicted from the simple combination of the individual risks (ACS, 1992).

Epidemiologic Studies

Occupational Studies

Production Workers   In a study of Dow Chemical Company workers in-volved in the production of 2,4-D (Bond et al., 1988), the SMR for lung cancer was 1.0 (eight observed versus 7.7 expected deaths, CI 0.5-2.0) (Table 7-3). When other Dow workers are used as a comparison group, the effect estimate is slightly higher, as might be expected from a more comparable, relatively healthy comparison group (i.e., less bias from the "healthy worker effect"). The SMR for all respiratory cancers (lung alone is not given) is 1.2 (nine observed versus 7.4 expected deaths, CI 0.6-2.3). The authors estimated lifetime cumulative expo-

TABLE 7-3 Selected Epidemiologic Studies—Lung Cancer

Reference	Study Population	Exposed Cases	Estimated Risk (95% CI)
Occupational Studies			
Bond et al., 1988	Dow 2,4-D production workers; 15 years latency	9	1.2(0.6-2.3)
	Low cumulative exposure	1	0.7
	Medium cumulative exposure	2	1.0
	High cumulative exposure	5	1.7
Bloemen, 1993	Dow 2,4-D production workers; update of Bond et al., 1988	9	0.8(0.4-1.5)
Coggon et al., 1986	MCPA production workers	101	1.2(1.0-1.4)
	Background exposure	39	1.0(0.7-1.4)
	Low-grade exposure	35	1.1(0.8-1.6)
	High-grade exposure	43	1.3(1.0-1.8)
Coggon et al., 1991	Phenoxy herbicide production workers	19	1.3(0.8-2.1)
		14	1.2(0.7-2.1)
Lynge, 1985	Danish phenoxy herbicide production workers - males	38	1.2
	- females	6	2.2
	Manufacture and packing only - males	11	2.1(1.0-3.7)
Lynge, 1993	Update of manufacturing subgroup - males	13	1.6(0.9-2.8)
Zober, 1990	TCDD reactor accident workers	6	1.6
	High exposure	4	2.0(0.6-5.2)
	Chloracne	6	1.8(0.7-4.0)
Manz et al., 1991	Phenoxy herbicide production workers	26	1.7(1.1-2.4)
Saracci, 1991	Herbicide spraying and production workers	173	1.0(0.9-1.2)
	Probably exposed subgroup	11	2.2 (1.1-4.0)
Bueno de Mesquita, 1993	Phenoxy herbicide workers	9	1.7(0.5-6.3)
Fingerhut et al., 1991	TCDD-exposed workers	89	1.1(0.9-1.4)
	≥ 1 year exposure; ≤ 20 years latency	40	1.4(1.0-1.9)
Kogevinas et al., 1993	Female herbicide spraying and production workers	2	1.4(0.2-4.9)
Axelson et al., 1980	Herbicide sprayers in Sweden	3	1.4(0.3-4.0)
Asp, 1994	Finnish herbicide applicators	37	1.0(0.7-1.4)
Blair, 1983	Licensed pesticide applicators in Florida, lawn and ornamental herbicides only	7	0.9(0.4-1.9)
Green, 1991	Herbicide sprayers in Ontario	5	1.1(0.4-2.5)
Bender, 1989	Herbicide sprayers in Minnesota	54	0.7(0.5-0.9)
Wiklund et al., 1989	Pesticide applicators in Sweden	38	0.5(0.4-0.7)
Swaen, 1992	Herbicide applicators	12	1.1(0.6-1.9)
Blair et al., 1993	U.S. farmers from 23 states		
	- white males	6,473	0.9(0.9-0.9)
	- nonwhite males	664	1.0(0.9-1.1)

TABLE 7-3 Continued

Reference	Study Population	Exposed Cases	Estimated Risk (95% CI)
Case-control studies			
McDuffie et al., 1990	Saskatchewan farmers applying herbicides	103	0.6
Environmental Studies			
Bertazzi et al., 1993	Seveso residents first ten years after accident		
	Zone A - males	2	0.8(0.2-3.4)
	Zone A - females	0	—
	Zone B - males	18	1.1(0.7-1.8)
	Zone B - females	0	—
	Zone R - males	96	0.8(0.7-1.0)
	Zone R - females	16	1.5(0.8-2.5)

sure to 2,4-D, and when the cohort was divided into three groups with a 15-year exposure lag with respect to this estimate, the SMRs were: low exposure, 0.7; medium exposure, 1.0; high exposure, 1.7. These subgroup SMRs were based on one, two, and five deaths, respectively; a test of the null hypothesis that there is no trend evidenced in these data has a p-value of 0.1.

Bloemen et al. (1993) updated a cohort mortality study of Dow Chemical Company production workers exposed to 2,4-D. This update added four additional years of follow-up for the 878 employees to the original study (Bond et al., 1988). Nine deaths from respiratory cancer were observed (SMR = 0.8, CI 0.4-1.5).

The mortality experience was evaluated for 754 male production workers at a Monsanto Company trichlorophenol plant at which an accident caused the release of TCDD in 1949 (Collins et al., 1993). One hundred and twenty two of these employees had developed chloracne as a result of the accident. Many of the employees in the plant were also exposed to another carcinogen, 4-aminobiphenyl, which causes bladder cancer in humans. Thirty eight deaths from respiratory cancer were observed (SMR = 1.1, CI 0.8-1.5).

Lung cancer mortality in a cohort employed in the production and spraying of MCPA and other phenoxy herbicides (Coggon et al., 1986) was close to that expected, with the national comparison population yielding a slight deficit in risk and the rural comparison a slight excess in risk (with national comparison: SMR = 0.9, CI 0.8-1.1; with rural comparison: SMR = 1.2, CI 1.0-1.4). When the cohort was subdivided by estimated level of exposure to phenoxy acids, weak evidence of an increase in risk with increase in exposure was observed (background exposure: SMR = 1.0 [CI 0.7-1.4]; low exposure: SMR = 1.1 [CI 0.8-1.6]; high exposure: SMR = 1.3 [CI 1.0-1.8]).

These figures, based on the rural comparison population, may suffer from the problem of noncomparability of indirectly standardized rates, but the authors do not provide data with which to perform the more appropriate internal analysis. Nevertheless, because these three categories are distinguished on "grade" or intensity of exposure and not on exposure duration, they most likely do not differ dramatically in underlying age distribution, so comparisons of the three SMRs are probably appropriate. When the cohort was subdivided by duration of potential exposure into three categories—less than one month, one to six months, and more than six months—the first of these groups contained only seven lung cancer deaths, and unstable risk estimates. When the <1 month and 1-6 month groups are combined into "short" duration, SMR = 1.2 (CI 0.8-1.6); for the "long" duration (>6 months), SMR = 1.3, (CI 1.0-1.7). The study included workers employed over a 29-year period, but maximum length of employment of individual workers was not reported. Note, however, that employment for more than six months does not necessarily imply substantial exposure and that this comparison may be affected by noncomparability of underlying age distributions, as discussed above.

Using very similar methods, Coggon et al. (1991) have reported on the mortality experience of the employees of four British factories where phenoxy herbicides and other chemicals were manufactured. When compared to either national or rural population, there was a slight excess of lung cancer mortality (SMR = 1.3, CI 0.8-2.1 with national rates; rural rates yield nearly identical results). However, when the analysis was restricted to those with any exposure above "background" levels, the risk dropped slightly (SMR = 1.2, CI 0.7-2.1), which is the opposite of what would be expected from a true association, because it would be expected that the overall association would be diluted by those with low exposure in the background group.

In a study of Danish phenoxy herbicide manufacturing workers (Lynge, 1985), the lung cancer incidence of the entire workforce was about that expected (SMR for males = 1.2, based on 38 observed cases; SMR for females = 2.2, based on six observed cases). However, when the cohort was restricted to those actually engaged in the manufacturing or packaging of phenoxy herbicides, the risk in men increased (SMR = 2.1, CI 1.0-3.7, based on 11 observed cases). There was only one female lung cancer case in these areas of the plant. These results were obtained without application of a latency period, but the author reports that the results were the same when a ten-year latency period was used. The excess lung cancer risk was present in both plants studied. The workers were generally recruited from the countryside where tobacco consumption was lower than the national average; however, no direct information on the smoking habits of the cohort was available. A review of the other occupational information for the lung cancer cases did not identify any known risk factors likely to explain the observed excess.

The study by Lynge was updated for an additional five years (Lynge, 1993). In the original study 4,461 eligible workers were identified (Lynge, 1985). Among 690 male employees in the specific departments in which phenoxy herbicides were manufactured and packaged, 13 cases of lung cancer were diagnosed, which yielded an SIR of 1.6 (CI 0.9-2.8). The risk of lung cancer was not elevated among female employees.

In a retrospective cohort mortality study of a population of chemical workers potentially exposed to TCDD in the production of hexachlorophene at a flavor and fragrance plant (Thomas, 1987), the SMR for lung cancer in white males was 1.2 (29 observed versus 25.1 expected deaths, CI 0.8-1.7). Because of the complex exposures of this cohort and the likelihood that only a small, unidentifiable fraction was exposed to TCDD, these results are of very limited usefulness in evaluating the associations under consideration.

After an industrial accident involving the release of TCDD, 78 deaths were observed in a 34-year period (Zober et al., 1990). With the small number of total deaths, the results concerning lung cancer (six deaths due to trachea, bronchus, or lung cancer) are inconclusive. In the most heavily exposed subgroup, there were four deaths from lung cancer, compared to 2.0 expected from national mortality rates (SMR = 2.0, CI 0.6-5.2). Among those with chloracne, lung cancer appeared somewhat elevated, although the sample size (3,589 person-years) precludes a precise estimate of this effect. Among those with chloracne, there were six deaths from lung cancer and 3.3 expected (SMR = 1.8, CI 0.7-4.0).

The workers in a Hamburg, Germany, herbicide production facility heavily contaminated with TCDD were studied by Manz et al. (1991) in the first few years of its operation. Two comparison groups were available for this study, the general population and a cohort of gas-company workers previously studied by the authors. The risk estimate for lung cancer was elevated compared to the gas company workers (SMR = 1.7, based on 26 observed and 15.6 expected deaths, CI 1.1-2.4). The gas worker's somewhat higher risk estimate was probably due to the "healthy worker effect." Smoking data were not available for all subjects, but in a subsample of 361 workers, 73 percent were self-reported smokers, compared to 76 percent of 2,860 gas workers who reported smoking. It is thus unlikely that smoking differentials could explain the observed excess of lung cancer.

Saracci et al. (1991) have reported on the mortality experience of a large international cohort that includes both production workers and herbicide sprayers. The degree of exposure to TCDD is more uncertain than that of the large U.S. study by Fingerhut and colleagues (1991) described below, in that some of the cohorts included in the Saracci study are of individuals either spraying or producing compounds, such as 2,4-D, MCPA, or 2-(4-chloro-2-methylphenoxy)-propanoic acid (MCPP), which are unlikely to contain significant quantities of

TCDD. Mortality from cancer of the respiratory tract was normal, based on 173 observed deaths (SMR = 1.0, CI 0.9-1.2).

The workers in two British herbicide production plants were not included in the above calculations, because job history information was not available. Nevertheless, the authors are confident that the majority of the subjects in these two plants were indeed exposed to phenoxy herbicides to some degree. An excess lung cancer mortality risk was observed (SMR = 2.2, CI 1.1-4.0, based on 11 observed cases). No smoking information is available (Saracci et al., 1991).

A cohort of production workers in the Netherlands (Bueno de Mesquita et al., 1993) showed no excess lung cancer deaths. Where results from two factories were combined, Factory A, where 2,4,5-T was produced, was the only source of the lung cancers that were reported.

A cohort study of cancer mortality was conducted among 701 women from seven countries, who were occupationally exposed to chlorophenoxy herbicides, chlorophenols, and dioxins (Kogevinas et al., 1993). Female workers on the IARC Registry who were ever employed in production or spraying of these chemicals were eligible for the study. Two deaths from lung cancer were observed, which yielded an SMR of 1.4 (CI 0.2-4.9). Both of these deaths occurred within the first ten years since first exposure.

In the NIOSH cohort (Fingerhut et al., 1991) of TCDD-exposed workers, an elevated risk of respiratory cancer was observed in those with more than one year of exposure and 20 years of latency (SMR = 1.4, CI 1.0-1.9, based on 43 observed deaths). An analysis of mortality according to duration of exposure in processes involving TCDD contamination shows increasing standardized rate ratios (SRR) with increasing duration of exposure for cancer of the trachea, bronchus, and lung (<1 year: SRR = 1.0; 1-5 years: SRR = 1.1; 5-15 years: SRR = 1.7; >15 years: SRR = 1.4; test for trend, p = .2). The increased risk for cancer of the lung is unlikely to be the result of excess cigarette smoking in the cohort. Workers from two of the plants were interviewed in 1987 and their smoking histories ascertained.

Summary of Production Worker Studies   Additional years of followup were added to several cohort studies of workers (Bloemen, 1993; Collins et al., 1993; Lynge, 1993). The additional person-years of observation and additional cases of respiratory cancer observed in these studies since the publication of *VAO*, do not materially change the results in any of these studies.

One might derive a pooled estimate of the lung cancer risk among production workers from the following studies (Table 7-3): Bond et al. (1988), Zober et al. (1990), Manz et al. (1991), Saracci et al. (1991), and Fingerhut et al. (1991). Of the six cohorts in these studies, there are three in which the committee is fairly confident that there was a substantial level of exposure to TCDD: those of Zober et al. (1990), Manz et al. (1991), and the high-exposure group of Fingerhut et al.

(1991). When just those three studies are combined, the pooled SMR is somewhat elevated: 1.4 (CI 1.2-1.8).

The studies of Coggon and Lynge are largely subsumed under the European registry of Saracci et al. and so should not be viewed as independent measurements of effect. Note, however, that certain findings in these two studies that are suggestive of an association with lung cancer are lost when the combined cohort of Saracci is presented. In the Coggon study (1986), weak evidence of a trend of increasing risk with increasing category of exposure was observed (see above). In the Lynge study (1985), an elevated risk of lung cancer was observed, and this elevation was consistent over the two plants studied. In addition, the rural population from which the workforce was derived would be expected to have had lower than average smoking rates, thus indirectly reducing the likelihood that the lung cancer excess could be explained by smoking.

Because many of the workers smoked and were exposed to other chemicals, it is not possible to rule out alternative explanations for this small excess risk. It is unlikely, however, that smoking explains the entire effect, since the studies of Fingerhut et al. (1991) and Manz et al. (1991) both found that smoking rates were only slightly different in samples of their study populations and in the comparison populations. Chemical production workers are often exposed to asbestos, which until recently was widely used wherever an industrial process involved high temperature. This well-known lung carcinogen might confound the observed association with herbicide and TCDD exposure in many of these studies. But it is also unlikely that asbestos could fully explain these findings, because the lung cancer risk from asbestos among chemical workers in general (as distinct from those whose occupations brought them into frequent and direct contact with the substance) is not elevated (Wong and Raabe, 1989). Thus, although tobacco and asbestos cannot be ruled out, the more likely explanation for the observed elevations in risk involves one or more agents associated with the production of phenoxy herbicides and related compounds.

Agricultural/Forestry Workers   Studies that compare the lung cancer experience of farmers as a group to that of other occupations or the general population show a consistent deficit of lung cancer among farmers. For example, studies by Burmeister (1981) and by Wigle et al. (1990) in North America, and by Wiklund (1983) in Sweden, provide strong evidence for a reduced risk of lung or respiratory cancer in farmers. A cohort study of Danish gardeners (Hansen et al., 1992) observed neither a deficit nor an excess of lung cancer.

In the United States, a recent PCMR study was performed for farmers in 23 states, using occupational information from death certificates (Blair et al., 1993). Because of the large population size, the confidence intervals are relatively narrow. Based on 6,473 deaths from lung cancer in white male farmers, the PCMR was significantly decreased, at 0.9 (CI 0.9-0.9). Based on 664 deaths in nonwhite male farmers, the PCMR was 1.0 (CI 0.9-1.1). The numbers of deaths in women of all races were small and nonsignificant. The PCMR for death from lung cancer was less than 1.0 in 18 of 23 states, a significant finding.

Several authors have attributed this observed deficit in lung cancer among male farmers to decreased smoking among this group, and there is evidence to support this supposition, at least in the United States (Sterling and Weinkam, 1976) and Sweden (Rylander, 1990). Another causal hypothesis that has been proposed is that farmers are exposed to high levels of bacterial endotoxins in a wide variety of organic dusts (Rylander, 1990); these biologically active compounds have been shown to retard cancer growth in laboratory animals and have been proposed as anticancer drugs (Engelhardt et al., 1991).

Several studies of cohorts whose members were engaged in agriculture-related activities have examined lung cancer risk, but the connection to herbicides is tenuous and does not add to the evidence of an association (Alavanja et al., 1988, 1989).

Herbicide and Pesticide Applicators Studies of pesticide applicators are more relevant than those studies just discussed, because it can be presumed that applicators had more sustained exposures to herbicides than did members of the other groups, and the types of herbicides and durations of exposure can often be quantified generally. There are several weaknesses in many of these studies, however, including a lack of individual estimates of exposure, the fact that many different kinds of herbicides were often used, and limited sample sizes.

Axelson and Sundell (1974) conducted a cohort study of herbicide sprayers who tended railroad rights-of-way in Sweden; the study initially covered the period 1957-72, and was extended until 1978 (Axelson et al., 1980). Based on follow-up through 1978, the results for lung cancer were ambiguous because of the very small numbers of both observed and expected cancers; for example, the SMR for lung cancer was 1.4 (CI 0.3-4.0), based on three observed cases for all types of exposure.

A cohort of Finnish workers who sprayed the herbicides 2,4-D and 2,4,5-T was followed by Riihimaki et al. (1982). Good employment records were available, and follow-up through 1980 was nearly complete. Additional strengths of this study include the apparent lack of confounding by other chemical exposures (although the authors do not explore what the cohort members did when they were not spraying) and the relatively high exposures that the subjects probably experienced during spraying seasons. No information on smoking habits for the cohort is available. By applying a ten-year latency period (the shortest latency for which data were provided), 12 lung cancer deaths were observed, compared to 11.1 expected (SMR = 1.1, CI 0.6-1.9). Lung cancer incidence for the period 1972-78, with ten-year latency applied, resulted in the SIR = 1.4 (nine cases observed versus 6.6 expected, CI 0.6-2.6) (Riihimaki et al., 1983).

Asp et al. (1994) extended this study by adding ten years of follow-up to the original eight years (Riihimaki et al., 1982, 1983). In both studies, the ten years following first exposure were not counted as time at risk, to allow time for disease to develop. The median duration of exposure was six weeks. While the number of respiratory cancer deaths among the 10+ years of latency group nearly tripled—from 12 to 33—the relative risk estimate of 1.1 was nearly unchanged, and the confidence interval narrowed (CI 0.7-1.5) with additional follow-up. The corresponding SIR, however, dropped to 1.0 based on 33 cases (CI 0.7-1.3).

In a study of licensed pesticide applicators in Florida (Blair et al., 1983), the overall lung cancer SMR was 1.4 (34 observed deaths versus 25.1 expected, CI 0.9-1.9). The risk estimate rose with the number of years licensed, from 1.0 for less than ten years licensed, to 1.6 for 10 to 19 years, to 2.9 for 20 years or more (in a test for trend, p = .13). Increased lung cancer SMRs were found for workers licensed to apply fumigants and to apply pesticides for termites and other wood-infesting organisms, general household pests, rodents, and lawn and ornamental pests. In applicators employed by a small group of firms that were licensed to treat lawns and ornamental plants, the SMR was not elevated (SMR = 0.9), but the numbers were small (seven observed deaths versus 7.6 expected, CI 0.4-1.9). However, workers were exposed to numerous chemicals, including some known carcinogens; individual exposure to phenoxy herbicides or to any TCDD-contaminated compound cannot be determined. It is unlikely that the elevated lung cancer risk in the entire cohort can be entirely attributable to smoking. The SMRs for other smoking-related diseases were depressed, the risk was related to duration of pesticide use, and implausibly high smoking prevalences would be necessary among this cohort to explain a lung cancer risk of this magnitude.

A cohort study by Green (1991) of right-of-way sprayers in Ontario, Canada, was based on records of spraying activities, but the number of subjects was small. Lung cancer mortality was essentially normal (five deaths versus 4.6 expected, RR = 1.1, CI 0.4-2.5), but the small numbers of observed deaths preclude strong conclusions. Minnesota highway workers (Bender et al., 1989) were at reduced risk of lung cancer (SMR = 0.7, CI 0.5-0.9), as were Swedish pesticide applicators (Wiklund et al., 1989); the standardized incidence ratio was 0.5 (CI 0.4-0.7), with 38 observed cases. No association with lung cancer was found when the cohort was subdivided by years since license or by year of birth.

Licensed herbicide applicators in the Netherlands were studied by Swaen et al. (1992). The study is about the same size as that of Riihimaki et al. (1982) in Finland and yielded similar results for lung cancer: 12 deaths observed compared to 11.2 expected (SMR = 1.1, CI 0.6-1.9).

Summary of Pesticide Applicator Studies   If the cohorts of Axelson (at second follow-up), Riihimaki (with minimum ten-year latency—all others have no latency restriction), Blair (lawn and ornamental sprayers only), and Green are considered roughly comparable studies of workers with likely exposure to phenoxy herbicides through manual spraying, the observed and expected deaths could be combined to yield a more precise estimate of risk. This yields 27 observed and 25.5 expected deaths and an SMR = 1.1 (CI 0.8-1.5).

Paper/Pulp Workers   Unlike the studies of farmers, the reports of paper worker are not consistent with respect to their estimates of lung cancer risk. Some studies do report an excess, although usually without adequate control for potential confounding by smoking (Solet et al., 1989; Jappinen and Pukkala, 1991), while others do not (Robinson et al., 1986; Henneberger et al., 1989).

Case-Control Studies

A case-control study that investigated lung cancer herbicide exposures was published by McDuffie et al. (1990). The occupational histories of chemical exposure for 273 male cases of primary lung cancer from the tumor registry in Saskatchewan, Canada, were compared to the histories of 187 male controls. Subjects were questioned about their use of many chemicals, including phenoxy herbicides. The response rate was rather low (74 percent), and duration of exposure appears not to have been considered in the exposure assessment. No association was found between reported use of phenoxy herbicides and lung cancer, either in the unadjusted analyses (OR = 0.5) or after controlling for cigarette smoking (OR = 0.6).

Environmental Studies

Studies of the population exposed to TCDD the 1976 industrial accident in Seveso, Italy, to TCDD include estimates of lung cancer risk (Bertazzi et al., 1989b, 1993; Pesatori et al., 1992). Ten years of follow-up for mortality and cancer incidence demonstrate an inconsistent pattern of lung cancer rates in the different exposed groups, as well as between males and females. People most heavily exposed (those living in Zone A at the time of the accident, but subsequently permanently evacuated) are too few in number (two observed lung cancer deaths in ten years) to provide any information. In Zone B, the lung cancer incidence in males was slightly elevated, based on 18 observed cases (RR = 1.1, CI 0.7-1.8), while there were no observed cases among women (expected number not given). The largest and least contaminated area, Zone R, was not found to have elevated lung cancer incidence rates in males (96 observed cases, RR = 0.8, CI 0.7-1.0), whereas a slight excess was observed in females (16 observed cases, RR = 1.5, CI 0.8-2.5).

Smoking is not likely to explain differences in lung cancer rates in people living in the zones around Seveso and the comparison population, because the latter consists of the residents of nearby towns that are economically and culturally similar to the contaminated region.

The Şeveso studies followed the population only until ten years after the accident. If the TCDD release did increase the risk for lung cancers, one might not expect to see the full impact on tumor incidence for some years to come. At least another ten years is needed before the impact of the accident on cancer incidence can be meaningfully assessed.

Vietnam Veterans Studies

Ranch Hands The follow-up study of Ranch Hand veterans is too small to evaluate excess cancer risks (Michalek et al., 1990). Lung cancer mortality was similar in Ranch Hands and the comparison group, although the study was based on only five Ranch Hand lung cancer deaths (incidence density ratio = 0.9, CI 0.3-2.1).

CDC The Vietnam Experience Study (Boyle et al., 1987) was too small to consider lung cancer risk; only one lung cancer death occurred in the comparison group of Vietnam era veterans.

DVA Studies Breslin et al. (1988) and Watanabe et al. (1991) have studied Army and Marine Vietnam veterans and Vietnam-era veterans, and both studies found a small increase in lung cancer risk in Army and Marine Corps veterans who served in Vietnam. For both groups combined, the PMR is 1.1 (CI 1.0-1.2), and the risk is only slightly higher in Marine than in Army veterans. No smoking data are available on this cohort, but other studies have suggested that the smoking habits of Vietnam and Vietnam-era veterans were not significantly different from each other.

Investigators at the DVA designed an additional PMR study based on deceased Army veterans who served in Military Region I (I Corps), where the majority of Marines were stationed (Bullman et al., 1990). Lung cancer risk was comparable in Army I Corps veterans and Army Vietnam-era veterans (PMR = 0.9, CI 0.8-1.1, based on 187 observed deaths).

The mortality experience of women who served in Vietnam has been studied by DVA investigators (Thomas et al., 1991). Lung cancer mortality was comparable or perhaps somewhat reduced in Vietnam veterans, although based on only eight lung cancer deaths in the exposed group; after adjusting for potential confounding factors, the relative risk was 0.6, CI 0.3-1.5.

The cancer mortality rates in 4,586 female Vietnam veterans were compared to the rates in 5,325 female veterans who served elsewhere (Dalager et al., 1995). This is an update of a previous study with four additional years of follow-up (Thomas et al., 1991). Based upon 15 cases of lung cancer, the adjusted SMR was 0.9 (CI 0.4-1.7). More than over 80 percent of the Vietnam cohort were nurses; therefore, their exposure to herbicides was probably low.

Twenty-two U.S. Army Chemical Corps units assigned to Vietnam between 1966 and 1971 have been followed for vital status through 1987 (Thomas and

Kang, 1990). In the final cohort of 894 men, there were only two deaths from lung cancer, against 1.8 expected based on the entire U.S. male population (SMR = 1.1, CI 0.1-4.0).

State Studies   Studies of Vietnam veterans in several states have examined lung cancer mortality rates. There include Wisconsin (Anderson et al., 1986a,b), Massachusetts (Kogan and Clapp, 1985, 1988), New York (Lawrence et al., 1985), and West Virginia (Holmes et al., 1986). In each case, lung cancer mortality rates were comparable between Vietnam veterans and Vietnam-era veterans.

A proportionate mortality study examining causes of death among veterans on Michigan's Vietnam-era Bonus list was recently reported (Visintainer et al., 1995). The cause-specific mortality rates among 3,364 Vietnam veterans were compared with the rates among 5,229 age-matched veterans who served else-where. There were 80 deaths from lung cancer among the Vietnam veterans (PMR = 0.9; CI 0.7-1.1).

Australian Vietnam Veterans   In a study that compared Australian Vietnam veterans to Australian Vietnam-era veterans who served elsewhere, the relative risk for lung cancer was 2.7 (CI 0.2-30.0) (Fett et al., 1987). This association is based on only two cases among the Vietnam veterans.

Summary of Veterans Studies   Current studies of lung cancer risk in veterans are of limited usefulness for evaluating the effect of herbicide exposure, either because the studies are too small or because it is not possible to identify those soldiers who were likely to have been exposed to herbicides.

Epidemiologic Studies of Laryngeal Cancer

In nearly all studies analyzing respiratory cancers, the authors either group all of the different types of cancer in this broad group together (ICD codes 161 to 165, which include trachea, bronchus, lung, larynx) or present data for the largest category within this group (ICD code 162, which includes trachea, bronchus, and lung). Cancers of the latter three sites are often simply called "lung cancer." In only a few cases are the data broken out to allow assessment of other respiratory sites.

Of note are five studies of production workers in which data for laryngeal cancer (ICD 161) are presented separately (Fingerhut et al., 1991; Bond et al., 1988; Coggon et al., 1986; Manz et al., 1991; Saracci et al., 1991). Although the numbers are too small to draw strong conclusions, the consistency of a mild elevation in relative risk is suggestive of an association for laryngeal cancer. Pooling all but the Coggon data (Coggon et al., 1986, 1991) yields an odds ratio of 1.8 (CI 1.0-3.2). Potential confounders of an occupational risk for this cancer include tobacco and alcohol consumption. As noted previously, these studies did not directly control for smoking, although its magnitude in Manz et al. (1991) and Fingerhut et al. (1991) is not likely to be large. There is no information on alcohol consumption in any of the studies.

Other than these studies of production workers, there is only one other study that reported separate results for cancer of the larynx. A PCMR study was performed for farmers in 23 states, using occupational information from death certificates (Blair et al., 1993). Based on 162 deaths from laryngeal cancer in white male farmers, the PCMR was significantly decreased, at 0.7 (CI 0.6-0.8). This was consistent with a significant decrease in lung cancer in the same subgroup. Based on 32 deaths from laryngeal cancer in nonwhite male farmers, the PCMR was 1.1 (CI 0.8-1.5). There were no deaths from this cancer in female farmers.

Summary

Among the many epidemiologic studies of respiratory cancers reviewed by the committee (see Table 7-3), positive associations were found consistently only when TCDD or herbicide exposures were probably high and prolonged. This was especially true in the largest, most heavily exposed cohorts of chemical production workers exposed to TCDD (Zober et al., 1990; Fingerhut et al., 1991; Manz et al., 1991; Saracci et al., 1991). Studies of farmers tended to show a decreased risk of respiratory cancers (perhaps due to lower smoking rates), and studies of Vietnam veterans were inconclusive. The committee concluded that the evidence for this association was limited/suggestive rather than sufficient, because of the inconsistent pattern of positive findings across populations with various degrees and types of exposure and because the most important risk factor for respiratory cancers—cigarette smoking—was not fully controlled for or evaluated in all studies. The update of scientific literature continues to support these conclusions.

Conclusions

Strength of Evidence in Epidemiologic Studies

There is limited/suggestive evidence of an association between exposure to the herbicides (2,4-D, 2,4,5-T and its contaminant, TCDD; cacodylic acid; and picloram) and respiratory cancers (lung, larynx, trachea). The evidence regarding association is drawn from occupational and other studies in which subjects were exposed to a variety of herbicides and herbicide components.

BONE CANCER

Background

According to the American Cancer Society, approximately 2,070 new cases of bone and joint cancer (ICD-9 170.0-170.9) were diagnosed in the United States in 1995, and some 1,280 persons died of this cancer (ACS, 1995). These cases are divided approximately equally between men and women. According to the committee's calculations, assuming that veterans have the same cancer rates as those of the general U.S. population, ten cases of bone cancer are expected among male Vietnam veterans and 0.1 among female veterans in 1995. For the year 2000, the expected numbers are 21 cases in male veterans and less than 0.05 cases in female veterans.

Primary bone cancers are among the least common malignancies. The bones are, however, a frequent site for secondary tumors of other cancers that have metastasized, meaning that they have spread from another site. Only the primary cancers are considered here.

Summary of *VAO*

Studies of bone cancer and herbicide exposure have included chemical production workers (Coggon et al., 1986; Bond et al., 1988; Zober et al., 1990; Fingerhut et al., 1991); agricultural workers (Burmeister, 1981; Wiklund, 1983; Ronco et al., 1992); and Vietnam veterans (Lawrence et al., 1985; Anderson et al., 1986a,b; Breslin et al., 1988). The studies regarding bone cancer were evenly distributed between positive and negative studies. Because of its rarity, this cancer is particularly difficult to study; very few of the studies were of sufficient size to have much statistical power, and the confidence limits were typically large. Case-control studies focusing on populations with potentially heavy exposure, such as production workers, might conceivably change this situation, but none had been published for bone cancer.

Update of the Scientific Literature

Bone cancer mortality was evaluated for a cohort of 754 white male employees of a Monsanto Company trichlorophenol plant at which an explosion occurred in 1949 (Collins et al., 1993). As a result of the accident, 122 employees developed chloracne. SMRs were calculated, based on a follow-up period through 1987 and using mortality rates in the local general population. Based on two observed cases of bone cancer, the SMR was 5.0 (0.6-18.1). The authors did not mention whether these two bone cancer cases had developed chloracne.

A PCMR study was performed for farmers in 23 states, using occupational information from death certificates (Blair et al., 1993). Based on 49 deaths from bone cancer in white male farmers, the PCMR was 1.3 (CI 1.0-1.8). The numbers of bone cancer were very small and nonsignificant in the other racial and gender groups: nonwhite males and white and nonwhite females.

Summary

The committee found only two new studies that reported bone cancer as an endpoint. These studies do not change the *VAO's* conclusions concerning bone cancer.

Conclusions

There is inadequate or insufficient evidence to determine whether an association exists between exposure to the herbicides (2,4-D, 2,4,5-T and its contaminant, TCDD; cacodylic acid; and picloram) and bone cancer. The evidence regarding association is drawn from occupational and other studies in which subjects were exposed to a variety of herbicides and herbicide components.

SOFT-TISSUE SARCOMAS

Background

According to the American Cancer Society, 6,000 new cases of soft-tissue sarcoma (STS) (ICD-9 171.0-171.9, 164.1) were diagnosed in the United States in 1995, and some 3,600 persons died of these cancers (ACS, 1995). New cases were slightly more common in men than in women, but similar numbers of deaths occurred. According to the committee's calculations, assuming that veterans have the same cancer rates as those of the general U.S. population, 65 cases of STS are expected among male Vietnam veterans and 0.1 among female veterans in 1995. For the year 2000, the expected numbers are 86 cases in male veterans and 0.2 in female veterans.

STSs arise in the soft somatic tissues that occur within and between organs. Three of the most common types of STS—liposarcoma, fibrosarcoma, and rhabdomyosarcoma—occur in similar numbers in men and women. Because of the diverse characteristics of STS, accurate diagnosis can be difficult.

A recent review of U.S. cancer registry data (the SEER program) clarifies many of the difficulties in the classification of the sarcomas (Mack, 1995), and underscores the challenges facing epidemiologic analyses of this cancer.

Summary of *VAO*

The strongest evidence for an association between STS and exposure to phenoxy herbicides comes from a series of case-control studies conducted in Sweden (Hardell and Sandstrom, 1979; Eriksson et al., 1981, 1990; Hardell and

Eriksson, 1988). The studies, involving a total of 506 cases, show an association between STS and exposure to phenoxy herbicides, chlorophenols, or both. The committee concluded that although these studies have been criticized, there is insufficient justification to discount the consistent pattern of elevated risks and the clearly described and sound methods employed. These findings are supported by a significantly increased risk in the NIOSH study (SMR = 9.2, CI 1.9-27.0) for the production workers most highly exposed to TCDD (Fingerhut et al., 1991), and a similar increased risk in the IARC cohort (SMR = 6.1, CI 1.7-15.5) for deaths that occurred between ten and 19 years after the first exposure (Saracci et al., 1991). These are the two largest, as well as the most highly exposed, occupational cohorts. Some studies in other occupational, environmental, and veterans groups showed an increased risk for STS, but the results were commonly nonsignificant, possibly because of small sample sizes (related to the relative rarity of STS in the population). An exception was the significantly elevated risk for males in Zone R of Seveso, which is consistent with the findings supporting an association.

Because of difficulties in diagnosing this group of tumors, the epidemiologic studies reviewed by the committee were inconsistent with regard to the specific types of tumors included in the analyses. The available data did not permit the committee to determine whether specific forms of STS are or are not associated with TCDD and/or herbicides. Therefore, the committee's findings relate to the class of STS as a whole.

Update of the Scientific Literature

Cancer mortality from STS was evaluated in the IARC cohort of 16,863 male and 1,527 female workers in ten countries, who were employed in the production or spraying of pesticides (Kogevinas et al., 1992). Exposure to chlorophenoxy herbicides and chlorophenols was evaluated on the basis of job histories and company questionnaires. Based on four deaths from STS, a nonsignificant twofold increased risk was observed for the total cohort. The deaths occurred ten to 19 years after first exposure (SMR = 6.1, CI 1.7-15.5).

A nested case-control study of STS within the IARC multicountry worker cohort has recently been published (Kogevinas et al., 1995). There were 11 cases of STS and five controls chosen per case. In the full cohort study, Saracci et al. (1991) had detected an elevated risk with a very crude exposure classification. A detailed exposure reconstruction was performed for all cases of STS and a set of controls by a team of industrial hygienists who did not know case or control status (Kauppinen et al., 1994). The team estimated cumulative exposures to TCDD and numerous phenoxy herbicides and related chemicals. There were associations between STS risk and exposure to "any phenoxy herbicide," "any dioxin," and several other definitions of exposure. The authors noted that because many of the workers had multiple exposures and few had single exposures, it is difficult to conclude with confidence that the risk is more strongly associated with any specific exposure in the broad class of phenoxy acids and related compounds. There was evidence of increasing risk with increasing cumulative exposure to several agents, including TCDD, and 2,4-D, a herbicide that does not contain TCDD.

Collins et al. (1993) point out that "All but one of the confirmed STS cases among more than 5000 workers in 12 plants mentioned in the Fingerhut et al. [(1991)] study occurred among the 754 persons in the [Monsanto] study," and, based on a detailed analysis of the exposure histories of the STS cases, argue that the TCDD is unlikely to be responsible and that 4-aminobiphenyl may be.

Several authors have added additional years of follow-up to occupational cohort studies (Bloemen et al., 1993; Lynge, 1993; Asp et al., 1994). Lynge (1993) found the risk of STS similar to that reported in the earlier study of this cohort of Danish herbicide manufacturers (Lynge, 1985). There were five cases of STS observed, versus 2.5 expected (relative risk = 2.0, CI 0.7 to 4.8). When the definition of exposure was restricted to those with at least one year of work in exposed areas, and a ten-year interval was applied between the start of exposure and the start of follow-up time considered to be at risk, there were 3 observed cases, compared to 0.5 cases expected (RR = 6.4, CI 1.3 to 18.7). These workers were engaged in the manufacture of 2,4-D and a related herbicide, 4-chloro-2-methylphenoxyacetic acid (MCPA), but not 2,4,5-T.

Despite additional follow-up, the Bloemen et al. (1993) study of 2,4-D workers was still of insufficient size to be useful for an evaluation of STS. This study was an extension of a cohort mortality study of 878 Dow Chemical Company workers exposed to 2,4-D (Bond et al., 1988). There were no deaths observed from this cancer, and considerably less than one case would have been expected.

Similarly, the Asp et al. (1994) study was too small to be useful for detecting an evaluation in risk of STS. This study was an update of a cancer incidence and mortality study of 1,909 herbicide applicators in Finland (Riihimaki et al., 1982, 1983). The authors noted that with 0.8 cases of STS expected, their study had sufficient power to detect only relative risks of 7.0 or greater with 90 percent confidence.

In the United States a PCMR study was performed for farmers in 23 states, using occupational information from death certificates (Blair et al., 1993). Based on 98 deaths from STS in white male farmers, the PCMR was 0.9 (CI 0.8-1.1). The numbers of deaths due to STS were small and nonsignificant in the other racial and gender groups: nonwhite males and white and nonwhite females.

The Bertazzi et al. (1993) study of cancer incidence at Seveso yielded results similar to those reported in earlier publications from this group and summarized in *VAO* (Bertazzi et al., 1989a,b; Pesatori et al., 1992). In the small, most heavily exposed group (Zone A), there were no cases of STS observed, when the class is defined as those tumors in ICD 171: "malignant neoplasms of connective and other soft tissues." There were two cases of "soft tissue sarcomas of parenchymal origin," which were not included in ICD 171 but which, by some classifications, belong in the group of tumors under consideration (Mack, 1995). It is difficult to evaluate this finding, because of the problem of estimating a comparable expected incidence for the same tumors, but the authors note that 1.4 cases would be expected in this cohort when cancers including ICD 171 and cancers of parenchymal origin are combined. In the larger but less exposed group from Zone B, there were again no cases of ICD 171 cancers observed, while about 0.5 cases were expected. Zone R is the largest group, with considerably lower exposures to TCDD on average. Two cases of STS (ICD 171) were observed in females (RR = 1.6, 95 percent CI 0.3-7.4). In males, six cases were observed, yielding an RR of 2.8 (95 percent CI 1.0-7.3). There appeared to be a trend in increasing risk with increasing duration of residence in Zone R.

A PMR study that examined the causes of death among veterans on the state of Michigan's Vietnam-era Bonus list was recently reported (Visintainer et al., 1995). The mortality rates of 3,364 Vietnam veterans were compared to the morality rates of 5,229 veterans who served elsewhere. Based on eight deaths from STS, the PMR was 1.1 (CI 0.5-2.2). No data were available to identify whether individual Vietnam veterans had been exposed to herbicides.

Summary

The reports issued since the publication of *VAO*, notably the Kogevinas et al. case control study (1995), provide additional evidence for an association between exposure to herbicides and STS.

Conclusions

Evidence is sufficient to conclude that there is a positive association between exposure to the herbicides (2,4-D, 2,4,5-T and its contaminant, TCDD; cacodylic acid; and picloram) and soft-tissue sarcoma. The evidence regarding association is drawn from occupational and other studies in which subjects were exposed to a variety of herbicides and herbicide components.

TCDD has been shown to have a wide range of effects in laboratory animals on growth regulation, hormone systems, and other factors associated with the regulation of activities in normal cells. In addition, TCDD has been shown to cause cancer in laboratory animals at a variety of sites. If TCDD has similar effects on cell regulation in humans, it is plausible that it could have an effect on human cancer incidence. TCDD administration increased fibrosarcoma formation in both rats and mice (NTP, 1982a,b). In contrast to TCDD, there is no convincing evidence of, or mechanistic basis for, the carcinogenicity in animals of any of the herbicides, although they have not been studied as extensively as TCDD.

SKIN CANCERS

Background

Skin cancers are generally divided into two broad categories—malignant melanomas and nonmelanotic skin cancers. According to the American Cancer Society, approximately 34,100 new cases of melanoma (ICD-9 172.0-172.9) were diagnosed in the United States in 1995, and some 7,200 persons died of this cancer (ACS, 1995). The incidence is similar in men and women, but men account for about 60 percent of deaths. Other skin cancers (basal-cell and squamous-cell carcinomas) led to about 800,000 new cases and 2,100 deaths. According to the committee's calculations, assuming that veterans have the same cancer rates as those of the general U.S. population, 486 cases of melanoma were expected among male Vietnam veterans and 1.1 among female veterans in the year 1995. For the year 2000, the expected numbers are 632 cases in male veterans and 1.3 in female veterans. No calculations were made for the very common and highly curable nonmelanotic skin cancers.

Epidemiologic Studies

Most of the epidemiologic studies reviewed in *VAO* did not find an excess risk of skin cancer among TCDD-exposed workers or veterans. These included studies of chemical production workers in the United States and other countries (Suskind and Hertzberg, 1984; Lynge, 1985; Coggon et al., 1986; Bond et al., 1988; Zober et al., 1990; Fingerhut et al., 1991; Manz et al., 1991; Saracci et al., 1991), agricultural workers (Burmeister, 1981; Alavanja et al., 1988; Wigle et al., 1990; Hansen et al., 1992; Ronco et al., 1992), pesticide applicators (Blair, 1983; Swaen et al., 1992), Seveso residents (Pesatori et al., 1992), and Vietnam veterans (Lawrence et al., 1985; Boyle et al., 1987; Breslin et al., 1988; CDC, 1988; Anderson et al., 1986a,b). The lack of association was also seen in a study in which the cohort observed consisted of those with chloracne (Moses et al., 1984). One exception is melanoma mortality following the Seveso accident. Bertazzi et al. (1989a,b) found an elevated risk in males from Zones B and R, but this was based on two and one melanoma deaths, respectively. In addition, the Ranch Hand study (Wolfe et al., 1990) found a relative risk of 1.5 (CI 1.1-2.0) for nonmelanomic skin cancer. One study of agricultural workers in Sweden (Wiklund, 1983) found an elevated risk for skin cancer excluding melanoma (RR = 1.1, 99 percent CI 1.0-1.2), but these results may be confounded by sun exposure in these groups.

One more recent study reviewed by this committee did find an excess risk of skin cancer (Lynge, 1993). Melanoma was studied in employees of two phenoxy herbicide manufacturing facilities in Denmark. There were 1,651 men and 468 women who were judged to have had potential exposure to phenoxy herbicides.

Based on four cases, a statistically significant increase in the risk of melanoma was observed in the subgroup of men who had been employed for at least one year, using a ten-year latency period (SIR = 4.3, CI 1.2-10.9). However, no information is given about the risk in men with less than 10 years of latency and expected numbers for women are not reported so observed elevated risk in the men with 10+ years of latancy cannot be put into context.

In the United States, a PCMR study was performed for farmers in 23 states, using occupational information from death certificates (Blair et al., 1993). Based on 244 deaths from melanoma in white male farmers, the PCMR was 1.0 (CI 0.8-1.1). Based on 425 deaths from other types of skin cancer in white male farmers, the PCMR was 1.1 (CI 1.0-1.2). The numbers for these two types of cancer were very small and nonsignificant for the other racial and gender groups: nonwhite males and white and nonwhite females.

The cancer incidence (including the rates of melanoma and other skin cancers) in the Seveso population was investigated for the first ten years after its potential exposure to TCDD (Bertazzi et al., 1993). No cases of melanoma were reported in Zones A or B. There was also no increase in the risk of nonmelanotic skin cancer in any of the zones. There was no increase in the risk of melanoma in men or women in Zone R, the least contaminated area. These risks were calculated based on only one or two cases, except for Zone R, there were larger numbers of both types of skin cancer.

Three other studies calculated SMRs for skin cancer, all of which were too small to have sufficient statistical power to give definitive results (Asp et al. 1994; Bueno de Mesquita et al., 1993; and Collins et al., 1993). These authors observed zero, one, and one cases of skin cancer, respectively.

Summary

Some of the studies have utilized melanoma as the end point of interest, whereas others have utilized skin cancer, which primarily reflects melanoma. While the studies are fairly evenly distributed between positive and negative studies, one recent study (Lynge et al., 1993) did find an excess risk of skin cancer. Another study also found a significant excess risk in men from the Seveso area (SMR = 3.3), based on only three cases (Bertazzi et al., 1989a,b). The committee felt that these studies, while not even suggestive evidence about an association, undermined the evidence of no association in *VAO*, and thus warranted changing skin cancer from the "limited/suggestive evidence of no association" category to the "inadequate/insufficient evidence to determine whether an association exists" category.

Conclusions

There is inadequate or insufficient evidence to determine whether an association exists between exposure to the herbicides (2,4-D, 2,4,5-T and its contaminant, TCDD; cacodylic acid; and picloram) and skin cancer. The evidence regarding association is drawn from occupational and other studies in which subjects were exposed to a variety of herbicides and herbicide components.

CANCERS OF THE FEMALE REPRODUCTIVE SYSTEM

Background

According to the American Cancer Society, new cases and deaths in the United States in 1995 for each of these cancers were as follows (ACS, 1995):

Site	New Cases	Deaths
Cervix	15,800*	4,800
Corpus uteri	32,800	5,900
Ovary	26,600	14,500
Other genital	5,700	1,200

*Excludes carcinoma in situ (65,000 cases of cervical cancer).

According to the committee's calculations, 1.6 cases of cancer of the uterine corpus were expected among female Vietnam veterans in 1995; For the year 2000, the expected number of cases is 2.8. For cervical cancer, 1.2 cases are expected among female Vietnam veterans in 1995; for the year and in 2000, the expected number of cases is 1.2 cases. For ovarian cancer, 1.5 cases were expected among female Vietnam veterans; for the year 2000, the expected number of cases is 1.9 cases.

Summary of VAO

Studies that examined exposure to herbicides and uterine and ovarian cancers were extremely limited. In a case-control study specifically designed to address the relation between herbicide exposure and risk of ovarian cancer, Donna et al. (1984) compared exposure histories among 60 women with ovarian cancer to controls (women with cancers at other sites, including breast, endometrium, cervix, and other organs). Overall, 18 women with ovarian cancer were classified as definitely or probably exposed, compared to 14 controls, giving an odds ratio of 4.4 (CI 1.9-16.1). These data provide the most direct evidence of an association between herbicides and ovarian cancer.

Bertazzi et al. (1989b) followed the Seveso population for ten years after the 1976 accident. If the TCDD did initiate cancers of female reproductive organs, the elapsed time is probably insufficient for these tumors to have come to clinical attention. In particular, women exposed to TCDD, during adolescence may be at increased risk for cancers that could not be detected for 20 or more years after the exposure.

Other studies examining the association between ovarian or uterine cancer and exposure to herbicides are Wiklund, 1983; Saracci et al., 1991; Ronco et al., 1992.

Update of the Scientific Literature

A cohort study of cancer incidence was conducted among employees of two phenoxy herbicide manufacturing facilities in Denmark (Lynge, 1993). This cohort included 1,071 women who were followed for the period from 1947 to 1987. A statistically significant increase in the risk of cervical cancer was found, based on seven cases (SIR = 3.2; CI 1.3-6.6).

A cohort study of cancer incidence and mortality was conducted among 701 women in the IARC cohort, who were occupationally exposed to chlorophenoxy herbicides, chlorophenols and dioxins (Kogevinas et al., 1993). Of these 701 women, 468 (66 percent) worked at two herbicide plants in Denmark, so there is considerable overlap with the cohort investigated by Lynge (1993). One death was observed from each of the following types of cancer: cervical cancer (SMR = 80); uterus nonspecified (SMR = 192); and ovary (SMR = 74).

Cancer incidence during the first ten years following exposure to TCDD was investigated in the Seveso cohort (Bertazzi et al., 1993). There were no significant increases in the rates of uterine cancer among female residents of Zones A, B, or R, based on two, two, and 21 cases, respectively; the relative risks were 2.6, 0.4, and 0.6, respectively. No cases of ovarian cancer were diagnosed among women in Zones A or B. Based on 20 cases, the relative risk for ovarian cancer in Zone R, the least contaminated area, was 1.1 (CI 0.7-1.7).

In the United States, a PCMR study was performed for farmers in 23 states, using occupational information from death certificates (Blair et al., 1993). Based on 21 deaths from cervical cancer in nonwhite female farmers, the PCMR was significantly elevated at 2.0 (CI 0.3-3.1). This may partially reflect the increased risk for this cancer type among both nonwhite women and women in the lower socioeconomic groups. Based on six deaths from cervical cancer in white female farmers, the PCMR was 0.9 (CI 0.3-2.0). The numbers of deaths from cancer of the uterine corpus were small and nonsignificant for both white and nonwhite female farmers.

The cancer mortality rates among 4,586 female Vietnam veterans were recently evaluated, as well as the rates among 5,325 female veterans who had served elsewhere (Dalager et al., 1995). Based on four cases of cancer of the uterine corpus, the relative risk for Vietnam veterans was 2.1 (CI 0.6-5.4), compared to that of the general U.S. population.

Summary

There has been considerable recent interest in the potential association of exposure to chlorinated hydrocarbons, including TCDD, and female reproductive cancers and other health outcomes in women. For example, teratogenic effects due to maternal exposures to TCDD have been well-documented in experimental animals (see Chapter 3). Endometriosis has recently been demonstrated in monkeys exposed to TCDD (Rier et al., 1993), and research on this disease has been proposed for women in the Seveso cohort (Bois and Eskenazi, 1994). The available epidemiologic evidence, however, is inconclusive. The committee concludes that more research is needed on populations of women with documented exposure to herbicides and TCDD.

Conclusions

There is inadequate or insufficient evidence to determine whether an association exists between exposure to the herbicides (2,4-D, 2,4,5-T and its contaminant, TCDD; cacodylic acid; and picloram) and uterine and ovarian cancers. The evidence regarding association is drawn from occupational and other studies in which subjects were exposed to a variety of herbicides and herbicide components.

BREAST CANCER

Background

Approximately 11 percent of U.S. women will develop breast cancer sometime during their lifetimes. Among U.S. women 40 to 55 years of age, breast cancer is the leading cause of death (U.S. DHHS, 1987). Rates of breast cancer increase rapidly up to the time of menopause. After menopause, incidence rates continue to increase with age but more slowly than before. Long-term increases in incidence rates have been observed. An analysis of SEER data indicates that the incidence of breast cancer increased 4 to 6 percent annually between 1980 and 1987. Only some of the increase can be attributed to more extensive screening and earlier diagnosis (Miller et al., 1991; Harris et al., 1992). Mortality patterns vary by age and race, with decreases seen among white women under age 65 and increases among older white women and black women of all ages (Miller et al., 1992). Earlier detection of tumors and improved treatments have kept increases in mortality lower than increases in incidence.

According to the committee's calculations, assuming that veterans have the same rates of cancer as those as the general U.S. population, 13.2 cases of breast cancer were expected among female Vietnam veterans in 1995. For the year 2000, the expected number of cases is 15.5.

Because of the public health significance of breast cancer, this discussion integrates the studies reviewed in *VAO* with those published more recently.

By far the most common histological type of breast cancer is adenocarcinoma, derived from the epithelium of breast ducts. Lobular carcinoma derived from gland lobule epithelium is a separate category (less than 5 percent of breast cancer). Lobular cancers are usually bilateral and grow very aggressively. Other malignant, although somewhat less invasive, cancers include medullary, mucinous, and tubular carcinomas. Noninvasive carcinomas are found in breast ducts (e.g., comedocarcinoma) and lobules. Intraductal papillomas, another histological variant, are nearly always benign and do not appreciably alter the overall statistics.

Risk factors for breast cancer include early age at menarche, late age at first birth and low parity (or nulliparity), late age at menopause, and family history of breast cancer and personal history of benign cystic breast disease (Henney and DeVita, 1987). Women living in the United States who are of northern European heritage have four to five times more breast cancer than women of Asian heritage living in Asian countries. Dietary factors have been postulated to modify risk, but only alcohol intake is consistently related to increased risk of breast cancer (Henderson, 1991). Investigations into the relationship between stress and breast cancer have not been conclusive. Age is an important modifier of risk, in that exposure to radiation between the onset of menses and first pregnancy creates a greater risk than a similar exposure at older ages.

Epidemiologic Studies

The data relating exposure to herbicides to cancer among women are extremely limited. The committee attempted to examine cancer among women separately from cancer among men. However, compared with the sparse data available for men, data for women are almost nonexistent.

Many studies have excluded women from analysis because of their small numbers in the groups under study. For example, in their follow-up of workers from 12 companies, Fingerhut et al. (1991) identified 67 women who were then excluded from the report. Likewise, Moses et al. (1984) excluded three women from their follow-up analysis of workers, and Zack and Suskind (1980) excluded the one woman who was living at the end of the study. Among the studies that were based on follow-up of workers, women contribute a minor portion of the data, and the results are accordingly even less precise than those reported for men.

Occupational Studies

Manz et al. (1991) describe a retrospective cohort of chemical workers employed in an herbicide plant in Hamburg, Germany. The standardized mortality ratio for breast cancer was elevated, at 2.2 (CI 1.0-4.1). This SMR, however, was based on only nine deaths. Only 7 percent of the women in this study worked in high-exposure departments, and the small number of women precluded separate examination of those with high exposure.

In a study focusing on all persons employed in the manufacture of phenoxy herbicides in Denmark before 1982, Lynge (1985) linked employment records for 1,069 women (contributing 17,624 person-years of follow-up) with the National Cancer Register. Thirteen cases of breast cancer were diagnosed, giving an SMR of 0.9.

As described in Chapter 6, Saracci et al. (1991) have established a study population comprising members of 20 cohorts from ten countries other than the United States who were likely to have had exposure to phenoxy herbicides or TCDD. Among the more than 18,000 workers included in this cohort, 1,527 were women. Follow-up continued for an average of 17 years. It is assumed that the follow-up rates were similar for women and for men, although details are not reported. Among the exposed women, there was one death from breast cancer— a lower mortality rate than expected. Among nonexposed women, four deaths were observed due to breast cancer. This mortality was not significantly different from that expected.

Additional data have been reported by Kogevinas et al. (1993), who identified and followed the subset of women in the IARC cohort who had been occupationally exposed to chlorophenoxy herbicides, chlorophenols, and dioxins (Saracci et al., 1991). Among the 701 women who were followed, 29 cases of cancer were diagnosed. Overall, no increase in total cancer was observed (SIR = 1.0, CI 0.6-1.4). Among those workers exposed to chlorophenoxy herbicides contaminated with TCDD, excess cancer incidence was observed, based on nine cases (SIR = 2.2, CI 1.0-4.2). However, no excess of breast cancer was observed among these 701 women; seven cases resulted in an SIR of 0.9 (CI 0.4-1.9). When the 169 women who were probably exposed to TCDD were analyzed separately, only one case of breast cancer was diagnosed (SIR = 0.9, CI 0.0-4.8).

Among women farm workers in Denmark, the standardized incidence ratios for breast cancer, ovarian cancer, and uterine cancer were all less than 1.0 (Ronco et al., 1992). There were 429 cases of breast cancer diagnosed, and the standardized incidence ratio of 0.8 was significantly less than unity. In this group, the standardized ratios for cervical cancer, uterine cancer, and ovarian cancer were all based on 100 or more cases, and all were significantly less than 1.0. The actual level of exposure of these women to herbicides is not defined, however, and it is possible that the reduced incidence of reproductive cancers reflects general patterns of female cancers seen elsewhere, in which rates are lower for rural than for urban populations.

In a similar occupational study based on census data for economically active women in Sweden (Wiklund, 1983), the SIR for breast cancer was 0.8. This result is not adjusted for reproductive risk factors for these cancers, and the actual exposures of interest are not defined.

In the United States, a PCMR study was performed using death certificate data from male and female farmers from 23 states (Blair et al., 1993). Occupation and industry data were coded based on the information listed on the death certificates. Based on the 71 deaths from breast cancer among white female farmers, the PCMR was 1.0 (CI 0.8-1.3). Based on 30 deaths from breast cancer among nonwhite female farmers, the PCMR was significantly decreased, at 0.7 (0.5-1.0).

In Seveso, one study includes cancer mortality among women (Bertazzi et al., 1989b). The ten-year mortality follow-up provides limited information for women in the high- and medium-exposure groups. Person-years of follow-up were 2,490 in Zone A (high exposure), 16,707 in Zone B, 114,558 in Zone R, and 726,014 in the reference area. There were only three deaths due to any cancer in females in Zone A; therefore, no conclusions are possible. Among the 14 deaths of Zone B women, 5 were due to breast cancer, resulting in a mortality ratio of 0.9 (CI 0.4-2.1). In Zone R, the least contaminated area, 28 women died from breast cancer, giving a significantly reduced estimated relative risk of 0.6 (CI 0.4-0.9).

Cancer incidence in the Seveso cohort during the first ten years following exposure to TCDD was investigated in the Seveso cohort (Bertazzi et al., 1993). One case of breast cancer was diagnosed among women in Zone A (RR = 0.5, CI 0.1-3.3). Among women in Zone B, there were 10 cases of breast cancer diagnosed (RR = 0.7, CI 0.4-1.4). Among women in Zone R, the least contaminated area, there were 106 cases of breast cancer diagnosed (RR = 1.1, CI 0.9-1.3).

Vietnam Veterans Studies

Thomas et al. (1991) assembled a list of female Vietnam veterans and followed them from 1973 to 1987. Cause-specific estimates of mortality risk among women Vietnam veterans relative to those for Vietnam-era veterans who served elsewhere were derived from proportional hazards multivariate models adjusted for rank (officer, enlisted), occupation (nurse, nonnurse), duration of service (at least ten years), age at entry to follow-up, and race. Of these women, 80 percent were classified as officers/nurses, and the majority served between three and 19 years. Slightly more than one-fourth of the cancer deaths were due to breast cancer among the Vietnam veterans. The relative risk was not significantly elevated (RR = 1.2, CI 0.6-2.5) compared to that among the other Vietnam-era veterans.

Cancer mortality rates among 4,586 female Vietnam veterans were recently compared with the rates among 5,325 female veterans who had served elsewhere (Dalager et al., 1995). This extended the follow-up of Thomas et al. (1991) an earlier study for four additional years, through 1991. There were 196 deaths observed among the Vietnam veterans. Based on 26 deaths from breast cancer among the Vietnam veterans, the relative risk was 1.0 (CI 0.6-1.8).

Summary

There have been a few occupational studies, two environmental studies, and two veterans studies of breast cancer among women exposed to herbicides and/or TCDD (Table 7-4). These include four recently published studies (Bertazzi et al., 1993; Blair et al., 1993; Dalager et al., 1995; and Kogevinas et al., 1993). Most of these studies reported a relative risk of approximately 1.0 or less, but it is uncertain whether or not the female members of these cohorts had substantial chemical exposure. TCDD appears to exert a protective effect on the incidence of mammary tumors in experimental animals (see Chapter 3), which is consistent with the tendency for the relative risks to be less than 1.0. In summary, however, the committee believes that there is insufficient evidence to determine whether an association exists between exposure to herbicides and breast cancer.

Conclusions

Strength of Evidence in Epidemiologic Studies

There is inadequate or insufficient evidence to determine whether an association exists between exposure to the herbicides (2,4-D, 2,4,5-T and its contaminant, TCDD; cacodylic acid; and picloram) and breast cancer. The evidence regarding association is drawn from occupational and other studies in which subjects were exposed to a variety of herbicides and herbicide components.

Biologic Plausibility

TCDD has been shown to have a wide range of effects in laboratory animals on growth regulation, hormone systems, and other factors associated with the regulation of activities in normal cells. Although animal data suggest TCDD may act as an antiestrogen, and it has been shown to inhibit growth of breast cancer cell lines in tissue culture, the extrapolation to prevention of breast cancers is plausible, but has not been clearly demonstrated in humans.

PROSTATE CANCER

Background

According to the American Cancer Society, approximately 132,000 new cases of prostate cancer (ICD-9 185) were diagnosed in the United States in 1992, and some 34,000 persons died of prostate cancer (ACS, 1992). According to the committee's calculations, assuming that veterans have the same cancer rates as those in the general U.S. population, 179 cases of prostate cancer were expected

TABLE 7-4 Selected Epidemiologic Studies—Breast Cancer

Reference	Study Population	Exposed Cases[a]	Estimated Risk (95% CI)[a]
Occupational			
Cohort studies			
Ronco et al., 1992	Danish family farm workers	429	0.8 ($p<.05$)
Wiklund, 1983	Swedish economically active agricultural workers	444	0.8 (0.7-0.9)[b]
Donna et al., 1984	Female residents near Alessandria, Italy		
Lynge, 1985	Danish production workers	13	0.9
Manz et al., 1991	German production workers	9	2.2 (1.0-4.1)
Kogevinas et al., 1993	701 women from IARC cohort	7	0.9 (0.4-1.9)
Saracci et al., 1991	IARC cohort	1	0.3 (0.01-1.7)
Blair et al., 1993	Female farmers from 23 states		
	-white	71	1.0 (0.8-1.3)
	-non-white	30	0.7 (0.5-1.0)
Environmental			
Bertazzi et al., 1993[c]	Seveso female residents —Zone A	1	0.5 (0.1-3.3)
	—Zone B	10	0.7 (0.4-1.4)
	—Zone R	106	1.1 (0.9-1.3)
Vietnam Veterans			
Thomas et al., 1991	Women Vietnam veterans	17	1.2 (0.6-2.5)
Dalager et al., 1995[d]	Women Vietnam veterans	26	1.0(0.6-1.8)

[a]Given when available.
[b]99% CI.
[c]This is further follow-up of women included in Bertazzi et al., 1989.
[d]This is further follow-up of women included in Thomas et al., 1991.

among male Vietnam veterans in 1995. For the year 2000, the expected number of cases is 855.

Because this type of cancer is of special interest to the DVA, this discussion integrates the studies reviewed in *VAO* with those published more recently.

One in 11 men develops prostate cancer, and it is the most common cancer in men (excluding skin cancers) and the second leading cause of cancer death (Pienta and Esper, 1993). Increased age is the major risk factor; more than 80 percent of cases occur in men over 65. The incidence of prostate cancer increases sharply at about age 40. Among men 65 and older, it occurs at higher rates than in any other cancer. With advancing age, the incidence of noninvasive prostate cancer increases. The percentage of these that undergo invasive transformation remains unknown. Prostate cancer occurs about twice as often in black men as in to white men. Incidence has increased since 1973 at an annual rate of about 3 percent for whites and about 2 percent for blacks. Between 1985 and 1989, the rate of increase for whites had reached 6 percent per year. Specific causes of prostate cancer are unknown, but associations have been observed with family history of prostate cancer, having had a vasectomy, hormonal factors, a high-fat diet, a history of untreated venereal diseases, multiple sex partners, cigarette smoking, certain occupations, and possibly exposure to ionizing radiation or cadmium (Nomura and Kolonel, 1991; Pienta and Esper, 1993). Improved detection accounts for some of the increase in incidence, but mortality rates are increasing as well. Early detection is the most important consideration for a cure. Hormonal treatment, radiation, and/or surgery remain the methods of choice.

Epidemiologic Studies

Occupational Studies

For prostate cancer, several studies have shown elevated risk in agricultural or forestry workers. Mortality was increased in studies of USDA agricultural extension agents (PMR = 1.5, CI 1.1-2.0) and forest and soil conservationists (PMR = 1.6, CI 1.1-2.0) (Alavanja et al., 1988, 1989). However, subsequent case-control analysis of these deaths showed no increased risk of prostate cancer for ever being an extension agent (OR = 1.0, CI 0.7-1.5) or a soil conservationist (OR = 1.0, CI 0.6-1.8), although the risk was elevated for forest conservationists (OR = 1.6, CI 0.9-3.0). The risk of prostate cancer was more highly elevated for those whose employment ended prior to 1960 and who had worked for at least 15 years as a conservationist (OR = 2.1 for forest workers and 2.9 for soil workers). A case-control study of white male Iowans who died of prostate cancer (Burmeister et al., 1983) found a significant association (OR = 1.2) with farming; this was not connected to a specific agricultural exposure. Higher relative risks were observed after restricting analysis to those born before 1890 (OR = 1.5) and for those age 65 or older (OR = 1.3).

A PCMR study was performed for farmers in 23 states, using occupational information from death certificates (Blair et al., 1993). Based on 3,765 deaths from prostate cancer in white male farmers (total N = 119,648), the PCMR was significantly increased, at 1.2 (CI 1.1-1.2). Based on 564 deaths from prostate cancer in nonwhite male farmers (total N = 11,446), the PCMR was also significantly increased at 1.1 (CI 1.1-1.2). This increased risk for prostate cancer was observed in 22 of the 23 states studied.

In a large cohort study of Canadian farmers, Morrison et al. (1993) found that an increased risk of prostate cancer was associated with herbicide spraying, and the risk was found to rise with increasing number of acres sprayed. For the entire cohort, the relative risk for prostate cancer and spraying at least 250 acres was 1.2 (CI 1.0-1.5). Adjustment for potential confounders showed no evidence of confounding for the association. Additional analyses were restricted to a one-third sample of farmers most likely to be exposed to phenoxy herbicides or other herbicides (RR = 1.3, CI 1.0-1.8 for ≥250 acres sprayed). To focus on farmers who were most likely to be exposed to herbicides, additional analyses were restricted to those with no employees (RR = 1.4, CI 1.0-1.9 for ≥250 acres sprayed); no customary expenses for assisting in work, which might include spraying (RR = 1.6, CI 1.1-2.2 for ≥250 acres sprayed); age between 45-69 years (RR = 1.7, CI 1.1-2.8 for ≥250 acres sprayed); and a combination of the three restrictions (RR = 2.2, CI 1.3-3.8 for ≥250 acres sprayed). For each of these comparisons, a statistical test for trend (increasing risk) over increasing number of acres sprayed was significant.

Other occupational and environmental studies of prostate cancer generally have been consistent. These include studies of chemical production workers in the United States and other countries (Bond et al., 1983; Lynge, 1985; Coggon et al., 1986; Zober et al., 1990), agricultural workers (Burmeister, 1981; Wigle et al., 1990; Ronco et al., 1992), pesticide applicators (Blair, 1983; Swaen et al., 1992), and paper and pulp workers (Robinson et al., 1986; Henneberger et al., 1989; Solet et al., 1989).

Cancer mortality was evaluated for employees of two Dutch companies that produced several chlorophenoxy herbicides; these men were a subgroup of the IARC Registry (Bueno de Mesquita et al., 1993). Mortality rates for 963 exposed and 1,111 nonexposed men were evaluated. Based on three deaths from prostate cancer among the exposed men, the SMR was 2.6 (CI 0.5-7.7).

The mortality experience was evaluated for employees of a Monsanto Company trichlorophenol plant, that had an accidental release of TCDD in 1949 (Collins et al., 1993). The mortality rates in 754 men with varying degrees of exposure to TCDD and 4-aminobiphenyl were compared to rates in the local population. Based on nine deaths from prostate cancer, the SMR was 1.6 (CI 0.7-3.0).

An 18-year prospective follow-up of cancer morbidity and mortality for 1,909 Finnish herbicide applicators was reported (Asp et al., 1994). These employees had previously been identified as being exposed to 2,4-D and 2,4,5-T for at least two weeks between 1955 and 1971 (Riihimaki et al., 1982). The median total duration of exposure was six weeks. Based on five deaths from prostate cancer, the SMR was 0.8 (CI 0.3-1.8). The SIR was 0.9 (CI 0.1-1.3) based on 6 cases.

Environmental Studies

Cancer incidence and mortality were described for the Seveso population in three previous studies (Bertazzi et al., 1989a,b; Pesatori et al., 1992). Cancer incidence for the first ten years after exposure to TCDD was thoroughly updated in the Seveso cohort (Bertazzi et al., 1993). In Zone A and Zone B (the more highly exposed areas), 4 cases of prostate cancer were diagnosed, and the relative risk was 1.4 (0.5-3.9) (Pesatori et al., 1992). In Zone R (the less exposed area), based on 16 cases of prostate cancer (Bertazzi et al., 1993), the relative risk was 0.9 (CI 0.5-1.5).

Vietnam Veterans Studies

Studies of prostate cancer among Vietnam veterans or following environmental exposures have not consistently shown an association (Anderson et al., 1986a,b; Breslin et al., 1988). However, prostate cancer is generally a disease of older men, and the risk among Vietnam veterans might not be detectable yet in epidemiologic studies.

A proportionate mortality study examining causes of death among veterans on the state of Michigan's Vietnam-era Bonus list was recently reported (Visintainer et al., 1995). The cause-specific mortality rates among 3,364 Vietnam veterans were compared with the rates among 5,229 age-matched veterans who had served elsewhere. There were 19 deaths from male genital cancer among the Vietnam veterans (PMR = 1.1, CI 0.6-1.7). Rates for prostatic cancer were not reported separately from testicular cancer.

Summary

Most of the agricultural studies indicate some elevation in risk of prostate cancer. One large, high-quality study in farmers showed an increased risk, and subanalyses in this study indicated that the increased risk is specifically associated with herbicide exposure (Morrison et al., 1993). In addition, a significantly increased risk of prostate cancer was observed in both white and nonwhite farmers in another large study (Blair et al., 1993). The three major studies of production workers (Fingerhut et al., 1991; Manz et al., 1991; Saracci et al., 1991) showed a small, but not statistically significant, elevation in risk. In the NIOSH study, the subcohort with at least 20 years latency and at least one year of exposure had a slightly increased risk, (SMR = 1.5, CI 0.7-2.9) (Fingerhut et al. 1991). Most of the studies used mortality as an outcome, so detection bias is not likely to explain these results. It should be noted, however, that most of the associations are relatively weak (RR < 1.5). Most Vietnam veterans have not yet reached the age when this cancer tends to appear. Results are summarized in Table 7-5.

TABLE 7-5 Selected Epidemiologic Studies—Prostate Cancer

Reference	Study Population	Exposed Cases[a]	Estimated Risk (95% CI)[a]
Occupational			
Cohort studies			
Fingerhut et al., 1991	NIOSH cohort	17	1.2 (0.7-2.0)
	≥20 year latency, ≥1 year exposure	9	1.5 (0.7-2.9)
Bond et al., 1988	Dow 2,4-D production workers	1	1.0 (0.0-5.8)
Coggon et al., 1986	British MCPA production workers	18	1.3 (0.8-2.1)
Lynge, 1985	Danish production workers	9	0.8
Manz et al., 1991	German production workers	7	1.4 (0.6-2.9)
Zober et al., 1990	BASF production workers	0	— (0-7.5)
Saracci et al., 1991	IARC cohort	30	1.1 (0.8-1.6)
Burmeister, 1981	Iowa farmers	1,138	1.1 (*p*<.01)
Morrison et al., 1993	Canadian farmers		
	Age 45-69 years, no employees, or custom workers, sprayed ≥250 acres	20	2.2 (1.3-3.8)
Ronco et al., 1992	Danish self-employed farm workers	399	0.9 (*p*<.05)
Wiklund, 1983	Swedish agricultural workers	3,890	1.0 (0.9-1.0)[b]
Blair, 1983	Florida pesticide applicators	2	0.5
Swaen et al., 1992	Dutch herbicide applicators	1	1.3 (0.0-7.3)
Solet et al., 1989	Paper and pulp workers	4	1.1 (0.3-2.9)
Robinson et al., 1986	Paper and pulp workers	17	1.2 (0.7-2.0)
Henneberger et al., 1989	Paper and pulp workers	9	1.0 (0.7-2.0)
Asp et al., 1994	Finnish herbicide applicators	5	0.8 (0.3-1.8)
Bueno de Mesquita et al., 1993	Dutch Production Workers	3	2.6 (0.5-7.7)
Blair et al., 1993	Farmers in 23 states -whites	3,765	1.2 (1.1-1.2)
	-nonwhites	564	1.1 (1.1-1.2)
Collins et al., 1993	Monsanto 2,4-D production workers	9	1.6 (0.7-3.0)
Case-control studies			
Burmeister et al., 1983	Iowa residents		1.2 (*p*<.05)
Alavanja et al., 1988	USDA agricultural extension agents		1.0 (0.7-1.5)
Alavanja et al., 1989	USDA forest conservationists		1.6 (0.9-3.0)
	Soil conservationists		1.0 (0.6-1.8)
Environmental			
Bertazzi et al., 1993	Seveso male residents - Zone R	16	0.9 (0.5-1.5)
Pesatori et al., 1992	Seveso male residents - Zones A and B	4	1.4 (0.5-3.9)

TABLE 7-5 Continued

Reference	Study Population	Exposed Cases[a]	Estimated Risk (95% CI)[a]
Vietnam veterans			
Breslin et al., 1988	Army Vietnam veterans	30	0.9 (0.6-1.2)
	Marine Vietnam veterans	5	1.3 (0.2-10.3)
Anderson et al., 1986b	Wisconsin Vietnam veterans	2	—
Visintainer et al., 1995	Michigan Vietnam veterans	19	1.1 (0.6-1.7)

[a]Given when available.
[b]99% CI.

Conclusions

There is limited/suggestive evidence of an association between exposure to the herbicides (2,4-D, 2,4,5-T and its contaminant, TCDD; cacodylic acid; and picloram) and prostate cancer. The evidence regarding association is drawn from occupational and other studies in which subjects were exposed to a variety of herbicides and herbicide components.

RENAL, BLADDER, AND TESTICULAR CANCERS

Background

Genitourinary cancers include renal (kidney), bladder, and testicular cancer, as well as prostate cancer. Cancers of the female reproductive organs are discussed in the section on female reproductive cancers. According to the American Cancer Society, approximately 50,500 new cases of bladder cancer (ICD-9 188.0-188.9) and 28,800 new cases of kidney and other urinary cancers (ICD-9 189.0, 189.1) were diagnosed in the United States in 1995, and some 11,200 and 11,700 men and women died of these cancers (ACS, 1995). These cases are slightly more common in men than in women. Unlike breast and cervical cancers, in situ bladder cancers, as well as invasive cancers, are included in these numbers (Miller et al., 1992). According to the committee's calculations, if veterans have rates similar to those of the U.S. population, 374 cases of bladder cancer and 307 cases of renal cancer were expected among male Vietnam veterans and 0.4 and 0.3, respectively, among female veterans in 1995. For the year 2000, the expected numbers are 777 cases of bladder cancer and 497 cases of renal cancer in male veterans and 0.7 cases and 0.6 cases, respectively, in female veterans. For testicular cancer, 117 cases were expected among male Vietnam veterans in 1995, and 86 cases are expected in the year 2000.

RENAL CANCER

Summary of *VAO*

Alavanja et al. (1988, 1989) found excess mortality due to renal cancer in studies of USDA agricultural extension agents (PMR = 2.0, CI 1.2-3.3) and forest and soil conservationists (PMR = 2.1, CI 1.2-3.3). In subsequent case-control studies of these deaths, comparing "ever" versus "never" being an extension agent resulted in a relative risk of 1.7 (CI 0.9-3.3). The relative risk for being a soil conservationist was 2.4 (CI 1.0-5.9) and for being a forest conservationist was 1.7 (CI 0.5-5.5). Other studies of renal cancer have generally produced inconclusive results, in some cases because of small sample sizes. These include studies of chemical production workers in the United States and other countries (Lynge, 1985; Coggon et al., 1986; Bond et al., 1988; Fingerhut et al., 1991; Manz et al., 1991; Saracci et al., 1991), agricultural workers (Burmeister, 1981; Wiklund, 1983; Ronco et al., 1992), pesticide applicators (Blair, 1983), paper and pulp workers (Robinson et al., 1986; Henneberger et al., 1989), the Seveso population (Pesatori et al., 1992), and Vietnam veterans (Anderson et al., 1986a,b; Breslin et al., 1988; Kogan and Clapp, 1985, 1988; Clapp et al., 1991).

Update of the Scientific Literature

A PCMR study was performed using death certificate data from male and female farmers from 23 states (Blair et al., 1993). Occupational data were coded, based on information on the death certificates, and nonfarmers in each state were used as the comparison group. There were 522 deaths due to renal cancer in white males, six deaths in white females, 30 deaths in nonwhite males, and six in nonwhite females. The PCMR among white males was marginally elevated at 1.1 (CI 1.0-1.2). The PCMRs among the other three groups were not significantly different from 1.0.

A case-control study of occupational risk factors and renal cell carcinoma included 365 cases identified from the Denmark Cancer Registry and from pathology records and 396 controls selected from the country's Central Population Registry (Mellemgaard et al., 1994). Detailed occupational histories were obtained, including exposure to herbicides and pesticides. Exposure histories were only considered positive if exposure had lasted more than one year. Based on 13 cases, the odds ratio for men for herbicide exposure was 1.7 (CI 0.7-4.3). Based on three cases, the odds ratio for herbicide exposure for women was 5.7 (CI 0.6-5.8). Because of the wide confidence limits, these data are highly uncertain.

Two other occupational studies reported too few cases of renal cancer to provide substantial information on risk (Asp et al., 1994; Bueno de Mesquita et al., 1993).

Cancer incidence during the first ten years after exposure to TCDD was investigated in the Seveso cohort (Bertazzi et al., 1993). There were no cases of renal cancer diagnosed in Zones A or B, the most heavily exposed areas. Based on ten cases of renal cancer in men in Zone R, the least exposed area, the relative risk was 0.9 (CI 0.4-1.7). Based on seven cases of renal cancer in women in Zone R, the relative risk was 1.2 (0.5-2.7).

A PMR study examining causes of death among veterans on the state of Michigan's Vietnam-era Bonus list was recently reported (Visintainer et al., 1995). This study compared 3,364 Vietnam veterans with 5,229 age-matched veterans who served elsewhere. Based on 21 cases of renal cancer among Vietnam veterans, the PMR was 1.4 (0.9-2.2).

Summary

The studies reviewed since the publication of *VAO* indicate marginally positive results. They are not, however, significant enough to suggest any change in the committee's view that there is inadequate or insufficient evidence to determine whether an association exists between exposure to herbicides and renal cancer.

Conclusions

There is inadequate or insufficient evidence to determine whether an association exists between exposure to the herbicides (2,4-D, 2,4,5-T and its contaminant, TCDD; cacodylic acid; and picloram) and renal cancer. The evidence regarding association is drawn from occupational and other studies in which subjects were exposed to a variety of herbicides and herbicide components.

BLADDER CANCER

Summary of *VAO*

For bladder cancer, Fingerhut et al. (1991) found a small excess in mortality in their study of chemical production workers exposed to TCDD. In the total cohort of 5,172 workers, there was an SMR of 1.6 (CI 0.7-3.0), based on nine cases. In workers with at least one year of employment and 20 years latency, there were four cases (SMR = 1.9, CI 0.5-4.8). Other studies of bladder cancer have produced inconclusive results. Occupational studies include studies of chemical production workers in the United States and other countries (Moses et al., 1984; Suskind and Hertzberg, 1984; Bond et al., 1988; Zober et al., 1990; Saracci et al., 1991), agricultural and forestry workers (Burmeister, 1981;

Alavanja et al., 1988, 1989; Green, 1991; Ronco et al., 1992), pesticide applicators (Blair, 1983), and paper and pulp workers (Robinson et al., 1986; Henneberger et al., 1989). Environmental studies of bladder cancer and herbicide or TCDD exposure include the Pesatori et al. (1992) study of Seveso residents and the Lampi et al. (1992) study of a Finnish community exposed to chlorophenols. Studies in Vietnam veterans examining bladder cancer include the Breslin et al. (1988) study of Army and Marine Corps Vietnam veterans and a study of veterans in Wisconsin (Anderson et al., 1986a,b). On the basis of this evidence, the committee concluded in *VAO* that there was limited/suggestive evidence of *no* association between exposure to herbicides and urinary bladder cancer.

Update of the Scientific Literature

As a subgroup of the IARC cohort, a cohort of workers was identified who manufactured chlorophenoxy herbicides in two factories in the Netherlands (Bueno de Mesquita et al., 1993). Among 963 exposed male workers, there was only one case of bladder cancer (SMR = 1.2, CI 0.0-6.7).

The mortality experience of 754 male production workers at a Monsanto Company plant was evaluated (Collins et al., 1993). One hundred and twenty-two of these workers had developed chloracne as a result of an accidental release of TCDD in 1949. Many of the employees studied were also exposed to 4-aminobiphenyl, a known bladder carcinogen. Based on 16 deaths due to bladder cancer, the SMR was 6.8 (CI 3.9-11.1). Eleven of these cases had documented exposure to 4-aminobiphenyl; therefore, TCDD exposure was not the primary suspected risk factor for them. The SMR was not significantly elevated for the other five cases non exposed to 4-aminobiphenyl.

An 18-year follow-up study of cancer incidence and mortality in 1,909 Finnish herbicide applicators was reported (Asp et al., 1994). These employees had previously been identified as having exposure to 2,4-D and 2,4,5-T (Riihimaki et al., 1982). The median total exposure to herbicides was six weeks. Based on 12 cases of bladder cancer, the SIR was 1.6 (CI 0.8-2.8).

In the United States, a PCMR study was performed for farmers in 23 states, using occupational information from death certificates (Blair et al., 1993). The number of bladder cancer cases among four subgroups of farmers were: 733 among white males, four among white females, 47 among nonwhite males, and three among nonwhite females. None of the four PCMR was not elevated. For example, the PCMR for white males was 0.9 (CI 0.9-1.0). Because of the large sample sizes, the confidence intervals were relatively narrow.

The cancer incidence for the first ten years after potential TCDD exposure was reported for the population in Seveso (Bertazzi et al., 1993). In Zone A, there were two and zero bladder cancers diagnosed in men and women, respectively. In Zone B, there were eight and one bladder cancers diagnosed in men and women, respectively. In Zone R, the least contaminated area, there were 39 and four bladder cancers diagnosed in men and women, respectively. None of these subgroups demonstrated a significant increase in relative risk. These results are very similar to the previous reports on bladder cancer incidence and mortality in the Seveso population (Bertazzi et al., 1989 a,b; Pesatori et al., 1992).

Summary

The additional evidence since publication of *VAO* does not warrant changing the conclusion on bladder cancer and herbicide exposure.

Conclusions

There is limited/suggestive evidence of no association between exposure to the herbicides (2,4-D, 2,4,5-T and its contaminant, TCDD; cacodylic acid; and picloram) and urinary bladder cancer. The evidence regarding association is drawn from occupational and other studies in which subjects were exposed to a variety of herbicides and herbicide components.

TESTICULAR CANCER

Summary of *VAO*

A case-control study of 137 testicular cancer cases and 130 hospital controls (Tarone et al., 1991) found an odds ratio of 2.3 (CI 1.0-5.5) for service in Vietnam. Risk for testicular cancer was not significantly elevated by service branch. In general, the other veteran studies and most of the occupational and environmental studies have shown no association between exposure and outcome, but the sample size of some of these studies may have been too small to detect an elevated risk. Other studies of testicular cancer have generally been inconsistent. These include studies of chemical production workers in the United States and other countries (Bond et al., 1988; Saracci et al., 1991), agricultural workers (Wiklund, 1983; Ronco et al., 1992), residents of Seveso (Pesatori et al., 1992), and Vietnam veterans (Anderson et al., 1986a,b; Boyle et al., 1987; Breslin et al., 1988; Watanabe et al., 1991).

Update of the Scientific Literature

A PCMR study was performed for farmers in 23 states, using occupational information from death certificates (Blair et al., 1993). Based on 32 deaths from testicular cancer in white male farmers, the PCMR was 0.8 (CI 0.6-1.2). Based on six deaths from testicular cancer in nonwhite male farmers, the PCMR was 1.3 (CI 0.5-2.9).

Cancer incidence during the first ten years after exposure to TCDD was investigated in the Seveso cohort (Bertazzi et al., 1993). There were zero and one cases (nonsignificant) of testicular cancer in Zone A and B, respectively. There were nine male cases in Zone R, the least contaminated area (RR = 1.4, CI 0.7-3.0).

A recent case-control study investigated the association between potential Agent Orange exposure and the risk of testicular cancer (Bullman et al., 1994). The subjects were chosen from the DVA's Agent Orange Registry; by definition, all of them were Vietnam veterans. This included 97 veterans with testicular cancer and 311 veterans with no clinical diagnosis recorded on the registry. Risk of testicular cancer was not significantly increased for ground troops, for combat duty, for service in the III Corps area (a heavily sprayed area), or for being close to other areas where Agent Orange was sprayed. Only Navy veterans had a statistically significant increased risk of testicular cancer (OR = 2.6, CI 1.1-6.2), based on 12 cases among 27 Navy veterans. Only one of these 27 Navy veterans served in the "brown water" Navy and may have had Agent Orange exposure due to spraying of riverbanks.

Summary

The new scientific evidence does not warrant changing the conclusions of *VAO* on testicular cancer and herbicide exposure.

Conclusions

There is inadequate or insufficient evidence to determine whether an association exists between the herbicides (2,4-D, 2,4,5-T and its contaminant, TCDD; cacodylic acid; and picloram) and testicular cancer. The evidence regarding association is drawn from occupational and other studies in which subjects were exposed to a variety of herbicides and herbicide components.

BRAIN TUMORS

Background

According to the American Cancer Society, approximately 17,200 new cases of brain and other nervous system cancers (ICD-9 191.0-191.9, 192.0-192.3, 192.8-192.9) were diagnosed in the United States in 1995, and some 13,300 persons died of these cancers (ACS, 1995). These cancers are slightly more common in men than in women. According to the committee's calculations, assuming that veterans have the same cancer rates as those in the general U.S. population, 226 cases of cancers of brain and nervous system were expected among male Vietnam veterans and 0.4 among female veterans in 1995. For the year 2000, the expected numbers are 268 cases in male veterans and 0.4 cases in female veterans.

Summary of *VAO*

A case-control study of gliomas and occupational exposure to chemical carcinogens was conducted in Italy (Musicco et al., 1988). Farmers had an increased risk of gliomas (RR = 1.6, CI 1.1-2.4) compared to all controls; this was found to be associated with the farmers' use of chemicals, including insecticides and herbicides. Another occupational study (Alavanja et al., 1988) found a PMR of 2.1 (CI 1.2-3.7) among USDA agricultural extension agents. A subsequent case-control analysis comparing "ever" versus "never" being an extension agent resulted in an OR of 1.0 (CI 0.4-2.4). A study of Wisconsin veterans (Anderson et al., 1986a) showed an excess risk (RR = 1.6, CI 0.9-2.7). On the other hand, no excess risk of central nervous system tumors has been found among other occupational groups or in other studies.

Other relevant reports on brain cancers included studies of chemical production workers in the United States and other countries (Lynge, 1985; Coggon et al., 1986; Bond et al., 1988; Fingerhut et al., 1991; Saracci et al., 1991), agricultural workers (Burmeister, 1981; Wigle et al., 1990; Morrison et al., 1992; Ronco et al., 1992), pesticide applicators (Blair, 1983; Swaen et al., 1992), paper and pulp workers (Robinson et al., 1986; Henneberger et al., 1989), the Seveso population (Bertazzi et al., 1989a,b; Pesatori et al., 1992), and Vietnam veterans (Lawrence et al., 1985; Anderson et al., 1986a,b; Boyle et al., 1987; Breslin et al., 1988; Thomas and Kang, 1990).

The only epidemiological study in *VAO* that had quantitative exposure measurements on serum TCDD levels was the NIOSH study of occupational workers, who had an estimated mean maximum TCDD level of 1,434 ppt (Fingerhut et al., 1991). Five deaths from brain cancer were observed, compared to an expected number of 7.3 deaths. For workers with more than 20 years latency, two such deaths were observed, compared to an expected number of 3.2.

Update of the Scientific Literature

Since *VAO*, a number of new studies on brain cancer have been published. A PCMR study was performed for farmers in 23 states, using occupational information from death certificates (Blair et al., 1993). No information on individual exposures to herbicides was available. Based on 447 deaths due to brain cancer in white male farmers, the PCMR was marginally increased at 1.2 (CI 1.1-1.3). Based on much smaller numbers of brain cancer deaths, the rates were not elevated in other race and gender groups.

In Finland, an 18-year prospective follow-up of cancer morbidity and mortality for 1,909 herbicide applicators was reported (Asp et al., 1994). These employees had previously been identified as being exposed to 2,4-D and 2,4,5-T for at least two weeks between 1955 and 1971 (Riihimaki et al., 1982). The median total duration of exposure was six weeks. Based on three deaths from brain cancer and eye cancer combined, the SMR was 1.2 (CI 0.3-3.6).

A cohort study of cancer mortality in Ireland was performed using occupation information on death certificates from the years 1971 to 1987 (Dean, 1994). There were 195 and 72 deaths due to brain cancer among men and women in farming occupations, respectively. These numbers were significantly less than the 226.1 and 90.5 deaths expected in men and women due to brain cancer. No specific information on herbicide use was available.

The cancer incidence for the first ten years after potential TCDD exposure was recently published for the Seveso population (Bertazzi et al., 1993). No cases of brain cancer were diagnosed among residents of the more highly contaminated areas (Zones A and B). In the less contaminated area, Zone R, six cases of brain cancer occurred in men (RR = 0.6, CI 0.3-1.4); and six cases of brain cancer occurred in women (RR = 1.4, CI 0.6-3.4).

A PMR study examining causes of death among veterans on the state of Michigan's Vietnam-era Bonus list was recently published (Visintainer et al., 1995). The mortality rates among 3,364 Vietnam veterans were compared with the rates among 5,229 veterans who served elsewhere. Based on 36 deaths due to brain cancer, the PMR was 1.1 (CI 0.8-1.5). There was no information on documented herbicide exposure among the Vietnam veterans.

The cancer mortality rates in 4,586 female Vietnam veterans were compared to the rates in 5,325 female veterans who served elsewhere (Dalager et al., 1995). More than 80 percent of the Vietnam veterans were nurses, so their exposure to herbicides was probably low. Based on four cases of brain cancer, the SMR was 1.4 (CI 0.4-3.7).

Summary

Although the number of cases of brain tumors is small in many studies, it is apparent that the risks associated with herbicide exposure are fairly evenly distributed around the null, and the confidence intervals are relatively narrow.

Conclusions

There is limited/suggestive evidence of no association between exposure to the herbicides (2,4-D, 2,4,5-T and its contaminant, TCDD; cacodylic acid; and picloram) and brain tumors. The evidence regarding association is drawn from occupational and other studies in which subjects were exposed to a variety of herbicides and herbicide components.

MALIGNANT LYMPHOMAS AND MYELOMA

Background

According to the American Cancer Society, approximately 60,900 new cases of lymphomas and myelomas were diagnosed in the United States in 1992, and 30,100 persons died from these cancers. These diseases are slightly more common in men than women. According to the committee's calculations, assuming that veterans have the same cancer rates as those in the general U.S. population, 94 new cases of Hodgkin's disease (HD), 380 new cases of non-Hodgkin's lymphoma (NHL), and 57 new cases of multiple myeloma (MM) were expected among male Vietnam veterans in 1995. Among women Vietnam veterans, a total of 0.8 of all these cancers were expected in 1995. For the year 2000, 109, 494, and 133 cases, respectively, are expected in male veterans and a total of 1.1 cases in female veterans.

NON-HODGKIN'S LYMPHOMA

Summary of *VAO*

Non-Hodgkin's lymphoma includes a group of malignant lymphomas—that is, neoplasms derived from lymphoreticular cells in lymph nodes, bone marrow, spleen, liver, or other sites in the body. One large, well-conducted case-control study in Sweden by Hardell et al. (1981) examined NHL and Hodgkin's disease together and found an odds ratio of 6.0 (CI 3.7-9.7) for exposure to phenoxy acids or chlorophenols, based on 105 cases. These results were replicated in further investigations of the validity of exposure assessment and other potential biases (Hardell, 1981). A more recent case-control study by Persson et al. (1989) showed increased risk for NHL in those exposed to phenoxy acids (OR = 4.9, CI 1.0-27.0), based on a logistic regression analysis of 106 cases. Other studies of farmers and agricultural workers are generally positive for an association between NHL and herbicides/TCDD; however, only some are statistically significant. All of the studies of U.S. agricultural workers reviewed showed elevated relative risks (although none was significant), and two National Cancer Institute studies of farmers in Kansas and Nebraska (Hoar et al., 1986; Zahm et al., 1990) show patterns of increased risk linked to use of 2,4-D. The CDC Selected Cancers Study found an increased risk of NHL in association with service in Vietnam; other studies of veterans, generally with small sample sizes, are consistent with an association. In contrast, studies of production workers—including the largest, most heavily exposed cohorts (Fingerhut et al., 1991; Saracci et al., 1991; Zober et al., 1990; Manz et al., 1991)—indicate no increased risk. Thus, unlike most of the other cancers studied in *VAO* the data did not distinguish between the effects of herbicides and TCDD; rather the data suggested that the phenoxy herbicides (including 2,4-D) rather than TCDD may be associated with non-Hodgkin's lymphomas.

Update of the Scientific Literature

Occupational Studies

Production Studies   Mortality from malignant lymphomas was examined in the IARC registry, which included 18,390 production workers or sprayers from 10 countries (Kogevinas et al., 1992). Exposure to chlorophenoxy herbicides and chlorophenols was evaluated from job histories and company records. Mortality from NHL among 13,898 workers who were classified as exposed or probably exposed to these chemicals was not elevated, based on 11 deaths (SMR = 1.0, CI 0.5-1.7). No difference in risk was seen in relation to potential exposure to TCDD, based on history of exposure to 2,4,5-T or 2,4,5-trichlorophenol.

A nested case-control study of 32 cases of NHL and 158 controls was performed, using the IARC registry (Kogevinas et al., 1995), which at the time contained information on 21,183 workers in 11 countries. Exposure to 21 chemicals or mixtures was estimated by industrial hygienists who evaluated individual job histories. None of the exposures was significantly associated with an increased risk of NHL, but there was a threefold increased risk in subjects with medium or high exposure to 2,4,5-T or TCDD. The odds ratio was 1.9 for any exposure to 2,4,5-T (CI 0.7-4.8) and 1.9 for any exposure to TCDD (CI 0.7-5.1). These results run counter to the trend discussed in *VAO* that suggested that 2,4-D rather than TCDD may be associated with NHL.

Two other studies focused on subgroups of production workers in the IARC registry. In the Netherlands, Bueno de Mesquita and colleagues (1993) demonstrated a nonsignificant increased risk of NHL among workers exposed to herbicides based on 2 deaths (SMR = 3.0, CI 0.4-10.8). In Denmark, Lynge (1993) found an increased but nonsignificant risk of NHL among male workers exposed to herbicides based on 10 incident cases (SIR = 1.7, CI 0.5-4.5), but no increase when men and women are combined (figures not given). Similarly, an update of mortality among 878 Dow Chemical workers exposed to 2,4-D demonstrated a nonsignificant increased risk of NHL, based on 2 cases (SMR = 2.0; CI 0.2-7.1) (Bloemen et al., 1993). All of these studies were limited by low statistical power.

Agricultural/Forestry Workers   The mortality experience from NHL was recently evaluated for 155,547 male farm operators in Saskatchewan, Manitoba, and Alberta (Morrison et al., 1994). Overall, the observed number of deaths from NHL was significantly lower than expected (SMR = 0.8, CI 0.7-0.9). There was no association between the number of acres sprayed with herbicides in 1970 and the relative risk of NHL. For farm operators who lived on the same farm in both 1971 and 1981, an increased risk of NHL mortality was associated with the number of acres sprayed with herbicides in 1970. The relative risk for the highest quartile of acres sprayed, 380 acres or more, was 2.1 (CI 1.1-3.9). The relative risk for the highest quartile of spraying for both 1970 and 1980, relative to farmers who reported no herbicide spraying in either 1970 or 1980, was 3.0 (CI 1.1-8.1). Because this was a cohort study and the health and agricultural data were collected by separate agencies, the risk of recall bias on the use of herbicides was reduced.

In the United States, a PCMR study was performed for farmers in 23 states, using occupational information from death certificates (Blair et al., 1993). Based on 843 deaths from NHL in white male farmers, the PCMR was significantly increased, at 1.2 (CI 1.1-1.3). Twenty states had two or more deaths from NHL; 15 of these states, a statistically significant proportion, had PCMRs greater than 1.0. The numbers of deaths due to NHL were small and did not significantly increase in other race and gender subgroups.

A cohort study of cancer mortality in Ireland was performed using occupational information on death certificates from the years 1971 to 1987 (Dean, 1994). Among men in farming occupations, there were 244 deaths due to all lymphomas combined, a significantly decreased risk compared to the 265.7 deaths expected. Among women in farming occupations, there were 84 deaths from all lymphomas, compared to 88.9 expected.

An 18-year follow-up study of cancer incidence in 1,909 Finnish herbicide applicators was recently reported (Asp et al., 1994). The median total duration of exposure to herbicides, including 2,4-D and 2,4,5-T, was six weeks. There was only one case of NHL diagnosed (SIR = 0.4, CI 0.0-2.0).

A recent Swedish case-control study compared the occupational histories of 93 men who were diagnosed with NHL between 1975 and 1984 with 204 male control subjects (Persson et al., 1993). Based on ten cases and 14 controls, logistic regression analysis revealed an odds ratio of 2.3 for a history of exposure to phenoxy herbicides for at least one year (90 percent CI 0.7-7.2). Work as a lumberjack was significantly associated with the risk of NHL (OR = 6.0, 90 percent CI 1.1-31.0), but there was no association with exposure to chlorophenols or creosote, which are used as wood preservatives.

Another Swedish case-control study compared the occupational histories of 105 cases who were diagnosed with NHL between 1974 and 1978 with 335 control subjects (Hardell et al., 1994). Previously published data (Hardell et al. 1981) that had combined both types of lymphomas was reanalyzed by removal of the data on Hodgkin's disease. Exposure to phenoxyacetic acids was reported by 25 cases and 24 controls (OR = 5.5, CI 2.7-11.0). Most of these 49 individuals had been exposed to a combination of 2,4-D and 2,4,5-T. Thirty-five cases and 35 controls reported exposure to chlorophenols (OR = 4.8, CI 2.7-8.8). An increased risk due to exposure to either class of chemical was found for all histological subtypes of NHL, according to the Rappaport classification.

A population-based case control study conducted in eastern Nebraska compared the occupational histories of 184 women diagnosed with NHL with 707 control subjects (Zahm et al., 1993). The risk of NHL was not increased in women who had ever lived or worked on a farm (OR = 1.0, CI 0.7-1.4). No class of herbicide, whether used on the farm or personally handled, was associated with a significantly increased risk of NHL. Only a few women, however, reported personally handling herbicides (four cases and 11 controls).

Environmental Studies

Cancer incidence during the first ten years after potential exposure to TCDD was investigated in the Seveso cohort (Bertazzi et al., 1993). No cases of NHL were found in the most heavily exposed population residing in Zone A; only 0.4 cases were expected. For women in Zone B, the relative risk of NHL was 0.9 (CI 0.1-6.4), based on one case. For men in Zone B, the corresponding relative risk was 2.3 (CI 0.7-7.4), based on three cases. Larger numbers of cases were found in the lower-exposed and much larger Zone R population. Relative risks for NHL were 1.2 (CI 0.6-2.3) in women, based on ten cases, and 1.3 (CI 0.7-2.5) in men, based on 12 cases.

Vietnam Veterans Studies

A PMR study that examined the causes of death among veterans on the state of Michigan's Vietnam-era Bonus list was recently published (Visintainer et al., 1995). The mortality rates of 3,364 Vietnam veterans were compared to the mortality rates of 5,229 veterans who served elsewhere. No data were available to identify whether individual veterans had been exposed to herbicides. Based on 32 deaths from NHL, the PMR was significantly increased, at 1.5 (CI 1.0-2.1).

Summary

The recent scientific literature continues to support the conclusion that there is a positive association between exposure to herbicides and non-Hodgkin's lymphoma.

Conclusions

Evidence is sufficient to conclude that there is a positive association between exposure to the herbicides (2,4-D, 2,4,5-T and its contaminant, TCDD; cacodylic acid; and picloram) and non-Hodgkin's lymphoma. The evidence regarding association is drawn from occupational and other studies in which subjects were exposed to a variety of herbicides and herbicide components.

HODGKIN'S DISEASE

Summary of *VAO*

Hodgkin's disease, also a malignant lymphoma, is a neoplastic disease characterized by painless, progressive enlargement of lymph nodes, spleen, and general lymphoid tissues. Fewer studies have been conducted of HD in relation to exposure to herbicides or TCDD than have been conducted of soft-tissue sarcoma or non-Hodgkin's lymphoma, but the pattern of results is strikingly consistent. The 60 HD cases in the study by Hardell et al. (1981) were later examined by Hardell and Bengtsson (1983), who found odds ratios of 2.4 (CI 0.9-6.5) for low-grade exposure to chlorophenols and 6.5 (CI 2.7-19.0) for high-grade exposures. The study by Persson et al. (1989) of 54 HD cases showed a large, but not statistically significant, OR of 3.8 (CI 0.5-35.2) for exposure to phenoxy acids. Furthermore, nearly all of the 13 case-control and agricultural worker studies show increased risk for HD, although only a few of these results are statistically significant for HD. As with NHL, even the largest studies of production workers exposed to TCDD do not indicate an increased risk. The few studies of HD in Vietnam veterans tend to show elevated risks; all but one are statistically insignificant.

Update of the Scientific Literature

Occupational Studies

Mortality from malignant lymphomas was examined in the IARC registry, which included 18,390 production workers or sprayers from ten countries (Kogevinas et al., 1992). Among the 13,898 workers classified as exposed or probably exposed to chlorophenoxy herbicides or chlorophenols, there were three deaths from HD (SMR = 0.6, CI 0.1-1.7). One of these deaths occurred in a female employee (Kogevinas et al., 1993).

In the United States, a PCMR study was performed for farmers in 23 states, using occupational information from death certificates (Blair et al., 1993). Based on 56 deaths due to HD among white male farmers, the PCMR was 1.0 (CI 0.8-1.3). The numbers of deaths due to HD were very small and nonsignificant for the other race and gender subgroups.

An 18-year follow-up study of cancer incidence in 1,909 Finnish herbicide applicators was recently reported (Asp et al., 1994). The median total duration of exposure to herbicides, including 2,4-D and 2,4,5-T, was six weeks. Two cases of HD were diagnosed (SIR = 1.7, CI 0.2-6.0).

A recent Swedish-case control study compared the occupational histories of 31 men who were diagnosed with HD with 204 male control subjects (Persson et al., 1993). Five cases and 14 controls reported a history of at least one year of exposure to phenoxy herbicides, which yielded a significantly increased adjusted odds ratio of 7.4 (90 percent CI 1.4-40.0).

Environmental Studies

Cancer incidence during the first ten years after exposure to TCDD was investigated in the Seveso cohort (Bertazzi et al., 1993). No HD cases were reported among residents in Zone A, which was the most heavily contaminated but had the smallest population. Among women in Zone B, one HD case occurred (RR = 2.1, CI 0.3-15.7); among men in Zone B, one HD case occurred (RR = 1.7, CI 0.2-12.8). Among women residents of Zone R, the zone with the lowest exposure, three cases of HD occurred (RR = 1.0, CI 0.3-3.2); there were four cases in men (RR = 1.1, CI 0.4-3.1). This study, which has one of the highest documented human exposures to TCDD, is limited by the relatively small size of the population in Zone A and by a short period of follow-up.

Vietnam Veterans Studies

A recent PMR study examined the causes of death among veterans on the state of Michigan's Vietnam-era bonus list (Visintainer et al., 1995). The mortality rates were compared between 3,364 Vietnam veterans and 5,229 veterans who served elsewhere. No data were available to identify whether individual veterans had been exposed to herbicides. Based on 20 deaths from HD, the PMR was not significantly elevated, at 1.1 (CI 0.7-1.8).

Summary

The recent scientific evidence continues to support the conclusions of a positive association between exposure to herbicides and Hodgkin's disease.

Conclusions

Evidence is sufficient to conclude that there is a positive association between exposure to the herbicides (2,4-D, 2,4,5-T and its contaminant, TCDD; cacodylic acid; and picloram) and Hodgkin's disease. The evidence regarding association is drawn from occupational and other studies in which subjects were exposed to a variety of herbicides and herbicide components.

MULTIPLE MYELOMA

Background

Because *VAO* classified multiple myeloma in the category of limited/suggested evidence of an association with exposure to herbicides, this discussion integrates the studies reviewed in *VAO* with those published more recently.

Multiple myeloma (MM) is characterized by proliferation of bone marrow stem cells that results in an excess of neoplastic plasma cells and the production of excess abnormal proteins, usually immunoglobulins. Identification of these proteins in the blood or urine (especially Bence-Jones protein) represents the best diagnostic feature of this disease. Multifocal aggregates of plasma cells in bone result in destructive "punched-out" bone lesions. Renal deposits of myeloma cells (interstitial infiltrates) occur in about 75 percent of cases.

The incidence of MM has changed little since 1973. The incidence is very low in people under age 40. Incidence reaches a peak at age 70 and older. Mortality rates have shown a small but steady increase of about 1.5 percent per year. Rates for blacks are about twice those for whites. Risk factors for MM remain unclear. Links to exposure to ionizing radiation have been suggested by studies of Japanese atomic bomb survivors (Higami et al., 1990), U.S. radiologists (Matanoski et al., 1975), and workers who made radium dials in watches (Stebbings et al., 1984). Increases in MM deaths have also been seen in those engaged in farming and agricultural work and in cases of nonspecific occupational exposure to metals, rubber, leather, paint, and petroleum (Riedel et al., 1991). The evidence for an association with immune suppressive diseases is mixed. One new study indicates an increased risk in association with such conditions as allergies, rheumatoid arthritis, and rheumatic fever (Riedel et al., 1991). This study also suggests that genetic factors may be involved (Riedel et al., 1991).

Epidemiologic Studies

A substantial number of studies have investigated associations between multiple myeloma and occupation or exposure to specific agents. Many of these studies have found an association with farming. Unfortunately, most such studies did not further investigate specific farm exposures. Among those studies that did, an association with herbicide use, exceeding that of the category of farming, was found in some but not all cases.

Occupational Studies

Production Workers Two studies dominate the data on the exposure of production workers to phenoxy acids and TCDD: a study by Fingerhut et al. (1991) in the United States and a study by Saracci et al. (1991) elsewhere. In the U.S. cohort (Fingerhut et al., 1991), 1,052 deaths occurred, five of which were due to MM; 3.0 deaths were expected (SMR = 1.6, CI 0.5-3.9). Three deaths occurred in the group with 20 years or more latency and with more than one year of exposure, yielding an SMR of 2.6 (CI 0.5-7.7). No MM deaths occurred in a separate study by Bond et al. (1988) of 878 2,4-D production workers at a Dow Chemical Company plant. The expected number of MM deaths, however, would have been less than 0.4.

Four MM deaths were reported in the Saracci et al. (1991) analysis of non-U.S. cohorts of workers engaged in the production and spraying of phenoxy herbicides or of compounds contaminated with TCDD. The SMR was 0.7 (CI 0.2-1.8). However, data on two of the 20 cohorts, comprising 3,544 of the 13,482 workers studied by Saracci et al., were published separately by Coggon et al. (1986). For this work force that manufactured or sprayed the phenoxy herbicide MCPA, Coggon and colleagues listed 5 deaths from MM, compared to 3.1 expected. One of these deaths was for an individual with only background exposure. The overall SMR was 1.6 (CI 0.5-3.8). The SMR for greater than 10 years latency was 2.3 and for the longest duration category, more than six months exposure, the SMR was 2.7. The apparent absence of MM deaths in the remainder of the Saracci group has no immediate explanation but may reflect a long latency for a cancer that occurs most commonly among the elderly (age 70 or older). Lynge (1993) found an increased risk of MM (SMR = 12.5, CI 0.6-45.1) among the women in a Danish cohort of production workers in the IARC registry, but there were no cases of MM among men. The observed elevated risk among women cannot be put into context because the expected number of cases for the entire cohort (men in particular) is not reported.

No MM deaths were observed in a group of workers exposed to TCDD from an accident that occurred in a BASF plant (Zober et al., 1990). However, fewer than 0.2 would be expected. A group of phenoxy herbicide production workers in the Netherlands was studied by Bueno de Mesquita et al. (1993). No MM deaths were observed; 0.8 was expected.

Summary of Production Worker Studies   There is some limited evidence in the Fingerhut and colleagues (1991) study of a relationship between exposure to TCDD and development of MM, which is not present in the Saracci et al. (1991) study. However, only seven or eight deaths from MM are known to have occurred among all U.S. and foreign chemical production workers. Further, uncertainties regarding exposure to TCDD exist in the study of Saracci and colleagues.

Agricultural/Forestry Workers   Table 7-6 summarizes the principal results of studies of MM and agricultural and forestry workers.

Multiple myeloma was investigated in analyses of the mortality of USDA forest and soil conservationists (Alavanja et al., 1989). The analyses produced a PMR of 1.3 (CI 0.5-2.8). There was a nonsignificant trend in increased risk of MM associated with duration of work as a conservationist. A similar analysis was conducted by Alavanja et al. (1988) of USDA agricultural extension agents, but the uncertainty introduced by other possible MM farm-related risk factors would apply; other potentially confounding risk factors are less likely with the forestry/soil conservationists.

Among studies of farming populations potentially exposed to herbicides was a nested case-control analysis of MM among subjects enrolled in the prospective, nationwide Cancer Prevention Study of the American Cancer Society (Boffetta et al., 1989). From an analysis of 282 MM cases and 1,128 controls, an odds ratio of 2.1 (CI 1.0-4.2) was obtained for any exposure to pesticides and herbicides. For herbicide use among farmers, the odds ratio was 4.3 (CI 1.7-10.9); farmers reporting no exposure to herbicides or pesticides had an odds ratio of 1.7 (CI 0.8-4.0). A logistic regression analysis with six occupations and 15 risk factors produced an odds ratio of 1.6 (CI 0.7-3.7) for herbicides/pesticides.

Burmeister (1981) found an increased SMR of 1.5 (p < .01) and an increased PMR of 1.3 (p < .01) among white male farmers in Iowa. The PMR for deaths among these under age 65 was substantially greater than for those 65 or older (1.7 versus 1.2). This difference might be due to such factors as a greater exposure of younger farmers to carcinogenic agents and a "healthy worker effect" for nonmalignant deaths among younger farmers. In an extension of this study, a case-control analysis was undertaken (Burmeister et al., 1983), using other causes of death, to evaluate the effect of herbicide usage. The overall odds ratio for farmers with MM was 1.5. The results showed odds ratios of 1.8, 2.7, and 2.4, respectively, for deaths of farmers born before 1890, from 1890 to 1900, and after 1900 in the 33 counties with highest herbicide use. The odds ratios for birth cohorts from 1890 to 1900 and after 1900 were statistically significant and lend support to an herbicide-related association, because younger farmers are more likely to have used herbicides than older farmers. Analyses also showed significantly increased odds ratios for counties that have high levels of egg-laying chickens, hog production, and insecticide use.

Among the more recent studies reviewed, Brown et al. (1993) is of particular importance. It is a case-control study of farm herbicide and pesticide use in Iowa. The area had been studied previously by Burmeister et al. (1981, 1983), but these studies lacked information on individual usage of specific pesticides. The newer study, which compared 173 white males who had been diagnosed with MM with 650 controls, found a relative risk of only 1.2 (CI 0.8-1.7) for farmers who reported using either herbicides or pesticides. This is to be compared with the earlier study by Burmeister et al. that found risks for farmers of 1.8 to 2.7, based on data from the counties with highest herbicide usage. Analyses by specific types of herbicides did not reveal any of them to be associated with a significantly increased risk of MM. A negative correlation was observed between MM risk and number of years farmed.

Cantor and Blair (1984) investigated the association of MM with farming and herbicide use in Wisconsin. Farmers had an odds ratio of 1.4 (CI 1.0-1.8) compared with nonfarmers. Among the 15 counties in which herbicides were

TABLE 7-6   Selected Epidemiologic Studies—Multiple Myeloma

Reference	Study Population	Exposed Cases[a]	Estimated Risk (95% CI)[a]
Occupational			
Cohort studies			
Fingerhut et al., 1991	NIOSH cohort	5	1.6 (0.5-3.9)
	20 years latency, 1+ years exposure	3	2.6 (0.5-7.7)
Saracci et al., 1991	IARC cohort	4	0.7 (0.2-1.8)
Alavanja et al., 1989	USDA forest/soil conservationists		1.3 (0.5-2.8)
Swaen et al., 1992	Dutch herbicide applicators	3	8.2 (1.6-23.8)
Asp et al., 1994	Finnish herbicide applicators	3	2.6 (0.5-7.7)
Semenciw et al., 1993	Farmers in Canadian prairie provinces	160	0.8 (0.7-1.0)
Dean, 1994	Irish farmers	170	1.0
Lynge, 1993	Danish production workers		
	Male	0	—
	Female	2	12.5 (1.5-45.1)
Blair et al., 1993	Farmers from twenty-three states		
	White males	413	1.2 (1.0-1.3)
	White females	14	1.8 (1.0-3.0)
	Non-white males	51	0.9 (0.7-1.2)
	Non-white females	11	1.1 (0.6-2.0)
	Farmers in central US states		
	White males	233	1.2
	White females	12	2.6
Case-control studies			
Boffetta et al., 1989	ACS Prevention Study II subjects	12	2.1 (1.0-4.2)
	Farmers using herbicides or pesticides	8	4.3 (1.7-10.9)
Burmeister et al., 1983	Iowa residents		
	Farmers in counties with highest herbicide usage		
	Born 1890-1900		2.7 ($p<.05$)
	Born after 1900		2.4 ($p<.05$)
Cantor and Blair, 1984	Wisconsin residents		
	Farmers in counties with highest herbicide usage		1.4 (0.8-2.3)
Morris et al., 1986	Residents of four SEER areas		2.9 (1.5-5.5)
Eriksson and Karlsson, 1992	Residents of northern Sweden	20	2.2 (1.0-5.7)
Pearce et al., 1986	Male residents of New Zealand		
	Use of agricultural spray	16	1.3 (0.7-2.5)
	Likely sprayed 2,4,5-T	14	1.6 (0.8-3.1)
LaVecchia et al., 1989	Residents of the Milan, Italy, area		
	Agricultural employment		2.0 (1.1-3.5)

TABLE 7-6 Selected Epidemiologic Studies—Multiple Myeloma

Reference	Study Population	Exposed Cases[a]	Estimated Risk (95% CI)[a]
Zahm et al., 1992	Eastern Nebraska users of herbicides		
	Male	8	0.6 (0.2-1.7)
	Female	10	2.3 (0.8-7.0)
	Eastern Nebraska users of insecticides		
	Male	11	0.6 (0.2-1.4)
	Female	21	2.8 (1.1-7.3)
Brown et al., 1993	Iowa male users of pesticides or herbicides	111	1.2 (0.8-1.7)
Environmental Studies			
Bertazzi et al., 1993	Seveso residents		
	Zone A - male	0	—
	Zone A - female	0	—
	Zone B - male	2	3.2 (0.8-13.3)
	Zone B - female	2	5.3 (1.2-22.6)
	Zone R - male	1	0.2 (0.0-1.6)
	Zone R - female	2	0.6 (0.2-2.8)

[a]Given when available.

used on the most acres, the odds ratio for farmers was also 1.4 (CI 0.8-2.3), suggesting no special herbicide-related risk.

A case-control study of herbicide and insecticide use by Nebraska residents presented some unusual results (Zahm et al., 1992). The odds ratios for use of either herbicides or insecticides was 0.6 for men. But, for women, the odds ratio for herbicide use was 2.3 (C.I = 0.8-7.0) and 2.8 (CI 1.1-7.3). The observed gender-related effect is interesting, but given that relatively few cases were considered, it may be the result of chance and requires confirmation by other studies. It is noteworthy that the comparison category, nonfarmers, contained only seven female cases.

In another U.S. study that examined farm use of herbicides in relation to the risk of cancer, Morris et al. (1986) used data from cancer registries in Washington, Utah, metropolitan Detroit, and metropolitan Atlanta. Results indicated an adjusted odds ratio of 2.6 (CI 1.5-4.6) for exposure to pesticides when data from all cases and controls were used. When only self-respondent interviews were used, the adjusted odds ratio was 2.9 (CI 1.5-5.5); the only other exposures with odds ratios in which the confidence intervals did not include 1.0 were to paints or solvents, metals, and carbon monoxide. The odds ratio for having lived on a farm was 1.3 (CI 1.0-1.6). Explicit exposure to herbicides gave an odds ratio of 4.8 but was based on only four cases.

A proportionate mortality study by Blair et al. (1993), which included 23 states, demonstrated a slightly increased risk of MM among white male farmers. Based on 413 deaths due to MM, the PMR was 1.2 (CI 1.0-1.3). However, no information was available on herbicide usage by individuals or groups. Twenty states had two or more deaths from MM; of these, 15 states had a PMR for MM that was greater than 1.0. This is a significant proportion of states. The numbers of deaths due to MM was small and nonsignificant in other racial and gender groups.

A cohort study of cancer mortality in Ireland was performed using death certificate information from the years 1971 to 1987 (Dean, 1994). There were 170 deaths due to multiple myeloma among men in farming occupations, which was less than the 177.9 deaths expected. There were 72 deaths due to MM among women in farming occupations, which was slightly more than the 67 deaths expected.

A cohort of 155,547 male farmers in Saskatchewan, Manitoba, and Alberta was followed from 1971 to 1987 (Semenciw et al., 1993). Based on 160 deaths due to MM, the SMR for farmers was significantly decreased at 0.8 (CI 0.7-1.0). There was a small, nonsignificant increase in risk of MM among farmers who had reported using herbicides in 1970.

In New Zealand, two studies by Pearce et al. (1985, 1986) found no evidence of an association between MM and herbicide exposure. In the initial study (Pearce et al., 1985), odds ratios for agricultural employment were 2.2 (CI 1.3-3.8) for MM cases identified at 20 to 64 years of age and 1.3 (CI 0.8-2.0) for cases identified over age 64, compared with correspondingly aged cases of other cancer in the New Zealand cancer registry during the period 1977-81. These odds ratios were the highest found in this study, which also considered NHL and HD, but no individual data on exposure to herbicides were given. However, in a follow-up case-control study (Pearce et al., 1986), interviews and a detailed questionnaire on use of herbicides were completed. The study produced an odds ratio of 1.7 (CI 1.0-2.9) for MM in relation to farming, an odds ratio of 1.3 (CI 0.7-2.5) for any agricultural use of chemical spray, and an odds ratio of 1.6 (CI 0.8-3.1) for spraying of specific plants on which phenoxy herbicides (specifically 2,4,5-T) are generally used. Potential exposure to chlorophenols found in wood preservatives used in fencing work gave an odds ratio of 1.6 (CI 0.9-2.7), and potential exposure in a sawmill gave an odds ratio of 1.4 (CI 0.5-3.9) for sawmill workers or timber merchants, although the odds ratio for explicit exposure to chlorophenols was 1.1 (CI 0.4-2.7), based on six cases.

Eriksson and Karlsson (1992) undertook a case-control study of MM in relation to occupation and exposures in northern Sweden between 1982 and 1986. An odds ratio of 1.7 (CI 1.2-2.6) was found for farmers and an odds ratio of 2.2 (CI 1.0-5.7) for exposure to phenoxy herbicides. An analysis by the number of days that phenoxyacetic acid was used showed no clear trend with exposure; the odds ratio for each of three exposure categories was 2.0 or greater.

In a multivariate analysis involving 22 exposure factors, the odds ratio for phenoxyacetic acids was 1.9 (CI 0.7-5.7). The multivariate analysis eliminated the raising of sheep, hogs, and poultry as risk factors and decreased the odds ratio for raising horses, cattle, and goats.

A case-control study of MM was undertaken in the region surrounding Milan, Italy, by LaVecchia et al. (1989). A multivariate regression analysis with terms for age, gender, area of residence, and smoking gave a relative risk of 2.0 (CI 1.1-3.5) among those employed in agriculture. An 18-year follow-up study of cancer incidence and mortality in 1,909 Finnish herbicide applicators was reported (Asp et al., 1994). These employees had previously been identified as having exposure to 2,4-D and 2,4,5-T (Riihimaki et al., 1983). The median total duration of exposure to herbicides was six weeks. Based on three deaths from MM, the SMR was 2.6 (CI 0.5-7.7). The SIR was 1.5 (CI 0.2-5.2) based on 2 cases.

A Dutch study by Swaen et al. (1992) observed three deaths from MM among licensed herbicide applicators (0.4 was expected), yielding an SMR of 8.2 (CI 1.6-23.8). Another small study of Canadian herbicide applicators (Green 1991) found no deaths from MM. However, only about 0.3 deaths would have been expected.

Summary of Agricultural/Forestry Worker Studies   Several studies of agricultural and forestry workers provide specific information on MM risk in relation to herbicide or pesticide exposure. Most studies demonstrated an odds ratio or SMR greater than 1.0, nine did so at a statistically significant level.

Paper/Pulp Workers   Three studies of pulp and paper workers observed that some cohort members may have had exposure to low levels of dioxins (Robinson et al., 1986; Henneberger et al., 1989; Solet et al., 1989). Grouping MM from these studies with lymphomas other than lymphosarcoma, reticulum cell sarcoma, and Hodgkin's disease resulted in a combined number of four cases; 4.4 were expected.

Environmental Studies

Cancer incidence for the Seveso cohort during the first ten years following exposure to TCDD was reported in more detail by Bertazzi et al. (1993). There were no cases of MM in Zone A. In Zone B, there were two cases of MM among men, a nonsignificant increase (RR = 3.2, CI 0.8-13.3). There were also two cases of MM among women in Zone B, a significant increase (RR = 5.3, CI 1.2-22.6). There was a deficit of MM cases in Zone R, the least exposed area, based on one case in men and two cases in women, (RR = 0.2 in men and 0.6 in women).

Vietnam Veterans Studies

The major study of multiple myeloma among veterans is the DVA's proportionate mortality study by Breslin et al. (1988). The authors found a PMR of 0.8 (CI 0.2-2.5) for Army Vietnam veterans and a PMR of 0.5 (CI 0.0-17.1) for Marine veterans (the latter was based on two cases). Each group was compared to Vietnam-era veterans of the same service. No MMs were noted in the CDC Vietnam Experience Study (Boyle et al., 1987) or the Air Force Ranch Hand study (Wolfe et al., 1990). Goun and Kuller (1986) reported that the odds ratio for MM among Pennsylvania Vietnam veterans was less than 1.0. The veteran studies are particularly limited, because of the small numbers of MM deaths in the few analyses that have been conducted and because they use such a broad exposure category: service in Vietnam. With the exception of the Ranch Hands, no definitively exposed groups were categorized.

Summary

Although multiple myeloma has been less extensively studied than the lymphomas, a consistent pattern of elevated risks appears in the studies. Several studies of agricultural and forestry workers provide information on MM risk in relation to herbicide or pesticide exposure. Most studies demonstrated an odds ratio or SMR greater than 1.0; nine did so at a statistically significant level. The committee determined that the evidence for this association was limited/suggestive, because the individuals in the existing studies (mostly farmers) have by the nature of their occupation probably been exposed to a range of potentially carcinogenic agents other than herbicides and TCDD. Multiple myeloma—like non-Hodgkin's lymphoma and Hodgkin's disease for which there is stronger epidemiologic evidence of an association—is derived from lymphoreticular cells, which adds to the biologic plausibility of an association.

The new data available on MM do not change the committee's view that there is a limited/suggestive association between exposure to herbicides and multiple myeloma.

Conclusions

There is limited/suggestive evidence of an association between exposure to the herbicides (2,4-D, 2,4,5-T and its contaminant, TCDD; cacodylic acid; and picloram) and multiple myeloma. The evidence regarding association is drawn from occupational and other studies in which subjects were exposed to a variety of herbicides and herbicide components.

LEUKEMIA

Background

According to the American Cancer Society, approximately 25,700 new cases of leukemia (ICD-9 202.4, 203.1, 204.0-204.9, 205.0-205.9, 206.0-206.9, 207.0-207.2, 207.8, 208.0-208.9) were diagnosed in the United States in 1995, and about 20,400 persons died of this cancer (ACS, 1995). It is somewhat more common among men than women. According to the committee's calculations, assuming that veterans have the same cancer rates as those in the general U.S. population, 205 cases of leukemia were expected among male Vietnam veterans and 0.4 among female veterans in 1995. For the year 2000, the expected numbers are 259 cases among male veterans and 0.5 cases among female veterans.

Summary of *VAO*

The epidemiologic evidence for an association between exposure to herbicides and leukemia comes primarily from studies of farmers and residents of Seveso, Italy. The observed overall relative risk for leukemia mortality and incidence in Seveso was elevated, but not significantly. The increase was significant, however, for cases who were in the most highly exposed zone and died five to ten years after the accident. A number of studies of farmers also show a consistently elevated risk of leukemia, but these results are not necessarily due to herbicide use, because confounding exposures were not controlled for adequately in the analyses. Also, when farmers are stratified by suspected use of herbicide, the incidence of leukemia is generally not elevated. Some studies of chemical workers found an increased risk of leukemia, but the number of cases was small in all of these studies.

The available data on Vietnam veterans are generally not conclusive, because the exposure data are inadequate for the cohort being studied. Small sample sizes weaken the studies of the Ranch Hands or Chemical Corps; therefore, excess risks are not likely to be detected.

Since no study has adequately differentiated between exposure solely to either herbicides or TCDD, or demonstrated a dose-response for any subtype of leukemia, it is not possible to attribute any symptom or subtype of leukemia as a result of exposure.

Update of Scientific Literature

Since the publication of *VAO*, a number of new studies have been published. There have been two reports on the female subgroup of the IARC registry, but they contain too few leukemia cases to allow for definite statements about risk. Kogevinas et al. (1993) reported one case of myeloid leukemia among 701 female production workers (not significant). Similarly, the 18-year follow-up of a cohort of 1,909 Finnish herbicide applicators reported two cases of leukemia (not significant) (Asp et al., 1994). Both of these studies have low statistical power. A cohort mortality study of 155,547 male farmers in Saskatchewan, Manitoba, and Alberta has been conducted over the period 1971-87 (Semenciw et al., 1994). The SMR for leukemia was 0.9, based on 357 cases, a significant decrease (CI 0.8-1.0). The risk of death from leukemia did not vary by herbicide use, based on reported numbers of acres sprayed with herbicides in 1970.

A cohort study of cancer mortality in Ireland was performed using death certificate information from the years 1971 to 1987 (Dean, 1994). Among men in farming occupations, there were 138 deaths due to lymphoid leukemia, 114 due to myeloid leukemia, and 46 due to monocytic and other leukemias. The corresponding numbers for women in farming occupations were 39, 37, and 24. None of these categories was significantly elevated.

In the United States, a PCMR study was performed for farmers in 23 states, using occupational information from death certificates (Blair et al., 1993). Based on 1,072 deaths from leukemia in white male farmers, the PCMR was significantly increased at 1.3 (CI 1.2-1.4). Twenty two states had two or more deaths from leukemia. Sixteen states had risks that were greater than 1.0. The numbers of leukemia deaths were small and the PCMRs were nonsignificant in other gender and racial groups.

Cancer incidence in the Seveso cohort during the first ten years following exposure to TCDD was investigated (Bertazzi et al., 1993). There were no cases of leukemia in Zone A. Among men in Zone B, there were two cases of leukemia (RR = 1.6, CI 0.4-6.5). Among women in Zone B, there were also two cases of leukemia (RR = 1.8, CI 0.4-7.3). In Zone R, where residents had much less potential for exposure to TCDD than in Zones A and B, there were eight cases of leukemia in men (RR = 0.9, CI 0.4-1.9) and three cases in women (RR = 0.4, CI 0.1-1.2).

A PMR study that examined the causes of death among veterans on the state of Michigan's Vietnam-era Bonus list was recently published (Visintainer et al., 1995). The mortality rates of 3,364 Vietnam veterans were compared with 5,229 veterans who served elsewhere. No data were available to identify whether individual Vietnam veterans had been exposed to herbicides. Based on 30 deaths from leukemia, the PMR was 1.0 (CI 0.7-1.5).

Summary

The committee concluded in VAO that there is inadequate or insufficient evidence to determine whether an association exists between exposure to herbicides and leukemia. The updated scientific studies do not provide enough information to change this classification.

Conclusions

There is inadequate or insufficient evidence to determine whether an association exists between exposure to the herbicides (2,4-D, 2,4,5-T and its contaminant, TCDD; cacodylic acid; and picloram) and leukemia. The evidence regarding association is drawn from occupational and other studies in which subjects were exposed to a variety of herbicides and herbicide components.

OVERALL SUMMARY FOR CANCER

Based on the occupational, environmental, and veterans studies reviewed, the committee has reached one of four standard conclusions about the strength of the epidemiological evidence regarding association between exposure to herbicides and/or TCDD and each of the cancers under study. As explained in Chapter 4, these distinctions reflect the committee's judgment that if an association between exposure and an outcome were "real," it would be found in a large, well-designed epidemiologic study in which exposure to herbicides or dioxin was sufficiently high, well-characterized, and appropriately measured on an individual basis. Consistent with the charge to the Committee by the Secretary of Veterans Affairs in Public Law 102-4, the distinctions between these standard conclusions are based on statistical association, not on causality, as is common in scientific reviews. The committee used the same criteria to categorize diseases by the strength of the evidence as were used in *VAO*.

Health Outcomes with Sufficient Evidence of an Association

In *VAO*, the committee found sufficient evidence of an association with herbicides and/or TCDD for three cancers: soft-tissue sarcoma, non-Hodgkin's lymphoma, and Hodgkin's disease. The recent scientific literature continues to support the classification of these three cancers in the category of sufficient evidence. Based on the literature, there are no additional cancers that satisfy the criteria necessary for this category.

Health Outcomes with Limited/Suggestive Evidence of Association

In *VAO*, the committee found limited/suggestive evidence of an association for three cancers: respiratory cancer, prostate cancer, and multiple myeloma. The recent scientific literature continues to support the classification of these three diseases in the category of limited/suggestive evidence. For outcomes in this category, the evidence must be suggestive of an association between herbicides and the outcome, but may be limited because chance, bias, or confounding could not be ruled out with confidence. Typically, at least one high-quality study indicates a positive association, but the results of other studies may be inconsistent.

Among the many epidemiologic studies of respiratory cancers (specifically cancers of the lung, larynx, and trachea), positive associations were found consistently only when TCDD or herbicide exposures were probably high and prolonged. This was especially true in the largest, most heavily exposed cohorts of chemical production workers exposed to TCDD (Zober et al., 1990; Fingerhut et al., 1991; Manz et al., 1991; Saracci et al., 1991). Studies of farmers tended to show a decreased risk of respiratory cancers (perhaps due to lower smoking rates), and studies of Vietnam veterans are inconclusive. The committee felt that the evidence for this association was limited/suggestive rather than sufficient, because of the inconsistent pattern of positive findings across populations with various degrees of exposure and because the most important risk factor for respiratory cancers—cigarette smoking—was not fully controlled for or evaluated in all studies.

Several studies have shown an elevated risk for prostate cancer in agricultural or forestry workers. In a large cohort study of Canadian farmers (Morrison et al., 1993), an increased risk of prostate cancer was associated with herbicide spraying, and the risk was shown to rise with increasing number of acres sprayed. The mortality risk was elevated in a study of USDA forest conservationists (PMR = 1.6, CI 0.9-3.0) (Alavanja et al., 1989), and a case-control study of white male Iowans who died of prostate cancer (Burmeister et al., 1983) found a significant association (OR = 1.2) that was not linked with any particular agricultural practice. These results are strengthened by a consistent pattern of elevated, though nonsignificant, risks in studies of chemical production workers in the United States and other countries, agricultural workers, pesticide applicators, paper and pulp workers, and the Seveso population. The most important recent study demonstrated a significantly increased risk of death from prostate cancer in both white and nonwhite farmers in 22 of the 23 states that were studied (Blair et al., 1993). Studies of prostate cancer among Vietnam veterans and studies of environmental exposures have not consistently shown an association. However, prostate cancer is generally a disease of older men, and the risk among Vietnam veterans would not be detectable in current epidemiologic studies. Because there was a strong indication of a dose-response relationship in one study and a consistent positive association in a number of others, the committee felt that the evidence for association with herbicide exposure was limited/suggestive for prostate cancer.

Multiple myeloma, a cancer of specific bone marrow cells, has been less extensively studied than other lymphomas, but a consistent pattern of elevated risks appears in the studies. Several studies of agricultural and forestry workers provide information on MM risk in relation to herbicide or pesticide exposure. Most demonstrated an odds ratio or SMR greater than 1.0; nine did so at a statistically significant level. The committee determined that the evidence for this association was limited/suggestive, because the individuals in the existing studies (mostly farmers) have by the nature of their occupation probably been exposed to a range of potentially carcinogenic agents other than herbicides and TCDD. Multiple myeloma—like non-Hodgkin's lymphoma and Hodgkin's disease, for which there is stronger epidemiologic evidence of an association—is derived from lymphoreticular cells, which adds to the biologic plausibility of an association.

Health Outcomes with Inadequate/Insufficient Evidence to Determine Whether an Association Exists

The scientific data for the remainder of the cancers reviewed by the committee were inadequate or insufficient to determine whether an association exists. For these cancers, the available studies are of insufficient quality, consistency, or statistical power to permit a conclusion regarding the presence or absence of an association. For example, studies fail to control for confounding or have inadequate exposure assessment. This category includes hepatobiliary cancers, nasal/nasopharyngeal cancer, bone cancer, female reproductive cancers (cervical, uterine, ovarian), breast cancer, renal cancer, testicular cancer, leukemia, and skin cancer. A recently published study reviewed by the committee (Lynge, 1993) contained enough evidence to warrant moving skin cancer from the "limited/suggestive evidence of no association" category to this one.

The scientific evidence for four cancers will be summarized here. Hepatobiliary cancer and nasopharyngeal cancer are of special interest to the Department of Veterans Affairs. The evidence for skin cancer will be presented because it has changed categories. Breast cancer also deserves attention, because of its public health importance.

There are relatively few occupational, environmental, and veterans studies of hepatobiliary cancer, and most of these are small in size and have not controlled for lifestyle-related factors. The estimated relative risk in the various studies range from 0.3 to 3.3, usually with broad confidence intervals. Given the methodological difficulties associated with most of the few existing studies, the evidence regarding hepatobiliary cancer is not convincing with regard to either an association with herbicides/TCDD or the lack of an association. The few studies that have been published since *VAO* do not change the conclusion that there is inadequate evidence to determine whether an association exists between exposure to herbicides and hepatobiliary cancer (Asp et al., 1994; Bertazzi et al., 1993; Blair et al., 1993; Collins et al., 1993; and Cordier et al., 1993).

There are only a few occupational studies, one environmental study, and one veterans study of nasal and/or nasopharyngeal cancer, including two recently published studies (Asp et al., 1994; and Bertazzi et al., 1993). The estimated relative risks in the various studies range from 0.6 to 6.7, usually with broad confidence intervals. The few studies published since *VAO* do not change the conclusion that there is inadequate evidence to determine whether an association exists between exposure to herbicides and nasal/nasopharyngeal cancer.

One recent study (Lynge et al., 1993) found an excess risk of skin cancer. Based on four cases, a statistically significant increase in the risk of melanoma was observed in the subgroup of men who had been employed for at least one year, using a ten-year latency period (SIR = 4.3, CI 1.2-10.9). However, no information is given about the risk in men with less than 10 years of latency and expected numbers for women are not reported so observed elevated risk in the men with 10+ years of latency cannot be put into context. Another study also found a significant excess risk in men from the Seveso area (SMR = 3.3), based on only three cases (Bertazzi et al., 1989a,b). The committee felt that these results, while not even suggestive evidence about an association, undermined the evidence of no association in *VAO*, and thus warranted changing skin cancer to the "inadequate/insufficient evidence to determine whether an association exists" category.

There have been a few occupational studies, two environmental studies, and two veterans studies of breast cancer among women exposed to herbicides and/or TCDD. These include four recently published studies (Bertazzi et al., 1993; Blair et al., 1993; Dalager et al., 1995; and Kogevinas et. al., 1993). Most of these studies reported a relative risk of approximately 1.0 or less, but it is uncertain whether or not the female members of these cohorts had substantial chemical exposure. For example, more than 80 percent of the women Vietnam veterans in the two studies were nurses (Thomas et al., 1991; Dalager et. al., 1995). There continues to be inadequate or insufficient evidence to determine whether an association exists between exposure to herbicides and breast cancer.

Health Outcomes with Limited/Suggestive Evidence of No Association

In *VAO*, the committee found a sufficient number and variety of well-designed studies to conclude that there is limited/suggestive evidence of no association between a small group of cancers and exposure to TCDD or herbicides. This group includes gastrointestinal tumors (colon, rectal, stomach, and pancreatic), brain tumors, and bladder cancer. The recent scientific evidence continues to support the classification of these cancers in this category. Based on the literature, there are no additional cancers that satisfy the criteria necessary for this category.

For outcomes in this category, several adequate studies covering the full range of levels of exposure that human beings are known to encounter are mutually consistent in not showing a positive association between exposure to herbicides and the outcome at any level of exposure. These studies have relatively narrow confidence intervals. A conclusion of "no association" is inevitably limited to the conditions, level of exposure, and length of observation covered by the available studies. In addition, the possibility of a very small elevation in risk at the levels of exposure studied can never be excluded.

Increased Risk in Vietnam Veterans

Although there have been numerous health studies of Vietnam veterans, most have been hampered by relatively poor or nonexistent measures of exposure to herbicides or TCDD, in addition to other methodologic problems. Most of the evidence on which the conclusions in this chapter are based comes from studies of people exposed to dioxin or herbicides in occupational and environmental settings, rather than from studies of Vietnam veterans. The committee found this body of evidence adequate for reaching the conclusions about statistical associations between herbicides and health outcomes in this chapter. However, the lack of adequate data on Vietnam veterans per se complicates the determination of the increased risk of disease among individuals exposed to herbicides during service in Vietnam. Given the large uncertainties that remain about the magnitude of potential risk from exposure to herbicides in the studies that have been reviewed, the inadequate control for important confounders, and the uncertainty about the nature and magnitude of exposure to herbicides in Vietnam (as discussed in Chapter 5), none of the ingredients necessary for a quantitative risk assessment is available. Thus, the committee cannot quantify the degree of risk likely to be experienced by veterans because of their exposure to herbicides in Vietnam. The available quantitative and qualitative evidence about herbicide exposure among various groups studied suggests that Vietnam veterans as a group (except those with documented high exposures, such as participants in Operation Ranch Hand) had lower exposure to herbicides and TCDD than did the subjects in many occupational and environmental studies. However, individual veterans who had very high exposures to herbicides could have risks approaching those in the occupational and environmental studies.

REFERENCES

Ablashi DV. 1978. Meeting report: international symposium on etiology and control of nasopharyngeal carcinoma. Cancer Research 38:3114-3115.

Alavanja MC, Blair A, Merkle S, Teske J, Eaton B. 1988. Mortality among agricultural extension agents. American Journal of Industrial Medicine 14:167-176.

Alavanja MC, Merkle S, Teske J, Eaton B, Reed B. 1989. Mortality among forest and soil conservationists. Archives of Environmental Health 44:94-101.

American Cancer Society (ACS). 1992. Cancer Facts and Figures: 1992. Atlanta: American Cancer Society.

American Cancer Society (ACS). 1995. Cancer Facts and Figures: 1995. Atlanta: American Cancer Society.

Andersen HC, Andersen I, Selgaard J. 1977. Nasal cancers, symptoms, and upper airway function in woodworkers. British Journal of Industrial Medicine 34:201-207.

Anderson HA, Hanrahan LP, Jensen M, Laurin D, Yick W-Y, Wiegman P. 1986a. Wisconsin Vietnam Veteran Mortality Study: Proportionate Mortality Study Results. State of Wisconsin, Department of Health and Social Sciences.

Anderson HA, Hanrahan LP, Jensen M, Laurin D, Yick W-Y, Wiegman P. 1986b. Wisconsin Vietnam Veteran Mortality Study: Final Report. State of Wisconsin, Department of Health and
Social Sciences.

Asp S, Riihimaki V, Hernberg S, Pukkala E. 1994. Mortality and cancer morbidity of Finnish
chlorophenoxy herbicide applicators: an 18-year prospective follow-up. American Journal of
Industrial Medicine 26:243-253.

Axelson O, Sundell L. 1974. Herbicide exposure, mortality and tumor incidence. An epidemiological
investigation on Swedish railroad workers. Scandinavian Journal of Work, Environment, and
Health 11:21-28.

Axelson O, Sundell L, Andersson K, Edling C, Hogstedt C, Kling H. 1980. Herbicide exposure and
tumor mortality: an updated epidemiologic investigation on Swedish railroad workers. Scandinavian Journal of Work, Environment, and Health 6:73-79.

Beasly RP, Hwang LY. 1984. Epidemiology of hepatocellular carcinoma. In: Vyas GN, Dienstag JL,
Hoofnagle JH, eds. Viral Hepatitis and Liver Disease. New York: Grune and Stratton.

Belamaric J. 1973. Intrahepatic bile duct carcinoma and C. sinensis infection in Hong Kong. Cancer
31:468-473.

Bender AP, Parker DL, Johnson RA, Scharber WK, Williams AN, Marbury MC, Mandel JS. 1989.
Minnesota highway maintenance worker study: cancer mortality. American Journal of Industrial Medicine 15:545-556.

Bertazzi PA, Zocchetti C, Pesatori AC, Guercilena S, Sanarico M, Radice L. 1989a. Mortality in an
area contaminated by TCDD following an industrial incident. Medicina Del Lavoro 80:316-
329.

Bertazzi PA, Zocchetti C, Pesatori AC, Guercilena S, Sanarico M, Radice L. 1989b. Ten-year mortality study of the population involved in the Seveso incident in 1976. American Journal of
Epidemiology 129:1187-1200.

Bertazzi A, Pesatori AC, Consonni D, Tironi A, Landi MT, Zocchetti C. 1993. Cancer incidence in a
population accidentally exposed to 2,3,7,8-tetrachlorodibenzo-para-dioxin [see comments]. Epidemiology 4:398-406. .

Blair A, Grauman DJ, Lubin JH, Fraumeni JF Jr. 1983. Lung cancer and other causes of death among
licensed pesticide applicators. Journal of the National Cancer Institute 71:31-37.

Blair A, Mustafa D, Heineman EF. 1993. Cancer and other causes of death among male and female
farmers from twenty-three states. American Journal of Industrial Medicine 23:729-742.

Bloemen LJ, Mandel JS, Bond GG, Pollock AF, Vitek RP, Cook RR. 1993. An update of mortality
among chemical workers potentially exposed to the herbicide 2,4-dichlorophenoxyacetic acid
and its derivatives. Journal of Occupational Medicine 35:1208-1212.

Boffetta P, Stellman SD, Garfinkel L. 1989. A case-control study of multiple myeloma nested in the
American Cancer Society Prospective Study. International Journal of Cancer 43:554-559.

Bois FY, Eskenazi B. 1994. Possible risk of endometriosis for Seveso, Italy, residents: An assessment of exposure to dioxin. Environmental Health Perspectives 102:476-477.

Bond GG, Ott MG, Brenner FE, Cook RR. 1983. Medical and morbidity surveillance findings among
employees potentially exposed to TCDD. British Journal of Industrial Medicine 40:318-324.

Bond GG, Wetterstroem NH, Roush GJ, McLaren EA, Lipps TE, Cook RR. 1988. Cause specific
mortality among employees engaged in the manufacture, formulation, or packaging of 2,4-
dichlorophenoxyacetic acid and related salts. British Journal of Industrial Medicine 45:98-105.

Boyle C, Decoufle P, Delaney RJ, DeStefano F, Flock MI, Hunter MI, Joesoef MR, Karon JM, Kirk
ML, Layde PM, McGee DL, Moyer LA, Pollock DA, Rhodes P, Scally MJ, Worth RM. 1987.
Postservice mortality among Vietnam veterans. Atlanta: Centers for Disease Control.

Breslin P, Kang H, Lee Y, Burt V, Shepard BM. 1988. Proportionate mortality study of U.S. Army
and U.S. Marine Corps veterans of the Vietnam War. Journal of Occupational Medicine 30:412-
419.

Brown LM, Burmeister LF, Everett GD, Blair A. 1993. Pesticide exposures and multiple myeloma in Iowa men. Cancer Causes and Control 4:153-156.

Bueno de Mesquita HB, Doornbos G, Van der Kuip DA, Kogevinas M, Winkelmann R. 1993. Occupational exposure to phenoxy herbicides and chlorophenols and cancer mortality in the Netherlands. American Journal of Industrial Medicine 23:289-300.

Bullman TA, Kang HK, Watanabe KK. 1990. Proportionate mortality among U.S. Army Vietnam veterans who served in military region I. American Journal of Epidemiology 132:670-674.

Bullman TA, Watanabe KK, Kang HK. 1994. Risk of testicular cancer associated with surrogate measures of Agent Orange exposure among Vietnam veterans on the Agent Orange Registry. Annals of Epidemiology 4:11-16.

Burmeister LF. 1981. Cancer mortality in Iowa farmers. 1971-1978. Journal of the National Cancer Institute 66:461-464.

Burmeister LF, Everett GD, Van Lier SF, Isacson P. 1983. Selected cancer mortality and farm practices in Iowa. American Journal of Epidemiology 118:72-77.

Burt RD, Vaughan TL, McKnight B. 1992. Descriptive epidemiology and survival analysis of nasopharyngeal carcinoma in the United States. International Journal of Cancer 52:549-556.

Cantor KP, Blair A. 1984. Farming and mortality from multiple myeloma: a case-control study with the use of death certificates. Journal of the National Cancer Institute 72:251-255.

Centers for Disease Control. 1988. Health status of Vietnam veterans. II. Physical health. Journal of the American Medical Association 259:2708-2714.

Centers for Disease Control. 1990. The association of selected cancers with service in the U.S. military in Vietnam. III. Hodgkin's disease, nasal cancer, nasopharyngeal cancer, and primary liver cancer. The Selected Cancers Cooperative Study Group [see comments]. Archives of Internal Medicine 150:2495-2505.

Clapp RW, Cupples LA, Colton T, Ozonoff DM. 1991. Cancer surveillance of veterans in Massachusetts, 1982-1988. International Journal of Epidemiology 20:7-12.

Coggon D, Pannett B, Winter PD, Acheson ED, Bonsall J. 1986. Mortality of workers exposed to 2 methyl-4 chlorophenoxyacetic acid. Scandinavian Journal of Work, Environment, and Health 12:448-454.

Coggon D, Pannett B, Winter P. 1991. Mortality and incidence of cancer at four factories making phenoxy herbicides. British Journal of Industrial Medicine 48:173-178.

Collins JJ, Strauss ME, Levinskas GJ, Conner PC. 1993. The mortality experience of workers exposed to 2,3,7,8-tetrachlorodibenzo-p-dioxin in a trichlorophenol process accident. Epidemiology 4:7-13.

Cordier S, Le TB, Verger P, Bard D, Le CD, Larouze B, Dazza MC, Hoang TQ, Abenhaim L. 1993. Viral infections and chemical exposures as risk factors for hepatocellular carcinoma in Vietnam. International Journal of Cancer 55:196-201.

Dalager MS, Kang HK, Thomas TL. 1995. Cancer mortality patterns among women who served in the military: the Vietnam experience. Journal of Occupational and Environmental Medicine 37:298-305.

Dean G. 1994. Deaths from primary brain cancers, lymphatic and haematopoietic cancers in agricultural workers in the Republic of Ireland. Journal of Epidemiology and Community Health 48:364-368.

Doll R, Matthews JD, Morgan LG. 1977. Cancers of the lung and nasal sinuses in nickel workers: a reassessment of the period risk. British Journal of Industrial Medicine 34:102-105.

Donna A, Betta P-G, Robutti F, Crosignanai P, Berrino F, Bellingeri D. 1984. Ovarian mesothelial tumors and herbicides: a case-control study. Carcinogenesis 5:941-942.

Elwood MJ. 1981. Wood exposure and smoking: association with cancer of the nasal cavity and paranasal sinuses in British Columbia. Canadian Medical Association Journal 124:1573-1577.

Engelhardt R, Mackensen A, Galanos C. 1991. Phase I trial of intravenously administered endotoxin (Salmonella abortus equi) in cancer patients. Cancer Research 51:2524-2530.

Eriksson M, Hardell L, Berg NO, Moller T, Axelson O. 1981. Soft-Tissue Sarcomas and Exposure to Chemical Substances: A Case-Referent Study. British Journal of Industrial Medicine 38:27-33.

Eriksson M, Hardell L, Adami HO. 1990. Exposure to dioxins as a risk factor for soft tissue sarcoma: a population-based case-control study [see comments]. Journal of the National Cancer Institute 82:486-490.

Eriksson M, Karlsson M. 1992. Occupational and other environmental factors and multiple myeloma: a population based case-control study. British Journal of Industrial Medicine 49:95-103.

Fett MJ, Nairn JR, Cobbin DM, Adena MA. 1987. Mortality among Australian conscripts of the Vietnam conflict era. II Causes of death. American Journal of Epidemiology 125:878-884.

Fingerhut MA, Halperin WE, Marlow DA, Piacitelli LA, Honchar PA, Sweeney MH, Greife AL, Dill PA, Steenland K, Suruda AJ. 1991. Cancer mortality in workers exposed to 2,3,7,8-tetrachlorodibenzo-*p*-dioxin. New England Journal of Medicine 324:212-218.

Gajwani BW, Devereaux JM, Beg JA. 1980. Familial clustering of nasopharyngeal carcinoma. Cancer 47:2325-2327.

Garry VF, Kelly JT, Sprafka JM, Edwards S, Griffith J. 1994. Survey of health and use characterization of pesticide appliers in Minnesota. Archives of Environmental Health 49:337-343.

Goun BD, Kuller LH. 1986. Final report: A case control mortality study on the association of soft tissue sarcomas, non-Hodgkin's lymphomas, and other selected cancers and Vietnam military service in Pennsylvania males. Pittsburgh: University of Pittsburgh.

Green LM. 1991. A cohort mortality study of forestry workers exposed to phenoxy acid herbicides. British Journal of Industrial Medicine 48:234-238.

Greenwald ED, Greenwald ES. 1983. Cancer Epidemiology. Hyde Park, N.Y.: Medical Examination Publishing.

Hansen ES, Hasle H, Lander F. 1992. A cohort study on cancer incidence among Danish gardeners. American Journal of Industrial Medicine 21:651-660.

Hardell L. 1981. Relation of soft-tissue sarcoma, malignant lymphoma and colon cancer to phenoxy acids, chlorophenols and other agents. Scandinavian Journal of Work, Environment, and Health 7:119-130.

Hardell L, Bengtsson NO. 1983. Epidemiological study of socioeconomic factors and clinical findings in Hodgkin's disease, and reanalysis of previous data regarding chemical exposure. British Journal of Cancer 48:217-225.

Hardell L, Eriksson M. 1988. The association between soft tissue sarcomas and exposure to phenoxyacetic acids: a new case-referent study. Cancer 62:652-656.

Hardell L, Sandstrom A. 1979. Case-control study: soft-tissue sarcomas and exposure to phenoxyacetic acids or chlorophenols. British Journal of Cancer 39:711-717.

Hardell L, Eriksson M, Degerman A. 1994. Exposure to phenoxyacetic acids, chlorophenols, or organic solvents in relation to histopathology, stage, and anatomical localization of non-Hodgkin's lymphoma. Cancer Research 54:2386-2389.

Hardell L, Eriksson M, Lenner P, Lundgren E. 1981. Malignant lymphoma and exposure to chemicals, especially organic solvents, chlorophenols and phenoxy acids: a case-control study. British Journal of Cancer 43:169-176.

Hardell L, Johansson B, Axelson O. 1982. Epidemiological study of nasal and nasopharyngeal cancer and their relation to phenoxy acid or chlorophenol exposure. American Journal of Industrial Medicine 3:247-257.

Hardell L, Bengtsson NO, Jonsson U, Eriksson S, Larsson LG. 1984. Aetiological aspects on primary liver cancer with special regard to alcohol, organic solvents and acute intermittent porphyria: an epidemiological investigation. British Journal of Cancer 50:389-397.

Harris JR, Lippman ME, Veronesi U, Willett W. 1992. Breast cancer (first of three parts). New England Journal of Medicine 327:319-328.

Henderson C. 1991. Breast cancer. In: Wilson JD, Braunwald E, Isselbacher KJ, Petersdorf RG, Martin JB, Faudi AS, Root RK, eds. Harrison's Principles of Internal Medicine. 12th ed. New York: McGraw-Hill.

Henle W, Henle G. 1981. The Epstein-Barr virus, its relation to Burkett's lymphoma and nasopharyngeal carcinoma. In: Burchenal JH, Oettgen HF, eds. Cancer: Achievements, Challenges, and Prospects for the 1980s. Vol I: New York: Grune & Stratton.

Henneberger PK, Ferris BG Jr, Monson RR. 1989. Mortality among pulp and paper workers in Berlin, New Hampshire. British Journal of Industrial Medicine 46:658-664.

Henney J, DeVita V. 1987. Breast cancer. In: Braunwald E, Isselbacher KJ, Petersdorf RG, Wilson JD, Martin JB, Fauci AS, eds. Harrison's Principles of Internal Medicine. 11th ed. New York: McGraw-Hill.

Higami Y, Shimokawa I, Iwasaki K, Matsuo T, Ikeda T, Mine M, Mori H. 1990. Incidence of multiple myeloma in Nagasaki City, with special reference to those subjected to atomic bomb exposure. Gan No Rinsho 36:157-162.

Higgenson J, Muir C. 1973. Epidemiology. In: Holland JF, Frei E, eds. Cancer Medicine. Philadelphia: Lea and Febiger.

Hoar SK, Blair A, Holmes FF, Boysen CD, Robel RJ, Hoover R, Fraumeni JF. 1986. Agricultural herbicide use and risk of lymphoma and soft-tissue sarcoma. Journal of the American Medical Association 256:1141-1147.

Hoffman RE, Stehr-Green PA, Webb KB, Evans RG, Knutsen AP, Schramm WF, Staake JL, Gibson BB, Steinberg KK. 1986. Health effects of long-term exposure to 2,3,7,8-tetrachlorodibenzo-p-dioxin. Journal of the American Medical Association 255:2031-2038.

Holmes AP, Bailey C, Baron RC, Bosenac E, Brough J, Conroy C, Haddy L. 1986. West Virginia Department of Health Vietnam-era Veterans Mortality Study, Preliminary Report. Charleston: West Virginia Department of Health.

Jappinen P, Pukkala E. 1991. Cancer incidence among pulp and paper workers exposed to organic chlorinated compounds formed during chlorine pulp bleaching. Scandinavian Journal of Work, Environment, and Health 17:356-359.

Kauppinen TP, Pannett B, Marlow DA, Kogevinas M. 1994. Retrospective assessment of exposure through modeling in a study on cancer risks among workers exposed to phenoxy herbicides, chlorophenols and dioxins. Scandinavian Journal of Work, Environment, and Health 20:262-271.

Kogan MD, Clapp RW. 1985. Mortality among Vietnam Veterans in Massachusetts, 1972-1983. Massachusetts Office of Commissioner of Veterans Services.

Kogan MD, Clapp RW. 1988. Soft tissue sarcoma mortality among Vietnam veterans in Massachusetts, 1972 to 1983. International Journal of Epidemiology 17:39-43.

Kogevinas M, Saracci R, Bertazzi PA, Bueno De Mesquita BH, Coggon D, Green LM, Kauppinen T, Littorin M, Lynge E, Mathews JD, Neuberger M, Osman J, Pearce N, Winkelmann R. 1992. Cancer mortality from soft-tissue sarcoma and malignant lymphomas in an international cohort of workers exposed to chlorophenoxy herbicides and chlorophenols. Chemosphere 25:1071-1076.

Kogevinas M, Saracci R, Winkelmann R, Johnson ES, Bertazzi PA, Bueno de Mesquita BH, Kauppinen T, Littorin M, Lynge E, Neuberger M. 1993. Cancer incidence and mortality in women occupationally exposed to chlorophenoxy herbicides, chlorophenols, and dioxins. Cancer Causes Control 4:547-553.

Kogevinas M, Kauppinen T, Winkelmann R, Becher H, Bertazzi PA, Bueno de Mesquita HB, Coggon D, Green L, Johnson E, Littorin M, Lynge E, Marlow DA, Mathews JD, Neuberger M, Benn T, Pannett B, Pearce N, Saracci R. 1995. Soft tissue sarcoma and non-Hodgkin's lymphoma in workers exposed to phenoxy herbicides, chlorophenols, and dioxins: two nested case-control studies. Epidemiology 6:396-402.

Kuratsune M, Nakamura K, Ikeda M, Hirohata T. 1986. Analysis of deaths seen among patients with Yusho. Dioxin '86 Symposium Abstracts. Fukuoka, Japan.

Lampi P, Hakulinen T, Luostarinen T, Pukkala E, Teppo L. 1992. Cancer incidence following chlorophenol exposure in a community in southern Finland. Archives of Environmental Health 47:167-175.

LaVecchia C, Negri E, D'Avanzo B, Franceschi S. 1989. Occupation and lymphoid neoplasms. British Journal of Cancer 60:385-388.

Lawrence CE, Reilly AA, Quickenton P, Greenwald P, Page WF, Kuntz AJ. 1985. Mortality patterns of New York State Vietnam veterans. American Journal of Public Health 75:277-279.

Luce D, Gerin M, Leclerc A, Morcet JF, Brugere J, Goldberg M. 1993. Sinonasal cancer and occupational exposure to formaldehyde and other substances. International Journal of Cancer 53:224-231.

Lynge E. 1985. A follow-up study of cancer incidence among workers in manufacture of phenoxy herbicides in Denmark. British Journal of Cancer 52:259-270.

Lynge E. 1993. Cancer in phenoxy herbicide manufacturing workers in Denmark, 1947-87—an update. Cancer Causes Control 4:261-272.

Mack TM. 1995. Sarcomas and other malignancies of soft tissue, retroperitoneum, peritoneum, pleura, heart, mediastinum, and spleen. Cancer 75:211-244.

Manz A, Berger J, Dwyer JH, Flesch-Janys D, Nagel S, Waltsgott H. 1991. Cancer mortality among workers in chemical plant contaminated with dioxin. Lancet 338:959-964.

Matanoski GM, Seltser R, Sartwell PE, Diamond EL, Elliott EA. 1975. The current mortality rates of radiologists and other physician specialists: specific causes of death. American Journal of Epidemiology 101:199-210.

Mayer RJ, Garnick MB. 1986. Liver Cancer. In: Holleb AI, ed. The American Cancer Society Cancer Book. Garden City, NY: Doubleday. 393-400.

McDuffie HH, Klaassen DJ, Dosman JA. 1990. Is pesticide use related to the risk of primary lung cancer in Saskatchewan? Journal of Occupational Medicine 32:996-1002.

McGee JOD, Isaacson PG, Wright NA, eds. 1992. Oxford Textbook of Pathology. Oxford: Oxford Medical.

Mellemgaard A, Engholm G, McLaughlin JK, Olsen JH. 1994. Occupational risk factors for renal-cell carcinoma in Denmark. Scandinavian Journal of Work, Environment, and Health 20:160-165.

Michalek JE, Wolfe WH, Miner JC. 1990. Health status of Air Force veterans occupationally exposed to herbicides in Vietnam II. Mortality. Journal of the American Medical Association 264:1832-1836.

Miller BA, Feuer EJ, Hankey BF. 1991. The increasing incidence of breast cancer: relevance of early detection. Cancer Causes and Control 2:67-74.

Miller BA, Ries LAG, Hankey BF, Kosary CL, Edwards BK, eds. 1992. Cancer Statistics Review: 1973-1989. Bethesda: National Cancer Institute. NIH Pub. No. 92-2789.

Morris PD, Koepsell TD, Daling JR, Taylor JW, Lyon JL, Swanson GM, Child M, Weiss NS. 1986. Toxic substance exposure and multiple myeloma: a case-control study. Journal of the National Cancer Institute 76:987-994.

Morrison HI, Semenciw RM, Morison D, Magwood S, Mao Y. 1992. Brain cancer and farming in western Canada. Neuroepidemiology 11:267-276.

Morrison H, Savitz D, Semenciw R, Hulka B, Mao Y, Morison D, Wigle D. 1993. Farming and prostate cancer mortality. American Journal of Epidemiology 137:270-280.

Morrison HI, Semenciw RM, Wilkins K, Mao Y, Wigle DT. 1994. Non-Hodgkin's lymphoma and agricultural practices in the prairie provinces of Canada. Scandinavian Journal of Work, Environment, and Health 20:42-47.

Moses M, Lilis R, Crow KD, Thornton J, Fischbein A, Anderson HA, Selikoff IJ. 1984. Health status of workers with past exposure to 2,3,7,8-tetrachlorodibenzo-*p*-dioxin in the manufacture of 2,4,5-trichlorophenoxyacetic acid: comparison of findings with and without chloracne. American Journal of Industrial Medicine 5:161-182.

Musicco M, Sant M, Molinari S, Filippini G, Gatta G, Berrino F. 1988. A case-control study of brain gliomas and occupational exposure to chemical carcinogens: the risks to farmers. American Journal of Epidemiology 128:778-785.

National Toxicology Program. 1982a. Carcinogenesis Bioassay of 2,3,7,8-tetrachlorodibenzo-*p*-dioxin (CAS No. 1746-01-6) in Osborne-Mendel Rats and B6C3F1 Mice (Gavage Study). Research Triangle Park, N.C.: NTP. NTP-80-31; NIH/PUB-82-1765.PC A09/MF A01.

National Toxicology Program. 1982b. Carcinogenesis Bioassay of 2,3,7,8-tetrachlorodibenzo-*p*-dioxin (CAS No. 1746-01-6) in Swiss Webster Mice (Dermal Study). Research Triangle Park, N.C.: NTP. NTP-80-31; NIH/PUB-82-1765.PC A09/MF A01.

Nicholson WJ. 1987. Report to the Workers' Compensation Board on Occupational Exposure to PCBs and Various Cancers. Industrial Disease Standards Panel Report No. 2. Toronto: Ontario Ministry of Labor.

Nomura AMY, Kolonel LN. 1991. Prostate cancer: a current perspective. American Journal of Epidemiology 13:200-227.

Pearce NE, Smith AH, Fisher DO. 1985. Malignant lymphoma and multiple myeloma linked with agricultural occupations in a New Zealand cancer registry-based study. American Journal of Epidemiology 121:225-237.

Pearce NE, Smith AH, Howard JK, Sheppard RA, Giles HJ, Teague CA. 1986. Case-control study of multiple myeloma and farming. British Journal of Cancer 54:493-500.

Percy C, Ries GL, Van Holten VD. 1990. The accuracy of liver cancer as the underlying cause of death on death certificates. Public Health Reports 105:361-368.

Persson B, Dahlander A-M, Fredriksson M, Brage HN, Ohlson C-G, Axelson O. 1989. Malignant lymphomas and occupational exposures. British Journal of Industrial Medicine 46:516-520.

Persson B, Fredriksson M, Olsen K, Boeryd B, Axelson O. 1993. Some occupational exposures as risk factors for malignant lymphomas. Cancer 72:1773-1778.

Pesatori AC, Consonni D, Tironi A, Landi MT, Zocchetti C, Bertazzi PA. 1992. Cancer morbidity in the Seveso area, 1976-1986. Chemosphere 25:209-212.

Pienta KJ, Esper PS. 1993. Risk factors for prostate cancer. Annals of Internal Medicine 118:794-803.

Riedel D, Pottern LM, Blattner WA. 1991. Etiology and epidemiology of multiple myeloma. In: Wiernick PH, Camellos G, Kyle RA, Schiffer CA, eds. Neoplastic Disease of the Blood and Blood-Forming Organs. New York: Churchill Livingstone.

Rier SE, Martin DC, Bowman RE, Dmowski WP, Becker JL. 1993. Endometriosis in rhesus monkeys (*Macaca mulatta*) following chronic exposure to 2,3,7,8-tetrachlorodibenzo-*p*-dioxin. Fundamental and Applied Toxicology 21:433-441.

Riihimaki V, Asp S, Hernberg S. 1982. Mortality of 2,4-dichlorophenoxyacetic acid and 2,4,5-trichlorophenoxyacetic acid herbicide applicators in Finland: first report of an ongoing prospective cohort study. Scandinavian Journal of Work, Environment, and Health 8:37-42.

Riihimaki V, Asp S, Pukkala E, Hernberg S. 1983. Mortality and cancer morbidity among chlorinated phenoxyacid applicators in Finland. Chemosphere 12:779-784.

Robinson CF, Waxweiler RJ, Fowler DP. 1986. Mortality among production workers in pulp and paper mills. Scandinavian Journal of Work, Environment, and Health 12:552-560.

Ronco G, Costa G, Lynge E. 1992. Cancer risk among Danish and Italian farmers. British Journal of Industrial Medicine 49:220-225.

Rylander R. 1990. Environmental exposure with decreased risks for lung cancer? International Journal of Epidemiology 19 (Suppl 1):S67-S72.

Saracci R, Kogevinas M, Bertazzi PA, Bueno de Mesquita BH, Coggon D, Green LM, Kauppinen T, L'Abbe KA, Littorin M, Lynge E, Mathews JD, Neuberger M, Osman J, Pearce N, Winkelmann R. 1991. Cancer mortality in workers exposed to chlorophenoxy herbicides and chlorophenols. Lancet 338:1027-1032.

Seidman H, Mushinski MH, Gelb SK, Silverberg E. 1985. Probabilities of eventually developing or dying of cancer: United States. Cancer 35:36-56.

Semenciw RM, Morrison HI, Riedel D, Wilkins K, Ritter L, Mao Y. 1993. Multiple myeloma mortality and agricultural practices in the prairie provinces of Canada. Journal of Occupational Medicine 35:557-561.

Semenciw RM, Morrison HI, Morison D, Mao Y. 1994. Leukemia mortality and farming in the prairie provinces of Canada. Canadian Journal of Public Health 85:208-211.

Solet D, Zoloth SR, Sullivan C, Jewett J, Michaels DM. 1989. Patterns of mortality in pulp and paper workers. Journal of Occupational Medicine 31:627-630.

Stebbings JK, Lucas HF, Stehney AF. 1984. Mortality from cancers of major sites in female radium dial workers. American Journal of Industrial Medicine 5:435.

Stehr PA, Stein G, Webb K, Schramm W, Gedney WB, Donnell HD, Ayres S, Falk H, Sampson E, Smith SJ. 1986. A pilot epidemiologic study of possible health effects associated with 2,3,7,8-tetrachlorodibenzo-*p*-dioxin contaminations in Missouri. Archives of Environmental Health 41:16-22.

Stehr-Green P, Hoffman R, Webb K, Evans RG, Knutsen A, Schramm W, Staake J, Gibson B, Steinberg K. 1987. Health effects of long-term exposure to 2,3,7,8-tetrachlorodibenzo-*p*-dioxin. Chemosphere 16:2089-2094.

Sterling TD, Weinkam JJ. 1976. Smoking characteristics by type of employment. Journal of Occupational Medicine 18:743-754.

Suskind RR, Hertzberg VS. 1984. Human health effects of 2,4,5-T and its toxic contaminants. Journal of the American Medical Association 251:2372-2380.

Swaen GMH, van Vliet C, Slangen JJM, Sturmans F. 1992. Cancer mortality among licensed herbicide applicators. Scandinavian Journal of Work, Environment, and Health 18:201-204.

Tarone RE, Hayes HM, Hoover RN, Rosenthal JF, Brown LM, Pottern LM, Javadpour N, O'Connoll KJ, Stutzman RE. 1991. Service in Vietnam and risk of testicular cancer. Journal of the National Cancer Institute 83:1497-1499.

Thomas TL. 1987. Mortality among flavour and fragrance chemical plant workers in the United States. British Journal of Industrial Medicine 44:733-737.

Thomas TL, Kang HK. 1990. Mortality and morbidity among Army Chemical Corps Vietnam veterans: a preliminary report. American Journal of Industrial Medicine 18:665-673.

Thomas TL, Kang H, Dalager N. 1991. Mortality among women Vietnam veterans, 1973-1987. American Journal of Epidemiology 134:973-980.

U.S. Department of Health and Human Services (DHHS). 1987. Vital Statistics of the United States. Washington: DHHS.

U.S. Department of Health and Human Services (DHHS). 1991. International Classification of Diseases, 9th revision, Clinical Modification. 4th ed. Washington: DHHS.

Visintainer PF, Barone M, McGee H, Peterson EL. 1995. Proportionate mortality study of Vietnam-era veterans of Michigan. Journal of Occupational and Environmental Medicine 37:423-428.

Watanabe KK, Kang HK, Thomas TL. 1991. Mortality among Vietnam veterans: with methodological considerations. Journal of Occupational Medicine 33:780-785.

Wigle DT, Semenciw RB, Wilkins K, Riedel D, Ritter L, Morrison HI, Mao Y. 1990. Mortality study of Canadian male farm operators: Non-Hodgkin's lymphoma mortality and agricultural practices in Saskatchewan. Journal of the National Cancer Institute 82:575-582.

Wiklund K. 1983. Swedish agricultural workers: a group with a decreased risk of cancer. Cancer 51:566-568.

Wiklund K, Dich J, Holm L-E, Eklund G. 1989. Risk of cancer in pesticide applicators in Swedish agriculture. British Journal of Industrial Medicine 46:809-814.

Wolfe WH, Michalek JE, Miner JC, Rahe A, Silva J, Thomas WF, Grubbs WD, Lustik MB, Karrison TG, Roegner RH, Williams DE. 1990. Health status of Air Force veterans occupationally exposed to herbicides in Vietnam. I. Physical health. Journal of the American Medical Association 264:1824-1831.

Wong O, Raabe GK. 1989. Critical review of cancer epidemiology in petroleum industry employees, with a qualitative meta-analysis by cancer site. American Journal of Industrial Medicine 15:283-310.

Yeh FS, Yu MC, Mo CC, Luo S, Tong MJ, Henderson BE. 1989. Hepatitis B virus, aflatoxins, and hepatocellular carcinoma in Southern Guangxi, China. Cancer Research 49:2506-2509.

Yu MC, Tong MJ, Coursaget P, Ross RK, Govindarajan S, Henderson BE. 1990. Prevalence of hepatitis B and C viral markers in black and white patients with hepatocellular carcinoma in the United States. Journal of the National Cancer Institute 82:1038-1041.

Zack JA, Suskind RR. 1980. The mortality experience of workers exposed to tetrachlorodibenzo-*p*-dioxin in a trichlorophenol process accident. Journal of Occupational Medicine 22:11-14.

Zahm SH, Weisenburger DD, Babbitt PA, Saal RC, Vaught JB, Cantor KP, Blair A. 1990. A case-control study of non-Hodgkin's lymphoma and the herbicide 2,4-dichlorophenoxyacetic acid (2,4-D) in eastern Nebraska. Epidemiology 1:349-356.

Zahm SH, Blair A, Weisenburger DD. 1992. Sex differences in the risk of multiple myeloma associated with agriculture (2). British Journal of Industrial Medicine 49:815-816.

Zahm SH, Weisenburger DD, Saal RC, Vaught JB, Babbitt PA, Blair A. 1993. The role of agricultural pesticide use in the development of non-Hodgkin's lymphoma in women. Archives of Environmental Health 48:353-358.

Zheng W, McLaughlin JK, Gao YT, Gao RN, Blot WJ. 1992a. Occupational risks for nasopharyngeal cancer in Shanghai. Journal of Occupational Medicine 34:1004-1007.

Zheng W, Blot WJ, Shu XO, Diamond EL, Gao YT, Ji BT, Fraumeni JF Jr. 1992b. A population-based case-control study of cancers of the nasal cavity and paranasal sinuses in Shanghai. International Journal of Cancer 52:557-561.

Zober A, Messerer P, Huber P. 1990. Thirty-four-year mortality follow-up of BASF employees exposed to 2,3,7,8-TCDD after the 1953 accident. International Archives of Occupational and Environmental Health 62:139-157.

8

Latency and Cancer Risk

One of the topics of special interest to the Department of Veterans Affairs (DVA) is the potential effect of herbicide exposure on cancer latency. The term "latency" is used in a variety of ways to denote the effect of the timing of exposure on the subsequent risk of disease. The importance of latency effects as well as other time-related factors, such as age at exposure, in determining cancer risk has long been recognized (Armenian, 1987). Some important practical questions at the heart of the investigation of these time-related factors are: (1) How long does it take after exposure to detect an increase in disease risk? (2) How long do the effects of exposure last? (3) How does the effect of exposure vary with the age at which it was received? and (4) Does a given carcinogen act at an early or late stage of the carcinogenic process?

Often, either because of poor exposure assessment or the desire to report a simple summary measure of association, measures of exposure such as ever/never exposed or cumulative exposure are used to summarize exposure histories. Although such measures can be useful for detecting whether there is or is not an association between exposure and disease, it is well-known that timing of exposure plays an important role in determining when and by how much the eventual disease risk is increased (or decreased) by the exposure.

In response to the DVA's request to explore latency issues related to Agent Orange, in this chapter the committee: 1) proposes a methodology to address the four questions listed above concerning the timing of herbicide exposure and the risk of cancer; 2) reviews the literature on herbicide exposure and cancers classified in sufficient and suggestive/limited categories for results that describe how timing of exposure affects the relative risk due to exposure; and 3) describes timing of exposure characteristics of the Vietnam veterans and summarizes the implications of these factors for their risk of cancer.

ANALYSIS OF LATENCY IN EPIDEMIOLOGIC STUDIES

In order to discuss latency issues, we need to establish what is meant by "the effect of exposure over time." First, for purposes of epidemiologic research and quantification, we are interested in the rate of disease among exposed individuals compared to the rate that would be expected if the subjects had not been exposed, as discussed more fully below. Thus, we are interested in the relative or excess rate of disease as the measure of comparison. Latency effects are essentially the change in *relative* or *excess* rates with "time since exposure." For exposures of short duration, time since exposure is easy to define. This is the case for environmental exposures from industrial accidents, such as the one that occurred in Seveso. If the exposure occurred over a long period of time (a protracted exposure), as with the production workers and pesticide applicators, the time since exposure is more difficult to quantify. Conceptually, we think of the effect of exposure at a particular time in the past as the resulting change in risk that today is ascribable to that exposure. Though perhaps overly simplistic, the effect of an entire exposure history can be usefully thought of as the sum of effects from exposure at each time point in the past.

In order to adequately study effects of protracted exposures, detailed exposure histories for each study subject, including the dates that the individual was exposed and, ideally, the level of exposure, are needed. Appropriate statistical methods have been developed for an investigation of the effect of exposure accrued as a function of time since that exposure (Thomas, 1983; Breslow and Day, 1987; Thomas, 1988), but these have not been used in the analysis of any of the herbicide-cancer studies.

In general, the ability to investigate the issues of timing of exposure in a given data set will depend on the quality of the exposure measure, the quality of the timing of exposure information, the number of people developing the disease of interest, and variation of exposure over time within the study group. These aspects of study quality are, of course, important in evaluating any epidemiologic investigation. But there are special problems that arise in the evaluation of time-related factors (Enterline and Henderson, 1973; Peto, 1985; Thomas, 1987).

Need to control for the effects of aging Progression along the time-since-exposure scale is paralleled by increasing age. Because the rate of most cancers increases dramatically with age, it is also true that for a given study group, the expected number of cancers per unit of time will increase with time since exposure, simply because the study group is aging. Thus, examination of absolute numbers of cases as time since exposure increases would be misleading. We would expect to see an increase even if there were no change due to the exposure.

Thus, it is standard epidemiologic practice to "normalize" the comparison by reference to an appropriate unexposed group. "Appropriate" in this context means a group with the same age structure at otherwise similar risk of disease as the study group so that we are measuring the effect of exposure in the development of cancers over and above those increases in disease rate that would be expected if the study group were simply aging with no exposure.

Correlation between various time factors It is important to keep in mind that duration of exposure, time since exposure, age of exposure, and exposure level itself may well be correlated with each other, so that an observed pattern for one of these factors may actually be due to correlation with one of the others. Thus, exploration of one factor within each level of the other, either by stratifying of the analysis or by modeling their effect, is commonly needed to disentangle the confounding of time-related variables. Realistically, however, most data sets do not have sufficient data to explore these issues, and for the most part, these considerations merely serve as a cautionary note in the interpretation of results. The following hypothetical situations help to illustrate how the various time-related factors are intertwined. For illustration, we refer to the exposure of interest as "the agent."

a) Two people are born in 1945. Both are continuously exposed to the agent for ten years. One person begins exposure at age 20 (continuing to age 30), and the other begins at age 30 (continuing to age 40). In 1995, at age 50, the first person has 30 years since his first exposure, whereas the second had only 20 years since first exposure. Thus, age at first exposure and time since first exposure, for a given duration of exposure, are linked.

b) One person begins exposure to the agent in 1970, a second starts in 1975. Both are the same age at first exposure and continue exposure until 1985. When evaluated in 1995, the first person has both a longer duration of exposure (15 vs. 10 years) and a longer time since first exposure (25 vs. 20 years), showing the link between those two factors for a given age at first exposure.

c) Two people are born in 1945. One starts exposure at age 20, the other at age 30. Both stop exposure at age 40. The first person has started at a younger age, has a longer duration of exposure, and a longer time since first exposure, showing that all three factors may be potentially linked.

d) Two people are both exposed at the same intensity, in the sense that the airborne concentration of the agent (e.g., in parts per million) is the same for both. The person with the longer duration of exposure will, by definition, have a higher cumulative exposure.

Although it is possible to construct counter-examples to the above, we believe these examples are fairly typical of what happens in many occupational settings and present them primarily to illustrate that interpreting an examination of the effects of one time-related factor may be difficult without information on the others.

Need for sufficient variation in time-related factors In evaluating the evolution of relative risk with time, the value of a study is limited by the amount of time that has elapsed along the time scale of interest. For instance, the ability to explore the pattern of relative risks as a function of time since exposure depends on the range of time since exposure among the study group. We note that this is not necessarily the "follow-up" time for the study group, although the amount of information about time-related factors increases with the amount of follow-up. Rather, it depends on the variation of the factors within the group. Thus, a case-control study with cases obtained over a short period of time may be very informative about latency effects if both cases and controls have a wide range of times of exposure.

Mortality and incidence studies for examining latency Generally, it is believed that carcinogenic agents increase the chance of cancer occurence but do not increase the likelihood of death once the cancer has occurred. If this is true, as we will assume, then studies of cancer incidence are preferable to those of mortality since exposure after the development of the cancer has no role in its etiology. In terms of the investigation of latency, the changes in relative risks with time since exposure will occur later for mortality studies compared to incidence studies, by an amount of time approximately equal to the average time from occurrence of the cancer to death. With the exception of Asp et al. (1994), the studies that reported latency results in the reviewed literature for the cancers we examined were mortality studies. We do not discuss this issue further in our description of the results, under the assumption that the exposure is associated with the cancer but does not change the risk of death once cancer occurs. However, it should be noted that mortality studies will result in a pattern of relative risks "shifted to the right" of the pattern that would have been observed in the corresponding incidence study. This phenomenon may also have implications for the number of "events" (deaths vs. cases) available for study at any given point in time, particularly for cancers with high survival rates. This, in turn, may have implications, especially in cohort studies, for statistical power.

Measurement errors that are time related In many instances, in epidemiologic studies, misclassification of exposed individuals as unexposed, and vice versa, tends to produce bias toward showing no association between exposure and disease when, in fact, an association may truly exist. This type of bias, called random misclassification, can generally be found when the misclassification of exposure status is unrelated to a person's ultimate disease status. In attempts to evaluate how time-related factors influence risk, this general principle still applies, but is far more complicated than in simple cases of classifying people as exposed or unexposed. Because of the complexity of the relationships, the effect of misclassification of time-related factors is difficult to predict in a straightforward, generalizable manner.

Questions Addressed by the Committee

For each question outlined in the introduction to this chapter, we discuss the measures that we are seeking in the reports of study results, how these measures are examined to address the particular question, the types of data a study would need in order to be informative about this question, and problems associated with the measures we have chosen.

How long does it take after exposure to see an increase in disease risk?

Measures of interest Relative risks for specific intervals of time since exposure are the appropriate measures of interest for this question. One must examine the pattern of relative risks, looking for the earliest indication of an increase in risk relative to the unexposed comparison group. For protracted exposures, it is sufficient to examine the relative risks by time-since-first-exposure because it is likely that the earliest detectable increase in relative risk is a manifestation of the earliest exposure. In fact, relative risks for specific times since first exposure are the only measures reported for the herbicide effects studies with protracted exposure.

Data requirements The critical data item for this measure is the date of first exposure. This is needed in order to determine the time that each subject spent in each time-since-first-exposure category. If full exposure histories are available, more sophisticated analyses are possible.

Potential problems with this approach The "earliest indication of an increase in relative risk" is not a fixed value, and it will be refined as more data are collected. First, it is likely that changes in risk occur continuously rather than suddenly jumping from "normal" to "above normal." Actual changes in relative risk probably would occur earlier than indicated by the analysis, but this would not be detectable. Second, "indication" necessarily means statistically detectable, and detectability is a function of the size of the particular data set as well as the magnitude of both the background level of risk and the relative increase in risk. In addition, the higher the quality of the exposure data, and the larger the exposure, the more likely the data would be to detect changes that occur earlier. In our evaluations, we determine the earliest increase in relative risk that can be detected based on the study results described in the literature. These are, of course, subject to change as more information becomes available.

How long does the effect of exposure last?

Measure of interest Relative risks for specific intervals of time since exposure are the major measures used to address this question. The pattern of relative risks must be examined for the latest indication that the relative risk is greater than one.

Data requirements Dates of each start and stop of exposure are required to answer this question. These are needed to classify the subjects' time spent in each time-since-exposure category. If full exposure histories are available, more sophisticated analyses are possible. However, if the critical issue is "time since exposure stopped," such multiple starts and stops will be difficult to analyze.

Potential problems with this approach If exposure is protracted, time since exposure must be analyzed in the proper time-dependent fashion (Clayton and Hills, 1993). This would apply to an examination of time since exposure stopped, when exposure is intermittent. Finally, a study group must have sufficient numbers of subjects with long times since exposure. Much longer time periods are needed than for addressing the previous question.

How does the effect of exposure vary with the age at which it was received?

Measures of interest Relative risks for exposure beginning at various ages are the critical measures needed to address this question. One must examine the pattern of relative risks associated with exposure beginning at various ages and compare the patterns of relative risks by time since exposure across age at exposure categories.

Data requirements Dates of exposure and date of birth are the critical data needed to construct these measures. These are needed to classify subjects as exposed or unexposed in each age category. The date of birth of study participants is generally known in epidemiologic studies. If level of exposure information is available, it would be used in preference to the simple exposed/unexposed categorization. For the relative risks stratified by time since exposure, the data requirements include those described above.

Potential problems with this approach The problems with this approach parallel those for the previous questions. Large studies with long follow-up are more likely than a small study to detect differential age effects. Sample size becomes a practical problem, as analysis within age groups requires more data than pooling all age groups within exposure categories. For examining time since exposure within age group, the comments about investigation of relative risk by time since exposure apply here as well. We found no studies that report the results needed to address this question for herbicides and cancer risk.

Does the exposure appear to act at an early or late stage of the carcinogenic process?

Measures of interest The key statistical measures needed to address this question are the relative risks by age at exposure and time since exposure or, alternatively, the parameters in one of several models of carcinogenesis. In the multistage model of carcinogenesis, a healthy cell is presumed to go through a series of stages before becoming a cancer cell (Armitage and Doll, 1961; Chu, 1987). This model predicts specific patterns of relative risks by age and time since exposure, depending on whether the agent acts on an early or late stage of the carcinogenic process (Whittemore, 1977; Thomas, 1988). Further, the parameters in the multistage model or other mechanistic models, such as the two-event "initiator-promoter" model of Moolgavkar and Venzon (1979), may be estimated from cohort data to distinguish early- and late-stage effects.

Data requirements To construct these measures, complete exposure histories and the date of birth are required. The study group must include subjects with protracted exposures, and there must be variation with respect to exposure histories.

Potential problems with this approach Estimation of the needed quantities requires large studies with high-quality exposure-history data.

RESULTS OF THE LITERATURE REVIEW OF HERBICIDE EXPOSURE AND CANCER

For the purposes of this discussion, the review of the literature on herbicide exposure and cancer was focused on cancers in the "sufficient" and "limited/suggestive" evidence of association categories in *VAO*— that is, those cancers for which there was some evidence of an association. These are soft-tissue sarcoma, non-Hodgkin's lymphoma, Hodgkin's disease, prostate cancer, respiratory cancer, and multiple myeloma. Although *VAO* and Chapter 7 of this report review the entire relevant literature on herbicide exposure, this chapter only discusses the articles that provide results that the committee believes reflect, with reasonable accuracy, the timing of herbicide exposure and that had sufficient cases to make some judgment about the patterns of relative risks reported.

Limitations of the Literature Review Approach

In Chapter 4, the committee considers the problem of using a literature review in order to determine whether an association exists between herbicides and disease. The committee concludes that for overall questions of association between exposure and disease, the published literature would adequately report results, whether "positive" or "negative," with respect to association from the studies that have been carried out to date. Thus, there should be little "publication bias," the tendency for positive results to be published more frequently than negative, in the review of the literature for association.

In a specific investigation of timing issues based on a review of the literature, the same question of publication bias needs to be addressed. That is, is it more likely that results of investigations of timing issues will be published depending on the outcome of those investigations? Unlike measures of association (in particular relative risk) that are universally reported, results of investigations of timing issues are not routinely reported. Indeed, although it is not possible to determine the reasons that timing was or was not reported, it is quite plausible that negative results (that is, no differential effect of timing) are less frequently reported than positive results. One likely scenario is that if no association is found between exposure and disease, then either timing issues were not investigated or were investigated and only "interesting" results (that is, large changes over time intervals) were reported, but "uninteresting" results (no association over all time intervals) were not reported. Thus, the committee recognizes that there is a potential for publication bias in our review.

Overview of the Findings

This focused review of the literature found few articles that were informative about timing of exposure. For soft-tissue sarcoma, non-Hodgkin's lymphoma, Hodgkin's disease, and multiple myeloma, the committee concluded that there was very little information about the timing of exposure and subsequent risk and therefore that no further discussion of latency issues and these cancers was warranted. The committee did find that there was enough information about timing of exposure and respiratory and prostate cancers to warrant reporting these results, with considerably more information about the former than the latter. Some of the available epidemiologic studies, particularly those of production workers, appear to have adequate variation in timing of exposure available, such that further analyses of timing issues may well provide additional insights about the relationship between herbicide exposure and cancer. However, even for these cancers, the reports of some potentially informative studies did not include latency results, so there is potential for publication bias. Also, both of these cancers are in the "limited/suggestive" evidence category, indicating that the committee believes that the evidence for association between herbicide exposure and these cancers is not conclusive. This view has not changed after this investigation of latency issues.

RESPIRATORY CANCER

Background

There is a substantial body of literature that explores issues of timing of exposure and respiratory cancer, because of its relatively high incidence and because numerous carcinogenic agents have been identified. We summarize some of the studies here to provide a background for the examination of these issues.

Gamma rays In an investigation of latency issues for radiation exposure in the atomic bomb survivors, it was found that the relative risk of respiratory cancer began to rise within five to ten years after exposure and reached a plateau about 15 years after exposure. After 30 years of exposure, there was no evidence of a decrease in relative risk (Land, 1987).

Radon daughters For miners exposed to radon daughters, the relative risk of lung cancer was seen to peak within five to ten years after first exposure, then slowly decline, although the risk still appears to be elevated even 30 years after exposure (Lubin et al., 1994; Thomas et al., 1994). In addition, the effect of exposure varies with age at exposure: a given exposure level results in a lower relative risk in older workers than it does in younger workers.

Smoking Based on an analysis of a large case-control study of lung cancer in five Western European countries, Brown and Chu (1987) reported that relative risks rise slowly after the start of cigarette smoking and fall quickly after quitting. Among ex-smokers, the relative risk continues to decline to about 50 percent of that of smokers by 12 years after cessation but then remains fairly constant (but still elevated relative to nonsmokers). Among continuing smokers, for the same cumulative amount smoked, the relative risk declines with age at start of smoking.

Arsenic In a cohort of workers from a copper smelter in Montana, relative risks were observed to increase with time after exposure, reaching a maximum between 15 and 20 years after exposure, after which they slowly declined (Breslow and Day, 1987). There was little change in relative risk with age at first exposure.

Asbestos In a cohort of workers exposed to high levels of asbestos only briefly during World War II, the relative risk rose sharply between five and ten years after exposure, after which the relative risk has remained constant up to 40 years after exposure (EPA, 1986). The relative risks are independent of age at exposure.

Nickel In a cohort study of nickel refiners in England and Wales, the relative risk for lung cancer peaks less than 20 years after exposure, then decreases sharply. After 50 years, however, the risk is still elevated, except in the low-exposure group. The relative risks are more or less constant across age at first exposure (Kaldor et al., 1986). It is interesting to note that in contrast to these results, the same author reported quite a different pattern of relative risks for nasal sinus cancer. It was found that the relative risks for nasal sinus cancer continued to increase slowly with time since exposure, but increase markedly with age at first exposure.

Thus, for all of these exposures, increases in relative risk either reached a plateau or peaked within 20 years after exposure. This indicates that the first detectable increases occurred somewhat earlier than this. The pattern of relative risks after reaching the peak and the pattern with age at exposure vary greatly across the agents, probably reflecting different mechanisms of action.

Review of the Herbicide Exposure and Respiratory Cancer Literature

Five studies have reported timing effects related to herbicide exposure and respiratory cancer. The National Institute for Occupational Safty and Health (NIOSH) study of chemical production workers gives the most detailed account of timing effects and exposure to TCDD. Fingerhut et al. (1991) report standardized mortality ratios (SMRs) for lung cancer of 0.8, 1.0, and 1.2 for 0-9, 10-19, and 20+ years since first exposure to TCDD based on a total of 85 cases. They further stratify time-since-exposure SMRs by duration of exposure category, as reproduced in Table 8.1. The increasing trend in SMR with increasing time since first exposure is somewhat consistent over the duration of exposure categories.

The mortality study of Dutch production workers, a subset of the International Agency for Research on Cancer (IARC) study, similarly reports respiratory cancer SMRs of 0.4, 0.4, and 1.6 for 0-9, 10-19, and 20+ years since first TCDD exposure. These results are based on nine cases, however—too few cases to yield statistically significant results (Bueno de Mesquita et al., 1993).

Assuming that the exposure to TCDD related to the Seveso accident was of relatively short duration, time since the accident is essentially time since exposure. The mortality study by Bertazzi et al. (1989a,b) provides some latency results for lung cancer mortality. Relative risks, compared to the surrounding unexposed population, are given by calendar periods 1976-81 and 1982-86 for males for Zones A, B, and R (see Chapter 7 for further details of this study). For those living in the area at the time of the accident, these correspond to 0-5 and 6-10 years since exposure to TCDD. Thus, assuming that the in-migrants represent a small proportion of the cohort, the calendar period relative risks will approximate time since exposure. The relative risks are summarized in Table 8.2. There are small, but consistent increases in relative risk with calendar period.

In an 18-year follow-up of Finnish herbicide applicators, Asp et al., (1994)

TABLE 8-1 NIOSH Study: Respiratory Cancer Relative Mortality by Time Since First Exposure and Duration of Exposure to TCDD

Time since first exposure	Duration of exposure to TCDD (Years)									
	<1		1-4		5-14		15+		Overall	
	Obs	SMR	Obs	SMR	Obs	SMR	Obs	SMR	Obs	SMR
0-9	3	77	3	95	1	79	0	0	7	84
10-19	6	69	5	79	9	180	1	137	21	101
20+	17	96	17	126	14	146	9	156	57	123
Total	26	86	25	109	24	151	10	154	85	112

SOURCE: Fingerhut et al., 1991, Table 4.

TABLE 8-2 Seveso Study: Lung Cancer Relative Mortality in Men by Calendar Period

Zone	Observed deaths	Relative Risk 1976-1981[a]	1982-1986[b]
A	2	(not given[c])	2.0
B	20	1.1	1.8
R	77	0.7	0.9

[a]Approximately 0-5 years since first exposure.
[b]Approximately 6-10 years since first exposure.
[c]Presumably 0 cases.

SOURCE: Bertazzi et al., 1989.

TABLE 8-3 Finnish Applicators Study: Respiratory Cancer Observed and Expected Deaths and SMRs for Men by Time Since First Exposure to Chlorophenoxy Herbicide

Time since first employment								
0-9 years			11-14 years			15+ years		
Obs	Exp	SMR	Obs	Exp	SMR	Obs	Exp	SMR
4	6.4	0.6	11	8.1	1.4	22	21.0	1.0

SOURCE: Asp et al., 1994, Table 3.

gives the respiratory cancer SMRs relative to the male Finnish age and calendar year specific rates by 0, 10, and 15 year "latency intervals." These correspond to 0+, 10+, and 15+ years since first exposure to chlorophenoxy herbicides. There were a total of 37 respiratory cancer deaths. By subtracting the given observeds and expecteds, the SMRs by time since first exposure can be computed. These are given in Table 8.3. These data do not indicate a trend in the SMRs.

Conclusions

Perhaps because respiratory cancers are the most common type of cancer in all of the cohort studies, there is more latency information available for them than for any other cancer. However, based on the review of the evidence in *VAO* and Chapter 7 of this report, respiratory cancer is in the "limited/suggestive" evidence category, indicating that the committee believes that the evidence for association between herbicide exposure and these cancers is not conclusive. Although investigation of latency effects could result in a change in association categorization, the fact that the committee reviewed the literature for latency effects does not imply an a priori belief on the part of the committee that the association is definitive.

How long does it take after exposure to see an increase in disease risk? The evidence in the literature suggests that the time from exposure to TCDD to increased risk of respiratory cancer occurs within ten years. This conclusion is based primarily on the NIOSH study (Fingerhut et al., 1991), because this study is the most informative about the changes in risk of respiratory cancer with time since first exposure to TCDD. The Seveso study (Bertazzi et al., 1989a,b) is also suggestive of an increase in relative risk five years after exposure, but the number of exposed cases is too small to rule out chance as a likely explanation for the observed increases. The other relevant studies have relatively few respiratory cancer cases but are consistent with this conclusion. It is unlikely that chance can explain these patterns of relative risk, given the numbers of cases and the consistency of the pattern across duration of exposure category.

Another explanation of the existing epidemiologic evidence is that TCDD exposure is not associated with respiratory cancer but is correlated with some other respiratory cancer risk factor, and that risk factor is related to the cancer and to TCDD exposure in a way that results in the observed pattern of relative risks with time since first exposure to TCDD. This explanation requires that the putative risk factor explain the observed increasing relative risk with duration as well as the time since first exposure pattern (see Table 8.1). Such a situation would occur if duration of TCDD exposure were correlated with duration of some other exposure that caused respiratory cancer, such as cigarette smoking or other chemical exposure. The committee is not aware of any evidence for this hypothesis but cannot discount it.

How long do the effects of exposure last? If there is, in fact, a causal association between TCDD exposure and respiratory cancer, the literature suggests that the risk is elevated at least five years after exposure, but we cannot determine how long it takes before the relative risks return to one, if they ever do. However, chance cannot be ruled out as a possible explanation for the observed pattern of relative risk.

This conclusion is based primarily on the Seveso mortality study (Bertazzi et al., 1989a,b) that reports a slight increase in the relative risk in the second five years after the accident (see Table 8.2), indicating that the risk continues to increase five years after exposure ends. All of the study groups that demonstrated latency results had protracted exposures. None of these report results of the type of analysis needed to address this question (see the previous section). However, although the NIOSH study does not directly address this issue, we can reasonably infer that the SMRs for time since exposure in the <1 year duration of exposure category closely track those of the time since first exposure. This is because subjects with less than one year of exposure were likely to have received all of their exposure in a single period of time. This will be less likely for subjects with longer duration of exposure because the possibility of "intermittent exposure" is greater. The SMRs, given in the first column of Table 8.1, appear to increase from <20 years to 20+ years since first exposure, but this is based on rather small numbers (nine cases in the <20 year group), and all the SMRs are less than one.

How does the effect of exposure vary with the age at which it was received? None of the available studies provides information on the variation of the effect of exposure with age.

Does the carcinogen appear to act at an early or late stage of the carcinogenic process? None of the available studies addresses this issue.

PROSTATE CANCER

Background

There are no environmental exposures other than herbicides associated with prostate cancer for which latency issues have been investigated.

Review of the Herbicide Exposure and Prostate Cancer Literature

The NIOSH study of chemical production workers exposed to TCDD (Fingerhut et al., 1991) reports SMRs for prostate cancer for 20+ years since first exposure by duration of exposure <1 and 1+ years as well as for the entire cohort (Fingerhut et al., 1991). These SMRs, with observed and expected numbers of deaths, are given in Table 8.4. Because numbers of observed and expected deaths

TABLE 8-4 NIOSH Production Workers Study: Prostate Cancer Observed, Expected and SMRs for Men by Time Since First Exposure and Duration of Exposure to TCDD

Entire cohort			20+ years since first exposure					
			< 1 year exposure			1+ years exposure		
Obs	Exp	SMR	Obs	Exp	SMR	Obs	Exp	SMR
17	13.9	122	2	3.0	67	9	5.9	152

SOURCE: Fingerhut et al., 1991, Table 2.

TABLE 8-5 NIOSH Production Workers Study:
Prostate Cancer Observed and Expected Numbers of
Deaths and SMRs by Time Since First Exposure to TCDD

Time since first exposure					
< 20 years			20+ years		
Obs	Exp	SMR	Obs	Exp	SMR
6	5.0	120	11	8.9	123

SOURCE: Derived from Fingerhut et al., 1991, Table 2.

are not given by duration of exposure for the entire cohort, it is not possible to compare the SMRs for <20 and 20+ years since first exposure within duration of exposure categories. Thus, the most informative comparison is based on SMRs for time-since-first exposure categories without respect to duration of exposure. The SMR for 20+ years since first exposure is obtained by summing the observed and expected numbers for the two duration categories. The SMR for <20 years since first exposure is obtained by subtracting the 20+ year numbers from the total. These are given in Table 8.5. While both are slightly elevated, there is no difference in the SMRs between the <20 and 20+ categories.

Assuming that the exposure to TCDD after the Seveso accident was of relatively short duration, time since the accident is essentially the same as time since exposure. The mortality study by Bertazzi et al. (1989a,b) provides results relevant to timing of exposure for prostate cancer mortality. Relative risks, compared to the surrounding unexposed population, are given by calendar periods 1976-81 and 1982-86 for males for Zones B and R. For those living in the area at the time of the accident, these time periods correspond to 0-5 and 6-10 years since exposure. Thus, assuming that inmigrants represent a small proportion of the cohort, the calendar-period relative risks will approximate the time since exposure. The relative risks are summarized in Table 8.6. There are too few cases (three) in Zone B to draw any conclusions about time since first exposure and changing risk patterns. In Zone R, there is a decrease in the relative risk with calendar period, although the small number of cases and the fact that this is a mortality rather than an incidence study preclude strong statements about the actual pattern of relative risks.

Conclusions

Our review of the literature yielded only two articles on prostate cancer with latency-related results and sufficient numbers of cases for statistical analysis. Prostate cancer is in the limited/suggestive evidence category, so it is important

TABLE 8-6 Seveso Study: Prostate Cancer Relative
Mortality in Men by Calendar Period

		Relative risk	
Zone	Observed deaths	1976-1981[a]	1982-1986[b]
A[c]	—	—	—
B	3	2.8	1.5
R	16	1.9	1.2

[a]Approximately 0-5 years since first exposure.
[b]Approximately 6-10 years since first exposure.
[c]Not provided.

SOURCE: Bertazzi et al., 1989.

to keep in mind that the committee believes that the evidence for association
between herbicide exposure and prostate cancer is not conclusive. Although
investigation of latency effects could result in a change in association categorization,
the fact that the committee reviewed the literature for latency effects does
not imply an a priori belief on the part of the committee that the association is
definitive.

How long does it take after exposure to see an increase in disease risk? The
inconsistent, limited data from the NIOSH study (Fingerhut et al., 1991) and the
Seveso study (Bertazzi et al., 1989a,b) do not indicate any increase in the relative
risk of prostate cancer with time since exposure to TCDD. Because the NIOSH
cohort was grouped into categories of <20 and 20+ years since first exposure,
they give no indication about changes in risk of prostate cancer within 20 years of
exposure. The Seveso study has too few cases of prostate cancer and too short an
observation period (up to ten years) to be informative on this question.

How long do the effects of exposure last? The available evidence is not informative
on this issue.

How does the effect of exposure vary with the age at which it was received?
None of the studies provides information on the variation of the effect of exposure
with age.

**Does the carcinogen appear to act at an early or late stage of the carcinogenic
process?** None of the studies addresses this issue.

RELEVANCE OF THE LATENCY ISSUE IN ASSESSING THE EFFECT OF HERBICIDES ON CANCER RISK IN VIETNAM VETERANS

One of the committee's tasks was to assess the likelihood that exposure to herbicides used in Vietnam resulted in or will result in increased risk of disease in Vietnam veterans. Currently, this needs to be inferred based on extrapolation from the findings about disease experience of other groups exposed to TCDD or herbicides generally. The validity of an extrapolation of this kind depends on the comparability of the groups upon which the extrapolation is based and (specific subgroups of) the Vietnam veterans. In particular, at the least, exposure status and level of exposure should be comparable. In addition, as we have discussed in this chapter, comparability with respect to timing of exposure may also be very important.

For the Vietnam veterans, assessing the extent of exposure and, in particular, identifying highly exposed individuals are perhaps the primary problems in assessing the relevance of findings in other groups to the risk of disease in veterans. This problem is discussed in Chapter 5. However, factors related to the timing of exposure may actually be determined with some accuracy. For an individual veteran, it is easy to ascertain the dates of service in Vietnam and the date of birth. Thus, although it is difficult to determine the exact dates of possible exposure, these dates put clear bounds on the number of years since first or last exposure. In fact, these limits bound the interval of potential exposure to a range that is adequate for categorization of time since exposure, given the accuracy level of epidemiologic studies. Thus, it is feasible to extrapolate from results on the timing of exposure from other study groups when determining the likely effect of exposure on groups of Vietnam veterans defined by age at exposure. Ideally, a table of relative risks by categories of time since exposure and age at exposure for a number of exposure-level categories, such as serum TCDD level, could be constructed. There is currently not enough information in the literature to estimate such relative risks. However, further analysis of existing studies with a focus on investigation of likely timing of exposure among Vietnam veterans may yield useful information.

REFERENCES

Armenian HK. 1987. Incubation periods in cancer epidemiology. Journal of Chronic Diseases 40:9-16.

Armitage P, Doll R. 1961. Stochastic Models for Carcinogenesis. In Proceedings of the 4th Berkeley Symposium on Mathematical Statistics and Probability (ed. J. Neyman). University of California Press.

Asp S, Riihimaki V, Hernberg S, Pukkala E. 1994. Mortality and cancer morbidity of Finnish chlorophenoxy herbicide applicators: an 18-year prospective follow-up. American Journal of Industrial Medicine 26:243-253.

Bertazzi PA, Zocchetti C, Pesatori AC, Guercilena S, Sanarico M, Radice L. 1989a. Mortality in an area contaminated by TCDD following an industrial incident. Medicina Del Lavoro 80:316-329.

Bertazzi PA, Zocchetti C, Pesatori AC, Guercilena S, Sanarico M, Radice L. 1989b. Ten-year mortality study of the population involved in the Seveso incident in 1976. American Journal of Epidemiology 129:1187-1200.

Breslow NE, Day NE. 1987. Statistical Methods in Cancer Research Vol II. The Design and Analysis of Cohort Studies. Lyon: International Agency for Research on Cancer. Oxford University Press.

Brown C, Chu K. 1987. Use of multistage models to infer stage affected by carcinogenic exposure: example of lung cancer and cigarette smoking. Journal of Chronic Diseases 40:171-180.

Bueno de Mesquita HB, Doornbos G, Van der Kuip DA, Kogevinas M, Winkelmann R. 1993. Occupational exposure to phenoxy herbicides and chlorophenols and cancer mortality in the Netherlands. American Journal of Industrial Medicine 23:289-300.

Chu K. 1987. A non-mathematical view of mathematical models of cancer. Journal of Chronic Diseases 40:163-170.

Clayton D, Hills M. 1993. Statistical Models in Epidemiology. Oxford University Press, New York.

Enterline P, Henderson V. 1973. Type of asbestos and respiratory cancer in the asbestos industry. Archives of Environmental Health 27:312-317.

Fingerhut MA, Halperin WE, Marlow DA, Piacitelli LA, Honchar PA, Sweeney MH, Greife AL, Dill PA, Steenland K, Suruda AJ. 1991. Cancer mortality in workers exposed to 2,3,7,8-tetrachlorodibenzo-p-dioxin. New England Journal of Medicine 324:212-218.

Kaldor J, Peto J, Easton D, Doll R, Hermon C, Morgan L. 1986. Models for respiratory cancer in nickel refinery workers. Journal of the National Cancer Institute 77:841-848.

Land C. 1987. Temporal distributions of risk for radiation-induced cancers. Journal of Chronic Diseases 40:45-58.

Lubin J, Boice J, Edling C, Hornung R, Howe G, Kunz E, Kusiak R, Morrison H, Radford E, Samet J, Tirmarche M, Woodward A, Xiang Y, Pierce D. 1994. Radon and Lung Cancer Risk: A Joint Analysis of 11 Underground Miners Studies. U.S. Department of Health and Human Services, Public Health Service, National Institutes of Health, Bethesda.

Moolgavkar S, Venzon D. 1979. Two-event models for carcinogenesis: incidence curves for childhood and adult tumors. Mathematical Biosciences 47:55-77.

Peto J. 1985. Some problems in dose-response estimation in cancer epidemiology. In Methods for Estimating Risk of Chemical Injury: Human and Non-Human Biota and Ecosystems (V. Voug, G. Butler, D. Hoel, D Peakall, eds). Wiley, New York.

Thomas DC. 1983. Statistical methods for analyzing effects of temporal patterns of exposure on cancer risks. Scandinavian Journal of Work, Environment, and Health 9:353-366.

Thomas DC. 1987. Pitfalls in the analysis of exposure-time-reponse relationships. Journal of Chronic Disease 40:70-78.

Thomas DC. 1988. Models for exposure-time-response relationships with applications to cancer epidemiology. Annual Review of Public Health 9:451-482.

Thomas DC, Pogoda J, Langholz B, Mack W. 1994. Temporal modifiers of the radon-smoking interaction. Health Physics 66:257-262.

U.S. Environmental Protection Agency. 1986. Airborne Asbestos Health Assessment Update. Environmental Criteria and Assessment Office, Research Triangle Park, N.C.

Whittemore AS. 1977. The age distribution of human cancer for carcinogenic exposures of varying intensity. American Journal of Epidemiology 106:418-432.

9

Reproductive Effects

INTRODUCTION

This chapter summarizes published scientific literature on exposure to herbicides and adverse reproductive and developmental effects. The literature discussed includes papers published since *VAO*. *VAO* included a number of environmental, occupational, and Vietnam veteran studies that evaluated herbicide exposure and the risk of adverse outcomes, including spontaneous abortion, birth defects, stillbirths, neonatal and infant mortality, low birthweight, and sperm quality and infertility. The report concluded that the evidence at that time was inadequate or insufficient to determine whether an association exists between exposure to herbicides and each of the above reproductive and developmental outcomes.

The primary emphasis of *VAO* and the present review is on the potential adverse reproductive effects of herbicide exposure for males, because the vast majority of the Vietnam veterans are men. Nevertheless, a brief discussion of the epidemiologic findings pertaining to female exposure is warranted because of the Department of Veterans Affairs' planned study of female Vietnam veterans and their reproductive health. Additionally, there is growing evidence from experimental animal research on female reproductive toxicity and developmental toxicity via in utero exposure to dioxin.

A number of studies have attempted to evaluate the potential association between herbicide exposure in women and the risk of adverse reproductive outcomes, including spontaneous abortion, stillbirth, preterm delivery, and birth defects (Hemminki et al., 1980; McDonald et al., 1987; Ahlborg et al., 1989;

Savitz et al., 1989; Fenster and Coye, 1990; Restrepo et al., 1990; Goulet and Theriault, 1991; Nurminen et al., 1994). The quality and results of these studies have been mixed. A major limitation of nearly all the studies is the determination of specific exposures. Many studies have defined exposure solely based on employment in agricultural occupations. Exposure to specific chemicals and other agents in these agricultural settings is usually not ascertained. Further, problems such as incomplete ascertainment of the outcome of interest, selection of inappropriate or no control groups, and failure to account for confounding factors have plagued some of this work. Improvements in study design, especially exposure assessment, should allow for a more definitive evaluation of the relationship between herbicide exposure and adverse reproductive outcomes among women.

The following sections will separately discuss specific categories of reproductive effects: fertility, spontaneous abortion, stillbirth, birth defects, and childhood cancer. Childhood cancer is discussed in this chapter rather than in Chapter 7, since many such cancers are related to preconceptual and in utero exposures. For most outcomes, a brief summary of the scientific evidence in *VAO* is presented, followed by an update of the recent scientific literature. A complete discussion of the evidence is presented for birth defects, because the committee has changed its assessment of this literature since *VAO*.

FERTILITY

Background

Male reproductive function is a complex system under the control of several components whose proper coordination are important for normal fertility. There are several components or endpoints related to male fertility, including reproductive hormones and sperm parameters. Only a brief description of male reproductive hormones will be given here; more detailed reviews can be found elsewhere (Yen and Jaffe, 1991; Knobil et al., 1994). The reproductive neuroendocrine axis involves the central nervous system, the anterior pituitary gland, and the testis. The hypothalamus integrates neural inputs from the central and peripheral nervous systems and regulates gonadotrophins (luteinizing hormone and follicle-stimulating hormone). Both of these hormones are necessary for normal spermatogenesis. Luteinizing hormone (LH) and follicle-stimulating hormone (FSH) are secreted in episodic bursts by the anterior pituitary gland into the circulation. LH interacts with receptors on the Leydig cells, which leads to increased testosterone synthesis. FSH and testosterone from the Leydig cells interact with the Sertoli cells in the seminiferous tubule epithelium to regulate spermatogenesis. Several agents, such as lead and dibromochloropropane (DBCP), have been shown to affect the neuroendocrine system (Ng et al., 1991; Whorton et al., 1979).

Summary of VAO

Only one occupational epidemiologic study is available for assessing the association between herbicide exposure and altered sperm parameters (sperm count, motility, morphology). This study of 2,4-D exposure did indicate an association with abnormal sperm morphology; however, given the small sample size and lack of additional studies, the evidence for determination of an association is considered inadequate. No studies were identified that examined occupational or environmental exposure and impaired fertility. One study of veterans reported an association with altered sperm measures (reduced sperm concentration and increased percentage of abnormal sperm), although there was no relationship to the number of children fathered, self-reported herbicide exposure, or the extent of combat experience. The paucity of occupational studies, lack of consistent findings in veterans studies, and methodologic problems in the studies reviewed do not permit a valid assessment of an increased infertility.

Update of the Scientific Literature

The Centers for Disease Control and Prevention (CDC) Vietnam Experience Study (VES) did not find any association between service in Vietnam and alterations in FSH, LH, and testosterone (Centers for Disease Control, 1989). The recent analysis of the Ranch Hand data indicated that FSH was not associated with estimated initial dioxin level (Roegner et al., 1991). There was a pattern of decreasing testosterone with increasing serum dioxin, although this was statistically nonsignificant.

NIOSH researchers conducted a cross-sectional study to evaluate the relationship between serum dioxin and serum testosterone and gonadotrophins in men previously occupationally exposed to dioxin and in a referent group (Egeland et al., 1994). The exposed group consisted of men who were either current or former employees at two of the 12 plants that are part of the NIOSH cohort study of dioxin-exposed workers. The plants manufactured 2,4,5-T from 1951 to 1969 in New Jersey and from 1968 to 1972 in the Missouri plant. A cross-sectional medical study was conducted in 1987, with a total of 586 workers identified. Among these men, 400 were considered eligible (143 died, 43 were not located). A total of 357 workers completed the interview, and 281 completed a medical exam (70 percent of eligible, 48 percent of original group). For comparison, age-, sex-, and race-matched neighborhood referents were identified and contacted. A total of 325 referents were interviewed, and 260 completed the medical exam. The original number of referents contacted was not stated. The interview included questions on medical history, demographics, and lifestyle factors. A random sample of the comparison subjects was chosen ($N = 99$), and their mean dioxin value (6.08 picograms/gram) was assigned to the 161 referent subjects without a serum measurement. A half-life decay model (7.1 year half-life; steady-state background = 6.08 picograms/gram) was used to estimate past dioxin levels. A single measurement of total serum testosterone, FSH and LH was taken for each subject. The strength of the relationship between serum dioxin and serum levels of testosterone, FSH, and LH were estimated by linear regression (continuous dioxin) and logistic regression (using quartiles of dioxin), adjusting for age, body mass index (BMI), diabetes, alcohol, smoking, and race.

The results of the linear regression analysis indicated that current serum dioxin was related to FSH, LH, and testosterone levels. Serum dioxin was positively related to FSH (b = .04) and LH (b = .03), and inversely related to testosterone (b = –.02). The regression coefficient b represents the unit increase or decrease in gonadotrophins and testosterone per unit increase in serum dioxin. The magnitude of the increases or decreases in hormones was thus rather small, compared to the normal range for these hormones in humans. The logistic regression analysis used serum dioxin categorized into quartiles and "high" LH and FSH and "low" testosterone. High LH was defined as >28 IU/liter (laboratory standard for normal range = 5-28 IU/liter) and high FSH as >31 IU/liter (normal range = 3-31 IU/liter). Low testosterone was defined as <10.4 nmol/liter (normal range = 9.4-34.7 nmol/liter). These cutoffs were at the 8th percentile of the LH and FSH distributions. The cutoff for low testosterone was set at the 8th percentile (<10.4 nmol/liter) to be consistent with FSH and LH. There was an association found between high LH and current serum dioxin (2nd dioxin quartile OR = 1.9; 3rd OR = 2.5; 4th OR = 1.9; p for trend = .03). For FSH, a pattern of increasing risk with increasing serum dioxin was also found, but the test for trend was not statistically significant (p = .10). The adjusted odds ratios for low testosterone were more elevated (2nd dioxin quartile = 3.9; 3rd = 2.7; 4th = 2.1), but again the trend test was not significant (p = .10). Similar estimates were obtained for half-life serum dioxin extrapolated to the time at which occupational exposure ended.

The results of this study indicated that estimated dioxin exposure levels were positively associated with LH and FSH levels and negatively associated with serum testosterone. The strengths of the study included the use of an occupational cohort with documented dioxin exposure and an attempt to control for potentially confounding factors. However, the cross-sectional nature of the study, the fact that only one serum hormone measurement was obtained, the imprecision of the effect estimates, the failure to detect a dose-response gradient, and the relatively low proportion of participating workers included in the analyses are of concern. The implications of some of these limitations on the interpretation of their findings are not straightforward. The authors argued that their single measurement results are likely to be conservative. Although this issue is not directly addressed in the original paper, the authors have argued in a Letter to the Editor in the *American Journal of Epidemiology* that any laboratory errors in the measurement of serum dioxin and hormones are unlikely to produce the results they obtained and that within- and between-assay variation was acceptable (Egeland et al., 1995). As to possible selection bias due to the poor response, no data exist to directly evaluate possible biasing effects on the odds ratio estimates.

As the authors correctly noted, the magnitude of the differences in hormone concentrations were small. Some of the men did have hormone levels that were either above (LH and FSH) or below (testosterone) the cutoff of the 8th percentile. A major issue in the interpretation of these findings, if real, is whether these changes in hormone concentration ascribed to dioxin have any implications for reproductive failure. Clearly, the hormonal changes are rather subtle and are well below levels expected to result in gonadal failure. Although the one study reviewed here suggested an association between TCDD exposure and changes in male reproductive hormones, there were a number of methodologic concerns with the study that do not permit definitive conclusions to be drawn.

Conclusions

Strength of Evidence in Epidemiologic Studies

There is inadequate or insufficient evidence to determine whether an association exists between exposure to the herbicides considered in the report and altered sperm parameters or infertility. The evidence regarding association is drawn from occupational and other studies in which subjects were exposed to a variety of herbicides and herbicide components.

Biologic Plausibility

Experimental animal evidence supports the notion that dioxin can alter testosterone synthesis, generally at relatively high doses, but does not provide direct clues as to the reproductive significance of hormone disregulation of the magnitude found in available studies.

SPONTANEOUS ABORTION

Background

Spontaneous abortion (or miscarriage), according to the World Health Organization (1977), is a "nondeliberate fetal death of an intrauterine pregnancy before 22 completed weeks of gestation, corresponding to a fetal weight of approximately 500 grams or more." Pregnancy losses prior to implantation (preimplantation) are not clinically detectable with current diagnostic procedures. The rate of early (postimplantation) detectable (but often unrecognized) pregnancy losses has been estimated to be approximately 30 percent (Wilcox et al., 1988).

Because preimplantation and early postimplantation losses are difficult to ascertain for epidemiologic studies of pregnancy loss, the appropriate epidemiologic endpoint for these studies is not all spontaneous abortions but rather all clinically recognized spontaneous abortions—those that come to the attention of a woman or her physician. All subsequent discussions of pregnancy loss, miscarriage, or spontaneous abortion refer to clinically recognized outcomes unless otherwise specified.

Approximately 10 to 15 percent of all clinically recognized pregnancies end in a clinically recognized loss. Of these clinically recognized pregnancy losses, 35 to 40 percent are losses of chromosomally abnormal embryos and fetuses (Kline et al., 1989). A wide range of maternal characteristics and exposures has been linked to miscarriage. However, two major risk factors have been established—advanced maternal age and history of previous miscarriage (Kline et al., 1989).

Summary of *VAO*

The studies involving occupational and environmental herbicide exposure generally reported no association with spontaneous abortion; however, these studies were inadequate with respect to sample size, elimination of potential bias, and assessment of exposure.

The available epidemiologic studies of veterans are generally limited by inadequate sample size, potential bias, and other methodologic problems. There are some suggestive findings indicating an increased risk for Vietnam veterans, including a possible dose-response gradient of increasing risk with increasing estimated (self-reported or inferred) Agent Orange exposure. Nonetheless, the inconsistency with environmental and occupational studies, the uncertainty of the methods of exposure determination, the marginal magnitude of the increased risk, and the failure to exclude chance are of enough concern that the evidence can be considered insufficient. Future analyses of the data for Ranch Hands, the Air Force personnel involved in handling and spraying herbicides, may contribute important evidence regarding an increased risk for spontaneous abortion among exposed Vietnam veterans.

Update of the Scientific Literature

The general introduction and review of the recently published Ranch Hand study of reproductive outcomes (Wolfe et al., 1995) can be found in the section on birth defects below. Overall, the conception and birth rates were similar for the Ranch Hands and the comparison veterans. There was a total of 157 (16 percent) spontaneous abortions among Ranch Hands and 172 (14 percent) among comparison veterans. The results by dioxin level showed only a weak increased relative risk estimates for the background (RR = 1.1; CI 0.8-1.5) and low-level (RR = 1.3; CI 1.0-1.7) categories and no association for the high-level category (RR = 1.0; CI 0.7-1.3).

The Ranch Hand study had some clear strengths. The AFHS cohorts were well defined and systematically followed, and health outcomes were carefully monitored. The Ranch Hands represent veterans with high potential for herbicide and dioxin exposure, and the use of serum dioxin assays has provided a direct estimate of exposure that is superior in some respects to the retrospective exposure assessment methods based on troop movement and spraying data.

Several aspects of how the study was conducted and how the data were analyzed deserve consideration. First, the difference in the number of original cohort subjects and those that were included in the final analyses raises the possibility of selection bias. The authors noted that those who volunteered for the study were more likely to have children with birth defects than those who did not volunteer. The impact on the risk ratio is not likely to be important, because this volunteerism was not associated with exposure. Nonetheless, there is no discussion of a comparison of the original cohort subjects and their children with those who were included in the final analyses, not just those who agreed to the serum dioxin assay. The complete exclusion of the subjects with serum dioxin sample measurements below the level of detectability, rather than their inclusion with the background or referent categories, does not appear justified.

Conclusions

Strength of Evidence in Epidemiologic Studies

There is inadequate or insufficient evidence to determine whether an association exists between exposure to the herbicides considered in this report and spontaneous abortion. The evidence regarding association is drawn from occupational and other studies in which subjects were exposed to a variety of herbicides and herbicide components.

STILLBIRTH

Background

The use of the terms "stillbirth" and "neonatal death" can be confusing and has differed in various epidemiologic studies. Stillbirth (or late fetal death) is typically defined as the delivery of a fetus occurring at or after 28 weeks of gestation and showing no signs of life at birth, although a more recent definition includes deaths among all fetuses weighing more than 500 grams at birth, regardless of gestational age at delivery (Kline et al., 1989). Neonatal death is usually defined as the death of a live-born infant within the first 28 days of life. Because there are no clear biological differences between late fetal deaths (stillbirths) and deaths in the early neonatal period, these are commonly referred to together as perinatal deaths (Kallen, 1988). Stillbirths occur in approximately 1 to 2 percent of all births (Kline et al., 1989). Among low-birthweight live- and stillborn infants (500-2,500 grams), placental and delivery complications such as abruptio placentae, placenta previa, malpresentation, and umbilical cord complications are the most common causes of perinatal mortality (Kallen, 1988). Among infants weighing more than 2,500 grams at birth, the most common causes of perinatal death are lethal congenital malformations and placental complications (Kallen, 1988).

Summary of VAO

A statistical association with stillbirth has not been reported in the available occupational and environmental epidemiologic studies. The majority of studies did not have adequate statistical power, and the assessment of exposure was incomplete. Some studies of veterans have reported an increased risk, whereas others have indicated no statistical association. Interpretation of these veteran studies is constrained by limited statistical power and most importantly, by uncertainty of correctly assigning herbicide exposure to study groups.

Update of the Scientific Literature

The general introduction and review of the recently published study of reproductive outcomes among the Ranch Hands is provided in the section on spontaneous abortion (Wolfe at al., 1995). With respect to stillbirth, a total of 14 (1.4 percent) Ranch Hand conceptions resulted in a stillbirth, compared with 13 (1.1 percent) comparison veteran conceptions. Elevated risk ratios were found for the background (RR = 1.8; CI 0.7-4.5) and low (RR = 1.8; CI 0.7-4.7) levels, although both estimates were nonsignificant and relatively imprecise. The risk ratio for the high level was 0.3 (CI 0.0-2.3), based on one stillbirth among Ranch Hands. Thus, study results indicated an association between TCDD levels and the risk of stillbirth among those Ranch Hand subjects with either *background* or *low* exposure levels. No association was seen among veterans in the high-exposure category. The evidence from the previous studies reviewed in *VAO* was mixed: some occupational, environmental, and Vietnam veteran studies suggested an increased risk of stillbirth, while other studies did not report an association.

Conclusions

Strength of Evidence in Epidemiologic Studies

There is inadequate or insufficient evidence to determine whether an association exists between exposure to the herbicides considered in this report and stillbirth. The evidence regarding association is drawn from occupational and other studies in which subjects were exposed to a variety of herbicides and herbicide components.

BIRTH DEFECTS

Background

The March of Dimes defines a birth defect as "an abnormality of structure, function or metabolism, whether genetically determined or as the result of an environmental influence during embryonic or fetal life" (Bloom, 1981). Other terms often used interchangeably with birth defects are "congenital anomalies" and "congenital malformations." Major birth defects are usually defined as those abnormalities that are present at birth and severe enough to interfere with viability or physical well-being. Major birth defects are seen in approximately 2 to 3 percent of live births (Kalter and Warkany, 1983). An additional 5 percent of birth defects can be detected with follow-up through the first year of life. Given the general frequency of major birth defects of 2 to 3 percent and the number of men who served in Vietnam (2.6 million), and assuming that they had at least one child, it has been estimated that 52,000 to 78,000 babies with birth defects have been fathered by Vietnam veterans, even in the absence of an increase due to exposure to herbicides or other toxic substances (Erickson et al., 1984a).

Epidemiologic Studies of Birth Defects

Because the publication of new data from the Ranch Hand study has caused the committee to change its conclusion about the strength of the evidence regarding the association between exposure to herbicides used in Vietnam and birth defects, the following material was included from *VAO* to present a complete picture about the evidence for the committee's conclusions. The section entitled "Ranch Hand Study," however, is based on the new information.

Occupational Studies

Four occupational epidemiology studies have examined the potential association between herbicide exposure of male workers and birth defects. The Townsend study (Townsend et al., 1982) of workers with potential dioxin exposure at a Dow Chemical plant did not find an increased risk of birth defects among dioxin-exposed workers (30 births with anomalies; 47/1,000 births) compared to unexposed workers (87 births with anomalies; 49/1,000 births; OR = 0.9, CI 0.5-1.4). A major limitation of this study is its limited statistical power to detect an elevated odds ratio for specific defects. The authors noted that the study had 26 percent power to detect a doubling of risk due to exposure for a group of indicator malformations (anomalies thought to be easily recognized and reported by the mother, such as an oral cleft, spina bifida, and Down's syndrome). An additional problem is that despite the use of these "indicator malformations," without medical records, validation of the accuracy of maternal self-report of birth defects is questionable for many conditions.

Two studies of workers from a 2,4,5-T plant in Nitro, West Virginia, did not report an association with birth defects among offspring (Moses et al., 1984; Suskind and Hertzberg, 1984). The relative risk estimates for any birth defect were 1.3 (CI 0.5-3.4) for Moses et al. and 1.1 (CI 0.5-2.2) from the Suskind and Hertzberg study. Both studies had limited statistical power, given the small number of subjects (204 exposed workers in the Suskind and Hertzberg study; 117 exposed workers in the Moses study). This is especially problematic for the evaluation of most specific birth defects. Both studies also relied on self-reports for the ascertainment of birth defects.

A study of 2,4,5-T sprayers found only a slightly elevated odds ratio for congenital anomalies (OR = 1.2, CI 0.5-3.0) associated with the spraying group (Smith et al., 1982). The study used self-administered questionnaires to determine outcomes. Like the other studies, it had limited power for the analysis of individual birth defects.

Environmental Studies

A variety of environmental studies have examined the relationship between herbicide exposure and prevalence of birth defects (Nelson et al., 1979; Gordon and Shy, 1981; Hanify et al., 1981; Mastroiacovo et al., 1988; Stockbauer et al., 1988; White et al., 1988; Fitzgerald et al., 1989; Jansson and Voog, 1989). Some studies reported a statistical association with specific birth defects (clubfoot, Fitzgerald et al., 1989; cleft lip with or without cleft palate, Gordon and Shy, 1981; heart, hypospadias, clubfoot, Hanify et al., 1981; oral clefts, Nelson et al., 1979), although others have not reported an association (Stockbauer et al., 1988; Fitzgerald et al., 1989; Jansson and Voog, 1989), including the Seveso study (Mastroiacovo et al., 1988). Interpretation of the results of these environmental studies is difficult, because most of the studies were inconsistent, were based on ecologic correlations, had inadequate statistical power, did not validate birth defects recorded from vital statistics or self-reports, and included both male and female exposures.

A recently published study from Vietnam evaluated the risk of birth defects among the offspring of mothers who resided in a village in the southern part of the country that had been sprayed during the conflict (Phuong et al., 1989); 81 cases of birth defects (diagnosis not specified) were identified. No differences were reported between cases and controls for the potentially confounding factors investigated. Strong associations were found for birth defects (calculated from data presented; OR = 3.8, CI 1.1-13.1). The paper is difficult to evaluate given the sparse details presented. Study design factors such as how birth defects were diagnosed and what types were detected, the size of the original case and control groups from which the final groups were sampled, the pattern of patient accrual for this hospital, the method of data collection, and how the potential herbicide spraying histories were determined were not specified. Finally, to put the study in the context of this review, the potential exposure 17 to 22 years earlier pertains to both the mother and the father.

Results from a number of other studies from Vietnam, both of sprayed villages in the southern part of the country and of veterans returning to the unsprayed northern regions, have been reported, mostly in a review by Constable and Hatch (1985). These studies indicate an increased risk of birth defects, including anencephaly, oral clefts, and a variety of other anomalies. Nonetheless, these studies generally suffer from poor reporting and a variety of methodologic problems such as limited control of confounding factors, use of a referral hospital, lack of comparison groups, uncertainty of exposure classification, and no validation of reported birth defects. Although the findings are suggestive of an association between herbicide spraying and birth defects, the available studies are insufficient to draw firm conclusions.

Vietnam Veterans Studies

As part of the CDC Vietnam Experience Study (1989), the reproductive outcomes and the health of children of male veterans were examined. The VES assessment included a telephone interview, a review of hospital birth defect records for a subsample of veterans who underwent a medical examination, and a review of the medical records of selected birth defects for all study subjects.

The interview data revealed that Vietnam veterans reported more birth defects (64.6 per 1,000 total births) among offspring than did non-Vietnam veterans (49.5 per 1,000 total births). The adjusted odds ratio estimate for congenital anomalies as a group was 1.3 (CI 1.2-1.4). When examined by specific defect category, elevated adjusted odds ratios were found for defects of the nervous system (OR = 2.3, CI 1.2-4.5); ear, face, neck (OR = 1.6, CI 0.9-2.8); and integument (OR = 2.2, CI 1.2-4.0). A small but statistically significant odds ratio of 1.2 (CI 1.1-1.5) was found for musculoskeletal defects. An analysis of specific defects considered by the investigators to be relatively common and reliably diagnosed was also conducted. Elevated (crude) odds ratios were reported for hydrocephalus (OR = 5.1, CI 1.1-23.1), spina bifida (OR = 1.7, CI 0.6-5.0), and hypospadias (OR = 3.1, CI 0.9-11.3). Vietnam veterans also reported having more children with multiple defects (OR = 1.6, CI 1.1-2.5) than non-Vietnam veterans. An analysis of Vietnam veterans' self-reported herbicide exposure found a dose-response gradient, with an adjusted odds ratio for birth defects of 1.7 (CI 1.2-2.4) at the highest level of exposure.

The VES also examined serious health problems in the veterans' children;

that is, the veterans were asked to report physician-diagnosed major health problems or impairments during the first five years of their children's lives. About half of the health conditions reported were respiratory disease (mostly asthma and pneumonia) and otitis media. For most of the conditions, the veterans reported more health conditions than non-Vietnam veterans (all conditions, OR = 1.3, CI 1.2-1.4). After excluding children with a serious health condition or either a birth defect or cancer, the overall crude OR was 1.2 (CI 1.1-1.3). Elevated crude odds ratios were found for anemias (OR = 2.0, CI 1.2-3.3), diseases of the skin (OR = 1.5, CI 1.1-1.9), rash (OR = 2.3, CI 1.1-4.9), and allergies (OR = 1.6, CI 1.2-2.1). Without medical records that validate for many of these types of common conditions and health problems, recall bias may be an explanation for many of these findings.

The CDC (1989) did conduct two substudies using hospital records to identify birth defects among the veterans' offspring. The first, the General Birth Defects Study (GBDS), compared the occurrence of birth defects recorded on hospital records for the children of Vietnam and of non-Vietnam veterans (130 cases and 112 cases, respectively) who participated in the medical examination component of the VES. For a variety of characteristics, there were no apparent differences between the group of men who participated in the exam and the total interview group. There was no difference in the prevalence of birth defects between the two groups of children (crude OR = 1.0, CI 0.8-1.3). There was a slight but nonsignificant excess for major birth defects (OR = 1.2, CI 0.8-1.9). When analyzed by organ system, only digestive system defects appeared to be elevated (OR = 2.0, CI 0.9-4.6), although the small number of defects precluded the analysis of several broad categories. The number of defects was also too small for the analysis of specific individual defects. An analysis by race did indicate an elevated odds ratio (3.4, CI 1.5-7.6) for black Vietnam veterans. An examination of the specific defects listed on hospital records for children of black veterans did not reveal any particular pattern. A comparison of interview and hospital records was also conducted to evaluate the extent of potential misclassification of veteran responses. In general, interview responses were not predictive of the presence of a defect for either veteran group. The agreement between interview and hospital records was slightly poorer for Vietnam veterans. For example, the positive predictive value of the interview response for the presence of a defect in the hospital record was 24.8 percent among Vietnam veterans and 32.9 percent among non-Vietnam veterans. Sensitivity was 27.1 percent among Vietnam veterans and 30.3 percent among non-Vietnam veterans. The kappa measure of agreement was also lower (20.9 percent versus 27.6 percent) among Vietnam veterans.

The second substudy, the Cerebrospinal Malformation (CSM) Study, involved the analysis of medical records for all cases of cerebrospinal malformations (spina bifida, anencephalus, hydrocephalus) and stillbirths reported by veterans in the interview study. The substudy found 26 cerebrospinal malformations (live and stillbirths) among children of Vietnam veterans and 12 among children of non-Vietnam veterans. No formal analysis of the difference in malformations between the veteran groups was conducted, because negative responses (i.e., children without a reported malformation) were not verified and the participation rates differed between groups (7.8 percent of Vietnam veterans and 22.1 percent of non-Vietnam veterans refused to participate).

The VES did find suggestive associations for birth defects. It is interesting to note that some potential associations were found for birth defects considered by the investigators to be "relatively common, easily diagnosed, and observable at birth" (CDC, 1989). These include hydrocephalus (OR = 5.1, CI 1.1-23.1) and hypospadias (OR = 3.1, CI 0.9-11.3). The GBDS did not replicate these findings, but this sample had limited power for the analysis of specific defects. Although associations were not found for all conditions, there was clearly a general pattern of a greater prevalence of birth defects in the offspring of Vietnam veterans, according to self-reports. The authors properly note the potential for recall bias as an explanation for the pattern of excess risk. As an attempt to evaluate recall bias, two record validation studies of birth defects were conducted. Overall, the GBDS did not find any association with an increased risk of birth defects among offspring of Vietnam veterans. However, this validation study had limited power to detect an increased risk for specific birth defects. The second validation substudy, the CSM review, was flawed by the differentially poor response rate among the non-Vietnam veteran group. This result and the fact that negative responses were not pursued discouraged the investigators from estimating the relative risk for cerebrospinal malformations.

Another important study of Vietnam veterans was the CDC Birth Defects Study (Erickson et al., 1984a,b). In this study, children with birth defects among 428 fathers who were reported to have been Vietnam veterans were compared to children with birth defects among 268 control fathers who were non-Vietnam veterans. The odds ratio for Vietnam veteran status in relation to any major birth defect among offspring was 1.0 (CI 0.8-1.1). Analysis of the Agent Orange exposure opportunity index (EOI; see *VAO* Chapter 6 for details) based on both military records and self-reports did not indicate a statistically significant trend of increasing risk of all types of birth defects (combined) with increasing levels of Agent Orange exposure. No association was noted between Vietnam veteran status or self-reported Agent Orange exposure and risk of fathering a child with multiple birth defects (OR = 1.1, CI 0.7-1.7). The odds ratios for Vietnam veteran status, self-reported Agent Orange exposure, and logistic regression coefficients for EOI based on self-report and military records for most of the 95 birth defect groups were not significantly elevated. Although the odds ratio for spina bifida was not elevated with Vietnam veteran status (OR = 1.1), the EOI indices showed a pattern of increasing risk. For example, the odds ratios for the EOI based on information obtained during the interview for low to high levels of exposure (levels 1 to 5) were 1.2 (CI 1.0-1.4), 1.5 (CI 1.1-2.1), 1.8 (CI 1.1-3.0), 2.2 (CI 1.2-4.3), 2.7 (CI 1.2-6.2). A similar pattern was found for cleft lip with/

without cleft palate— namely, EOI-1 (OR = 1.2, CI 1.0-1.4), EOI-2 (OR = 1.4, CI 1.0-1.9), EOI-3 (OR = 1.6, CI 1.0-2.6), EOI-4 (OR = 1.9, CI 1.0-3.6), and EOI-5 (OR = 2.2, CI 1.0-4.9). The category "specified anomalies of nails" had an increased odds ratio for Vietnam veteran status and elevated coefficients (not statistically significant) for the two exposure indices. The category "other neo-plasms" was related to the EOI based on the father's self-reported Agent Orange exposure. This group included a variety of congenital neoplasms such as cysts, teratomas, and benign tumors. In an attempt to search for a Vietnam veteran birth defect "syndrome," pairs and triplets of defects were examined for combinations that yielded significant differences in the distribution among Vietnam veterans and controls. According to the authors, these analyses did not produce any important associations or patterns among defect combinations.

The results of this study were generally negative; that is, there was not a general pattern of increased risk for birth defects among the offspring of Vietnam veterans. However, the analysis of the Agent Orange EOIs based on military records found a significant trend for increased risk for spina bifida with increased exposure. As the authors note, this finding must be viewed with caution, because a related defect, anencephalus, was not found to be associated with a significant EOI trend. Another positive association was noted for cleft lip without cleft palate, where a significant regression coefficient was found for the EOI index based on the father's interview. No association was found for the EOI from military records.

The CDC Birth Defects Study has many strengths, including the use of a population-based registry system with careful classification of birth defects for analysis. The statistical power of the study was excellent for many major birth defects. Use of the Agent Orange EOIs is an attempt to refine exposure assess-ment procedures compared to measures used in most other studies. The study did have several important limitations. First, the response rates among cases and controls were problematic, with approximately 56 percent of eligible case and control fathers interviewed. Examination of the nonparticipation group revealed lower participation among persons classified as "nonwhite." The analyses by race did not find important differences, but the potential for bias should not be overlooked. Another problem relates to the fact that case births occurred from 1968 through 1980, but interviews took place during 1982 and 1983, up to 14 years after the birth. To minimize the potential recall bias induced by this long lag period, controls were matched on year of birth.

Aschengrau and Monson (1990) studied late adverse pregnancy outcomes among 14,130 obstetric patients who delivered at Boston Hospital for Women from August 1977 to March 1980. History of the fathers' military service in Vietnam was determined from Massachusetts and national military records by using the husbands' names and Social Security numbers. The likelihood of combat experience, based on branch of service and military occupation, was used to estimate potential herbicide exposure. The analyses compared the risk of malformations among children of 107 Vietnam veterans to that for children of 1,432 men without known military service; the risk in 313 non-Vietnam veterans compared to the men without military service; and the risk in the Vietnam veterans compared with the non-Vietnam veterans. There was a slight, nonsignificant increase in the odds ratio for all congenital anomalies for Vietnam veterans compared to men without known military service (OR = 1.3, CI 0.9-1.9) and for Vietnam veterans compared with non-Vietnam veterans (OR = 1.2, CI 0.8-1.9). For major malformations, the odds ratio was elevated for Vietnam veterans compared with men without military service (OR = 1.8, CI 1.0-3.1), but the ratio decreased for Vietnam veterans compared with non-Vietnam veterans (OR = 1.3, CI 0.7-2.4). Only slight increases were found for the analysis of minor malformations and "only normal variants." Although based on small numbers, the analyses of 12 malformation groups found that children of Vietnam veterans, compared to children of men with no known military service, had an increased risk of malformations of the nervous system, cardiovascular system, genital organs, urinary tract, and musculoskeletal system. Confidence intervals were not presented with the odds ratio estimates, but it was noted that they included 1.0, so elevated risks were not significantly increased. Further examination of specific anomaly diagnoses for the 18 infants of Vietnam veterans with major malformations did not reveal any pattern of association with potential herbicide exposure.

Although the study did find a positive association between paternal military service in Vietnam and the risk of major malformations in offspring, the authors suggest cautious interpretation of their findings, given the small number of subjects in many of the comparisons involving specific groups of birth defects. Additionally, it was noted that some of the malformations observed can also be due to maternal and delivery factors (endocrine condition and fetal presentation). An important problem relates to misclassification of herbicide exposure due to equating exposure to service in Vietnam.

Two state health surveys of veterans (Iowa and Hawaii) did not indicate an increased prevalence of birth defects (Rellahan, 1985; Wendt, 1985), but a survey in Maine did report an increased risk of birth defects among veterans (Deprez et al., 1991). The limitations of these general survey studies affect their usefulness in this evaluation.

As part of the National Vietnam Veterans Birth Defects/Learning Disabilities Registry and database, a joint project of the Association of Birth Defect Children and the New Jersey Agent Orange Commission, a self-administered questionnaire was sent to Vietnam veterans to inquire about birth defects and a variety of conditions and disabilities in the children of Vietnam veterans and non-Vietnam veterans (Lewis and Mekdeci, 1993). A preliminary analysis indicated no differences in birth defects between the two groups; however, for a variety of conditions, including allergies, frequent infections, benign tumors, cysts, and chronic skin disorders, the veterans showed a higher frequency. The possibility of recall bias and the self-selected nature of the registry are of concern. Nonetheless, a carefully designed and comprehensive epidemiologic study with review of medical records could address the possibility of an association with some of these childhood health conditions.

A study of birth defects among offspring of Australian Vietnam veterans was conducted using a total of 8,517 matched case-control pairs, with 127 infant cases and 123 infant controls having a father who served in Vietnam (Donovan et al., 1984). There were 202 cases and 205 controls whose fathers were in the Army but did not serve in Vietnam. The adjusted odds ratio for birth defects among children of Vietnam veterans versus all other men was 1.02 (CI 0.8-1.3). Analysis of subgroups based on the type of Army veteran (Australian Regular Army enlistees, National Service draftees) did not detect any increased odds ratios for these comparisons. There was a slight, statistically nonsignificant increase in the odds ratio for National Service Vietnam veterans versus those who did not serve in Vietnam (OR = 1.3, CI 0.9-2.0). The risk was independent of the length of Vietnam service and the time between service and conception. Analyses by diagnostic group (central nervous system, cardiovascular, oral clefts, hypospadias, musculoskeletal, dislocation of hip, chromosomal anomalies) did not show an excess risk for Vietnam veterans. However, two defects had odds ratios above 1.5 (statistically nonsignificant)—ventricular septal defects (OR = 1.8) and Down's syndrome (OR = 1.7).

Overall, this study was negative; that is, there was no evidence of an increased risk of fathering a child with a congenital anomaly for Australian Army veterans who served in Vietnam. As indicated by the upper confidence limit (1.3), this study had adequate power to rule out an odds ratio greater than 1.3 for congenital anomalies. Assessment of potential Agent Orange exposure in this study is limited, because "history of service" in Vietnam was used as the primary "exposure" variable. This uncertainty is further compounded by potential differences in the location and nature of service of Australian veterans in Vietnam and their resultant herbicide exposure.

The Australian study of veterans living in Tasmania reported more congenital anomalies among the 357 Vietnam veterans than among the comparison families (Field and Kerr, 1988). The authors suggested that the results indicated a pattern of association with congenital heart disease and anomalies of the central nervous system. As described earlier in the section on spontaneous abortion, there are several notable problems with this study, including inadequate presentation of results, potential selection bias, self-reported health outcomes, and using service in Vietnam as a surrogate for herbicide exposure.

Ranch Hand Study   The latest report from the Air Force Health Study (AFHS) of Operation Ranch Hand veterans ("Ranch Hands") and their children was published in 1995 (Wolfe et al., 1995). The Air Force released a first report on the analysis of reproductive effects in 1982, and this report was reviewed in *VAO* (AFHS, 1992). The original study cohort comprised 1,098 Ranch Hands who regularly handled and sprayed herbicides in Southeast Asia from 1962 to 1971 ("exposed cohort") and a comparison group of 1,549 Air Force veterans who were in Southeast Asia at the same time but presumably were not exposed to herbicides. In 1987, 995 Ranch Hands (91 percent of original study group) and 1,299 comparison veterans (84 percent of original group) participated in a physical exam and agreed to provide serum samples for the dioxin assay. A total of 872 Ranch Hands (79 percent of original cohort, 88 percent of 1987 cohort) and 1,036 comparison subjects (67 percent of original group, 80 percent of 1987 cohort) were available for analysis, after exclusion of samples that were unreliable because of laboratory error or that had dioxin levels below the level of detection or above an upper threshold for background (10 parts per trillion [ppt]) for comparison subjects. Of the 872 Ranch Hands, 454 had 1,006 self-reported conceptions and 419 fathered 792 liveborn infants during their service in Vietnam or until January 1990. Of the 1,036 comparison veterans, 570 had 1,235 conceptions and 531 fathered 981 liveborn infants during this period.

The initial dioxin level was estimated from the current level using a first-order decay rate model with a fixed 7.1-year half-life estimate. The referent group for the Ranch Hands included the conceptions and offspring of comparison men with "background" levels ($\leq$10 ppt, N = 570, mean = 3.9ppt). Ranch Hands with levels at background were analyzed as a separate stratum (N = 179), since the authors felt this group included a mixture of exposed and unexposed veterans, given their mean level of 6.1 ppt and uncertainties in dioxin elimination. The other strata used in the analysis included Ranch Hand "low" (current $\leq$10 ppt and initial $\leq$ 110 ppt, N = 119) and Ranch Hand "high" (current $\leq$10 ppt and initial >110 ppt, N = 156). The 110 ppt level was chosen because it is the median estimated initial dioxin level at the time of conception of the Ranch Hands with levels greater than 10 ppt. As the authors point out, this cutoff is arbitrary, with no assumed biologic meaning. Reproductive outcomes of comparison veterans with a current dioxin levels of greater than 10 ppt were not analyzed, because the investigators suspected that these may reflect dioxin exposure after service in Vietnam.

The reproductive and developmental outcomes included in the analyses included spontaneous abortion (miscarriage, fetal death less than 20 weeks gestation), stillbirth (fetal death 20 weeks or greater gestation), and birth defects. All conceptions reported by the men, their wives, or their partners were verified through medical records and vital statistics review. The proportion of adverse outcomes verified by specific sources was not stated. This may be important, given the known limitations of vital statistics records for the identification and classification of certain pregnancy outcomes.

Stratified analyses were performed, adjusting for six covariates, including father's race, mother's smoking and drinking during pregnancy, mother's and father's age at birth or conception, and father's military occupation (officer, enlisted flyer, enlisted nonflyer). In addition, adjustment was made for history of spontaneous abortion prior to service in Southeast Asia. The authors noted that the adjustment of father's military occupation was performed because it may serve as a proxy for education and occupation is associated with dioxin level. Adjustment for occupation may, in fact, lead to some degree of "overadjustment" owing to the high correlation between occupation and exposure potential. Comparison of the adjusted estimates with the unadjusted risk ratio estimates derived from the data provided in the paper showed little difference, indicating that the adjustment for military occupation did not materially affect the results.

The validation of self-reported birth defects in this study was systematic and of high quality. Although the etiology of most birth defects remains unknown, the study accounted for an array of factors controlled for in most previous studies of birth defects. Considering all birth defects combined, there was a slightly higher proportion of defects among Ranch Hand children than among comparison children (22.3 percent versus 20.8 percent). No general pattern of increasing risk with increasing dioxin levels was found. A small increased RR of 1.3 (CI 1.0-1.6) was found for the low-dioxin category. There was a slightly higher prevalence of major birth defects among Ranch Hand children compared to comparison children (7.4 percent versus 5.7 percent). There was an elevated risk ratio for the low-level category (RR = 1.7; CI 1.1-2.7), although a dose-response gradient was not evident, with an RR of 1.1 for background (0.6-1.8) and 1.2 (CI 0.8-2.1) for the high-level category. The analysis of birth defect groups yielded a total of 11 increased and five decreased risk ratios for the low- and high-level comparisons with the referent category. For example, the analysis of circulatory system and heart defects found risk ratios of 2.3 for low and 0.9 for high levels. Genital defects had risk ratios of 1.8 for low and 1.2 for high; urinary system defects had risk ratios of 2.0 for low and 2.1 for high. Examination of specific defects included in this larger defect grouping did not show any specific associations or patterns. Interestingly, neural tube defects (spina bifida, anencephaly) were in excess among offspring of Ranch Hands, with four total (rate of five per 1,000), in contrast to none among the comparison infants (exact p = .04). The four cases were distributed as two spina bifida in the high-level category, one anencephaly and one spina bifida in the low-dioxin category. There was no clear pattern of association with developmental disabilities in terms of specific delays in development or hyperkinetic syndrome, although the low-level stratum for specific delays in development had a risk ratio of 1.5 (CI 1.0-2.3).

Summary

The recently published results of the analysis of birth defects among the offspring of Ranch Hands suggest the possibility of an association between dioxin exposure and risk of neural tube defects. These findings require a consideration of the current evidence for an association between herbicides and neural tube defects and an increased risk among Vietnam veterans exposed to herbicides. Table 9.1 includes a summary of the studies that have reported results specifically for neural tube defects (typically anencephaly and/or spina bifida), including studies in *VAO* and more recent publications. Unfortunately, some studies (e.g., Seveso), particularly the occupational and environmental studies, do not have results specific for individual birth defects, usually because of the small number of cases. A number of studies of veterans appear to show an elevated relative risk for either service in Vietnam or estimated exposure to herbicides or dioxin and neural tube defects (anencephaly and/or spina bifida) in their offspring. Many of the estimates are imprecise, and chance cannot be ruled out. Nonetheless, the pattern of association warrants further evaluation. The CDC Birth Defects Study (Centers for Disease Control, 1988), the CDC Vietnam Experience Study (Centers for Disease Control, 1989), and the Ranch Hand Study (Wolfe et al., 1992) are of the highest overall quality. The CDC VES cohort study found that more Vietnam veterans reported that their children had a central nervous system anomaly (OR = 2.3; 95 percent CI 1.2-4.5) than did non-Vietnam veterans (Centers for Disease Control, 1989). The odds ratio for spina bifida was 1.7 (CI 0.6-5.0). A substudy was conducted in an attempt to validate the reported cerebrospinal defects (spina bifida, anencephaly, hydrocephalus) by examination of hospital records. A difference was detected, but its interpretation was limited by differential participation between the veteran groups and failure to validate negative reported—i.e., the veterans not reporting their children having a birth defect. Thus, the issue of a recall bias remains a major concern with this study.

The CDC Birth Defects Study utilized the population-based birth defects registry system in the metropolitan Atlanta area (Centers for Disease Control, 1988). There was no association between overall Vietnam veteran status and the risk of spina bifida (OR = 1.1, CI 0.6-1.7) or anencephaly (OR = 0.9, CI 0.5-1.7). However, the exposure opportunity index based on interview data was associated with an increased risk of spina bifida; for the highest estimated level of exposure (EOI-5), the OR was 2.7 (CI 1.2-6.2). There was no similar pattern of association for anencephaly. This study has a number of strengths, including the use of a population-based birth defects registry system and adjustment for a number of potentially confounding factors. Two study limitations include the relatively low response proportions among the case and control subjects (approximately 56 percent) and the lag between birth and interview for some cases and controls.

Thus, all three epidemiologic studies (Ranch Hand, VES, CDC Birth Defects Study) suggest an association between herbicide exposure and an increased risk of spina bifida in offspring. Although the studies were judged to be of relatively high quality, they suffer from methodologic limitations, including possible recall bias, nonresponse bias, small sample size, and misclassification of exposure. In addition, the failure to find a similar association with anencephaly, an embryologically related defect, is of concern.

TABLE 9-1 Epidemiologic Studies—Neural Tube Defects

Reference	Description	N	OR/RR (95% CI)
Occupational No specific results for neural tube defects			
Environmental			
Hanify et al., 1981	Anencephaly	10	1.4 (0.6-3.3)
	Spina bifida	13	1.1 (0.6-2.3)
Stockbauer et al., 1988	TCDD soil contamination in Missouri		
	Central nervous system defects	3	3.0 (0.3-35.9)
Vietnam veterans			
Erickson, 1984a,b	Birth Defects Study		
	Vietnam veteran: spina bifida	19	1.1 (0.6-1.7)
	Vietnam veteran: anencephaly	12	0.9 (0.5-1.7)
	EOI-5: spina bifida	19[a]	2.7 (1.2-6.2)
	EOI-5: anencephaly	7[a]	0.7 (0.2-2.8)
CDC, 1989	Vietnam Experience Study Interview study		
	Spina bifida	9	1.7 (0.6-5.0) among Vietnam veterans
		5	among non-Vietnam veterans
	Anencephaly	3	among Vietnam veterans
		0	among non-Vietnam veterans
Australian veterans	Birth defects and father's Vietnam service (Australia)		
Health Studies, 1983	Neural tube defects	16	0.9
AFHS, 1995	Follow-up of Air Force Ranch Hands		
	Neural tube defects		4 among Ranch Hand[b] 0 among comparison

NOTE: N = number of exposed cases; OR/RR = Odds Ratio/Relative Risk; CI = Confidence Interval; SIR = Standardized Incidence Ratio.

[a]Number of Vietnam veterans fathering a child with a neural tube defect given any exposure opportunity index score.
[b]Four neural tube defects among Ranch Hand offspring include 2 spina bifida (high dioxin level), 1 spina bifida (low dioxin), and 1 anencephaly (low dioxin). Denominator for Ranch Hand group is 792 liveborn infants.

Conclusions

Strength of Evidence in Epidemiologic Studies

There is limited/suggestive evidence of an association between exposure to the herbicides considered in this report and spina bifida. There is inadequate or insufficient evidence to determine whether an association exists between exposure to the herbicides and all other birth defects. The evidence regarding association is drawn from occupation and other studies in which subjects were exposed to a variety of herbicides and herbicide components.

Biologic Plausibility

Laboratory studies of the potential developmental toxicity, specifically birth defects, of TCDD and herbicides as a result of exposure to adult male animals are too limited to permit conclusions.

Risk in Vietnam Veterans

Since the strongest associations are from studies of.Vietnam veterans and there are some data suggesting that the highest risks were for those veterans estimated to have had exposure to Agent Orange (e.g., Ranch Hands), it therefore follows that there is limited/suggestive evidence for an increased risk in Vietnam veterans of spina bifida in offspring.

CHILDHOOD CANCER

Background

In most epidemiologic studies, childhood cancer usually refers to cancer diagnosed from birth through age 15. Childhood cancers are usually classified by primary anatomic site or tumor cell type. The distribution of childhood cancers by type includes leukemia (23 percent), lymphoma (13 percent), central nervous system (19 percent), neuroblastoma (8 percent), soft-tissue sarcoma (7 percent), kidney (6 percent), bone (5 percent), retinoblastoma (3 percent), liver (1 percent), and other (8 percent). There are approximately 6,500 new cases of cancer diagnosed each year in the United States in persons under age 15 (Young et al., 1986). About 2,200 deaths each year result from childhood cancer. Compared with adult cancers, relatively little is known about the etiology of most childhood cancers, and especially about potential environmental risk factors.

Summary of *VAO*

There are no available occupational and environmental epidemiologic studies of herbicide exposure that address childhood cancer as an outcome. Two studies of Vietnam veterans found some suggestion of an increased risk of cancer among offspring. The evidence is, however, inadequate, given the lack of other studies, failure to exclude chance and bias, and problems with herbicide exposure assessment.

Update of Scientific Literature

A mortality study conducted as part of the continuing follow-up of the possible health effects of the Seveso accident (see Chapter 6 for general description), suggested an increased risk of leukemia among children and young adults under age 20 (Bertazzi et al., 1992). This report led to a more detailed incidence study of cancer among young persons in the Seveso study groups (Pesatori et al., 1993). Specifically, the population for these analyses included subjects who were living in the study accident zones (A, B, R) and a reference (noncontaminated) area on the day of the accident and were between 0 and 19 years old during the first ten years afterward. Cases were identified from linkage of the study population subjects with the hospital discharge data from the Lombardy region. Medical records were reviewed to confirm diagnoses. The follow-up period was from 1977 through 1986. Owing to the small number of subjects in Zones A and B, the three zones were combined for analysis. Poisson regression was used to compare the risk of cancer in the exposed study group (Zones A, B, and R) relative to the risk in the unexposed group.

The vital status ascertainment and follow-up of the subjects was excellent, with vital status determined for 99 percent of the study group. At the end of follow-up, 95 percent of subjects were still living in the Lombardy area. A total of 17 cancers were found in the exposed study group from Zones A, B, and R. A total of 62 cases were detected in the reference population. Among the 17 cases, one was from zone A (the most exposed, 0.2 expected), two from Zone B (1.9 expected), and 14 were from Zone R (the least exposed). The overall relative risk was 1.2 (95 percent CI 0.7-2.1; 17 observed, 13.6 expected). When analyzed by site or type of cancer, there was a nearly fivefold increased risk of thyroid cancer (RR = 4.6; CI 0.6-32.7). Among hematological malignancies, a relative risk of 2 was found for Hodgkin's disease (CI 0.5-7.6), and a nearly threefold increased risk of myeloid leukemia was observed (3 observed, 1.1 expected; RR = 2.7; CI 0.7-11.4). An excess was also found for ovarian cancer (two observed versus none expected). No cancer was found among the 186 children who had chloracne diagnosed after the accident (expected = 0.2).

As the authors acknowledged, the study had a number of limitations. A major concern was the small number of subjects, as reflected in the wide confidence intervals associated with the relative risk estimates. This forced the investigators to combine the three exposed zones into one group for analysis. A serious concern with the Seveso studies in general is the fact that exposure is ecological, and all subjects were assigned to one of three exposure groups based on area of residence.

Thus, results from the Seveso study suggest an increased risk of some types of childhood cancer among potentially exposed residents. As described in *VAO* report, the CDC Vietnam Experience Study found an elevated relative risk estimate for childhood leukemia (OR = 1.6; CI 0.6-4.0) (Centers for Disease Control, 1989). The specific types of leukemia found were not reported.

Conclusions

Strength of Evidence in Epidemiologic Studies

There is inadequate or insufficient evidence to determine whether an association exists between exposure to the herbicides considered in this report and childhood cancer. The evidence regarding association is drawn from occupational and other studies in which subjects were exposed to a variety of herbicides and herbicide components.

CONCLUSIONS FOR REPRODUCTIVE EFFECTS

Strength of Evidence in Epidemiologic Studies

There is limited/suggestive evidence of an association between exposure to the herbicides considered in this report and spina bifida.

There is inadequate or insufficient evidence to determine whether an association exists between exposure to the herbicides and infertility, spontaneous abortion, stillbirth, birth defects (other than spina bifida), and childhood cancer.

Biologic Plausibility

Experimental animal evidence indicates that dioxin can alter gonadotrophin and testosterone levels, but generally at relatively high doses. Laboratory studies of herbicides and male-mediated developmental endpoints such as birth defects and cancer are too limited to permit conclusions.

Increased Risk of Disease among Vietnam Veterans

Since there are some data suggesting that the highest risks occur in those veterans estimated to have had exposure to Agent Orange (e.g., Ranch Hands), it therefore follows that there is limited/suggestive evidence for an increased risk of spina bifida among offspring of Vietnam veterans.

Given the large uncertainties that remain about the magnitude of potential risk of infertility, spontaneous abortion, stillbirth, birth defects (other than spina bifida), and childhood cancer from exposure to herbicides in the studies that have been reviewed, it is not possible for the committee to quantify the degree of risk likely to be experienced by Vietnam veterans because of their exposure to herbicides in Vietnam.

REFERENCES

Ahlborg G, Hogstedt C, Bodin L, Barany S. 1989. Pregnancy outcome among working women. Scandinavian Journal of Work, Environment, and Health 15:227-233.

Air Force Health Study. 1992. An Epidemiologic Investigation of Health Effects in Air Force Personnel Following Exposure to Herbicides. Reproductive Outcomes. Brooks AFB, TX: Armstrong Laboratory. AL-TR-1992-0090.

Air Force Health Study. 1995. An Epidemiologic Investigation of Health Effects in Air Force Personnel Following Exposure to Herbicides. 1992 Followup Examination Results. 10 vols. Brooks AFB, TX: Epidemiologic Research Division. Armstrong Laboratory.

Aschengrau A, Monson RR. 1990. Paternal military service in Vietnam and the risk of late adverse pregnancy outcomes. American Journal of Public Health 80:1218-1224

Australia Department of Veterans Affairs. 1983. Case-Control Study of Congenital Abnormalities and Vietnam Service. Canberra, Australia: Department of Veterans Affairs.

Bertazzi PA, Zocchetti C, Pesatori AC, Guercilena S, Consonni D, Tironi A, Landi MT. 1992. Mortality of a young population after accidental exposure to 2,3,7,8-tetrachlorodibenzo dioxin. International Journal of Epidemiology 21:118-123.

Bloom AD, ed. 1981. Guidelines for Studies of Human Populations Exposed to Mutagenic and Reproductive Hazards. White Plains, New York: March of Dimes Foundation.

Centers for Disease Control. 1988. Health status of Vietnam veterans. III. Reproductive outcomes and child health. Journal of the American Medical Association 259:2715-2717.

Centers for Disease Control. 1989. Health status of Vietnam veterans. Vietnam Experience Study. Atlanta: U.S. Department of Health and Human Services. Vols. I-V, Supplements A-C.

Constable JD, Hatch MC. 1985. Reproductive effects of herbicide exposure in Vietnam: recent studies by the Vietnamese and others. Teratogenesis, Carcinogenesis, and Mutagenesis 5:231-250.

Deprez RD, Carvette ME, Agger MS. 1991. The health and medical status of Maine veterans: a report to the Bureau of Veterans Services Commission of Vietnam and Atomic Veterans.

Donovan JW, MacLennan R, Adena M. 1984. Vietnam service and the risk of congenital anomalies: a case-control study. Medical Journal of Australia 140:394-397.

Egeland GM, Sweeney MH, Fingerhut MA, Wille KK, Schnorr TM, Halperin WE. 1994. Total serum testosterone and gonadotropins in workers exposed to dioxin. American Journal of Epidemiology 139:272-281.

Egeland GM, Sweeney MH, Fingerhut MA, Wille KK, Schnorr TM, Halperin WE. 1995. Reply to letter to the editor. American Journal of Epidemiology 141:477-478

Erickson J, Mulinare J, Mcclain P, Fitch T, James L, McClearn A, Adams M. 1984a. Vietnam Veterans' Risks for Fathering Babies with Birth Defects. Atlanta: U.S. Department of Health and Human Services, Centers for Disease Control.

Erickson JD, Mulinare J, Mcclain PW. 1984b. Vietnam veterans' risks for fathering babies with birth defects. Journal of the American Medical Association 252:903-912.

Fenster L, Coye MJ. 1990. Birthweight of infants born to Hispanic women employed in agriculture. Archives of Environmental Health 45:46-52.

Field B, Kerr C. 1988. Reproductive behaviour and consistent patterns of abnormality in offspring of Vietnam veterans. Journal of Medical Genetics 25:819-826.

Fitzgerald EF, Weinstein AL, Youngblood LG, Standfast SJ, Melius JM. 1989. Health effects three years after potential exposure to the toxic contaminants of an electrical transformer fire. Archives of Environmental Health 44:214-221.

Gordon JE, Shy CM. 1981. Agricultural chemical use and congenital cleft lip and/or palate. Archives of Environmental Health 36:213-221.

Goulet L, Theriault G. 1991. Stillbirth and chemical exposure of pregnant workers. Scandinavian Journal of Work, Environment, and Health 17:25-31.

Hanify JA, Metcalf P, Nobbs CL, Worsley KJ. 1981. Aerial spraying of 2,4,5-T and human birth malformations: an epidemiological investigation. Science 212:349-351.

Hemminki K, Mutanen P, Luoma K. 1980. Congenital malformations by the parental occupation in Finland. International Archives of Occupational and Environmental Health 46:93-98.

Jansson B, Voog L. 1989. Dioxin from Swedish municipal incinerators and the occurrence of cleft lip and palate malformations. International Journal of Environmental Studies 34:99-104.

Kallen B. 1988. Epidemiology of Human Reproduction. Boca Raton: CRC Press.

Kalter H, Warkany J. 1983. Congenital malformations. Etiologic factors and their role in prevention (first of two parts). New England Journal of Medicine 308:424-491.

Kline J, Stein Z, Susser M. 1989. Conception to Birth: Epidemiology of Prenatal Development. New York: Oxford University Press.

Knobil E, Neill JD, Greenwald GS, Markert CL, Pfaff DW, (eds). 1994. The Physiology of Reproduction. New York: Raven Press.

Lewis W, Mekdeci B. 1993. Birth Defect/Learning Disabilities Registry and Database. New Jersey Agent Orange Commission, Association of Birth Defect Children. Submitted to the Institute of Medicine Committee to Review the Health Effects in Vietnam Veterans of Exposure to Agent Orange.

Mastroiacovo P, Spagnolo A, Marni E, Meazza L, Bertollini R, Segni G, Borgna-Pignatti C. 1988. Birth defects in the Seveso area after TCDD contamination [published erratum appears in JAMA 1988:260(6):792]. Journal of the American Medical Association 259:1668-1672.

McDonald AD, McDonald JC, Armstrong B. 1987. Occupation and pregnancy outcome. British Journal of Industrial Medicine 44:521-526.

Moses M, Lilis R, Crow KD, Thornton J, Fischbein A, Anderson HA, Selikoff IJ. 1984. Health status of workers with past exposure to 2,3,7,8-tetrachlorodibenzo-p-dioxin in the manufacture of 2,4,5-trichlorophenoxyacetic acid: comparison of findings with and without chloracne. American Journal of Industrial Medicine 5:161-182.

Nelson CJ, Holson JF, Green HG, Gaylor DW. 1979. Retrospective study of the relationship between agricultural use of 2,4,5-T and cleft palate occurrence in Arkansas. Teratology 19:377-383.

Ng TP, Goh HH, Ng YL, Ong HY, Ong CN, Chia KS, Chia SE, Jeyaratna M. 1991. Male endocrine functions in workers with moderate exposure to lead. British Journal of Industrial Medicine 48:485-491.

Nurminen T, Rantala K, Kurppa K, Holmberg PC. 1994. Agricultural work during pregnancy and selected structural malformations in Finland. Epidemiology 1: 23-30

Pesatori AC, Consonni D, Tironi A, Zocchetti C, Fini A, Bertazzi PA. 1993. Cancer in a young population in a dioxin-contaminated area. International Journal of Epidemiology 22:1010-1013.

Phuong NTN, Thuy TT, Phuong PK. 1989. An estimate of reproductive abnormalities in women inhabiting herbicide sprayed and non-herbicide sprayed areas in the south of Vietnam, 1952-1981. Chemosphere 18:843-846.

Rellahan W. 1985. Aspects of the Health of Hawaii's Vietnam-era Veterans. Honolulu: Hawaii State Department of Health, Research and Statistics Office.

Restrepo M, Munoz N, Day NE, Parra JE, Hernandez C, Brettner M, Giraldo A. 1990. Prevalence of adverse reproductive outcomes in a population occupationally exposed to pesticides in Colombia. Scandinavian Journal of Work, Environment, and Health 16:232-238.

Roegner RH, Grubbs WD, Lustik MB, Brockman AS, Henderson SC, Williams DE, Wolfe WH, Michalek JE, Miner JC. 1991. An Epidemiologic Investigation of Health Effects in Air Force Personnel Following Exposure to Herbicides. Serum Dioxin Analysis of 1987 Follow-up Examination Results. NTIS AD A-237-516 through AD A-237-524: San Antonio: Armstrong Laboratory, Brooks Air Force Base.

Savitz DA, Whelan EA, Kleckner RC. 1989. Effect of parents' occupational exposures on risk of stillbirth, preterm delivery, and small-for-gestational-age infants. American Journal of Epidemiology 129:1201-1218.

Smith AH, Fisher DO, Pearce N, Chapman CJ. 1982. Congenital defects and miscarriages among New Zealand 2,4,5-T sprayers. Archives of Environmental Health 37:197-200.

Stockbauer JW, Hoffman RE, Schramm WF, Edmonds LD. 1988. Reproductive outcomes of mothers with potential exposure to 2,3,7,8-tetrachlorodibenzo-p-dioxin. American Journal of Epidemiology 128:410-419.

Suskind RR, Hertzberg VS. 1984. Human health effects of 2,4,5-T and its toxic contaminants. Journal of the American Medical Association 251:2372-2380.

Townsend JC, Bodner KM, Van Peenen PFD, Olson RD, Cook RR. 1982. Survey of reproductive events of wives of employees exposed to chlorinated dioxins. American Journal of Epidemiology 115:695-713.

Wendt AS. 1985. Iowa Agent Orange survey of Vietnam veterans. Iowa State Department of Health.

White FMM, Cohen FG, Sherman G, McCurdy R. 1988. Chemicals, birth defects and stillbirths in New Brunswick: associations with agricultural activity. Canadian Medical Association Journal 138:117-124.

Whorton MD, Milby TH, Krauss RM. 1979. Testicular function in DBCP exposed pesticide workers. Journal of Occupational Medicine 21:161-166.

Wilcox AJ, Weinberg CR, O'Connor JF, Baird DD, Schlatterer JP, Canfield RE, Armstrong EG, Nisula BC. 1988. Incidence of early loss of pregnancy. New England Journal of Medicine 319:189-194.

Wolfe WH, Michalek JE, Miner JC, Roegner RH, Grubbs WD, Lustik MB, Brockman AS, Henderson SC, Williams DE. 1992. The Air Force health study: an epidemiologic investigation of health effects in Air Force personnel following exposure to herbicides, serum dioxin analysis of 1987 examination results. Chemosphere 25:213-216.

Wolfe WH, Michalek JE, Miner JC, Rahe AJ, Moore CA, Needham LL, Patterson DG Jr. 1995. Paternal serum dioxin and reproductive outcomes among veterans of Operation Ranch Hand. Epidemiology 6:17-22.

World Health Organization. 1977. Recommended definitions, terminology and format for statistical tables related to the perinatal period and use of a new certificate for cause of perinatal deaths (modifications recommended by FIGO as amended October 14, 1976). Acta Obstetrica et Gynecologica Scandinavica 56:247-253.

Yen SC, Jaffe RB. 1991. Reproductive Endocrinology. Philadelphia: WB Saunders Company.

Young JL, Ries LG, Silverberg E, Horm JW, Miller RW. 1986. Cancer incidence, survival, and mortality for children younger than age 15 years. Cancer 58:598-602.

10

Neurobehavioral Disorders

INTRODUCTION

Neurologic problems in clinical medicine cover a wide variety of disorders. The nervous system is anatomically and functionally divided into central and peripheral subsystems. The central nervous system (CNS) includes the brain and spinal cord, and CNS dysfunction can be subdivided into two general categories: neurobehavioral and motor/sensory. Neurobehavioral difficulties involve two primary categories: cognitive decline, including memory problems and dementia; and neuropsychiatric disorders, including neurasthenia (a collection of symptoms including difficulty concentrating, headache, insomnia, and fatigue), depression, posttraumatic stress disorder (PTSD), and suicide. Other CNS problems can be associated with motor difficulties, characterized by problems such as weakness, tremors, involuntary movements, incoordination, and gait/walking abnormalities. These are usually associated with subcortical or cerebellar system dysfunction. The anatomic elements of the peripheral nervous system (PNS) include the spinal rootlets that exit the spinal cord, the brachial and lumbar plexus, and the peripheral nerves that innervate the muscles of the body. PNS dysfunctions, involving either the somatic nerves or the autonomic system, are known as neuropathies.

Neurologic dysfunction can be further classified, based on anatomic distribution, as either global or focal; temporal onset, as acute, subacute, or chronic; or temporal course, as transient or persistent. For example, global cerebral dysfunction may lead to altered levels of consciousness, whereas focal lesions cause isolated signs of cortical dysfunction, such as aphasia. Acute onset of motor/coordination disturbances leads to symptoms that develop over minutes or hours, whereas subacute onset occurs over days or weeks and chronic onset over months or years. Finally, transient peripheral neuropathies resolve spontaneously, whereas persistent ones may lead to chronic deficits. In the original report, *VAO*, attention was deliberately focused on persistent neurobehavioral dysfunction. In the present report, all new data pertinent to clinical neurobehavioral dysfunction are reviewed; in addition, at the specific request of the Department of Veterans Affairs (DVA), earlier data relating to transient acute and subacute peripheral neuropathy are reexamined.

Case identification in neurology is often difficult. Despite advances in neuroimaging, many types of neurologic alterations are biochemical and show no abnormalities on scanning tests. The nervous system is not usually accessible for biopsy, so pathologic confirmation is not feasible for many neurologic disorders. Behavioral and neurophysiologic changes can be partly or largely subjective and, even when objectively documented, may often be reversible. Timing is important in assessing the effect of chemical exposures on neurologic function. Some symptoms of neurologic importance will appear acutely but be short-lived, whereas others will appear slowly and be detectable for extended periods. These caveats must be considered in the design and critique of epidemiologic studies evaluating an association between exposure to any chemical agent and neurologic or neurobehavioral dysfunction.

Many reports have addressed the possible contribution of herbicides and pesticides to nervous system dysfunction, and reported abnormalities have ranged from mild and reversible to severe and long-standing. These assessments have been conducted in three general settings, related to occupational, environmental, and Vietnam veteran exposures (see Table 10-1). Several case reports of patients ingesting 2,4-dichlorophenoxyacetic acid (2,4-D) are mentioned under environmental exposures. This chapter reviews reports of neurologic alterations associated with exposure to herbicides, TCDD (2,3,7,8-tetrachlorodibenzo-*p*-dioxin), or other compounds used in herbicides in Vietnam. The chapter emphasizes the small number of cross-sectional studies with comparison samples in which both exposed and unexposed persons were neurologically assessed by systematic physical examinations and/or ancillary tests, such as neuropsychological evaluations or EMG measurements.

The potential neurotoxicity of TCDD and herbicides in animal studies has not been thoroughly investigated (see Chapter 3). A large number of acute and subchronic toxicity studies have been conducted with TCDD, but the majority of these studies were not designed specifically to investigate neurotoxicity. Available data imply that CNS alterations or changes in the responsiveness of neurochemical processes in the CNS may be associated with lethal or near-lethal dose levels of TCDD in some animal species; however, the changes observed may also be regulatory responses occurring secondary to changes induced in other organ systems. TCDD concentrations in the brain after systemic exposure are low, and are quite similar among rodent species. Relatively little work has been done to

TABLE 10-1 Selected Neurobehavioral Studies of Herbicide Exposure

Study Group	N	Tests of Neurological Dysfunction	Exposure Measures	Comparison Group
Environmental				
Peper et al., 1993	19 German residents exposed to 2,3,7,8-TCDD	Neuropsycholog-ical battery and symptom questionnaires	Serum TCDD	None
Occupational				
Zober et al., 1994	158 German BASF employees	Medical record review	Chloracne and TCDD levels	161 reference comparisons
Baader and Bauer, 1951	10 pentachloro-phenol plant workers	Record review Clinical evaluation	No	None
Goldstein et al., 1959	2 farmers 1 bookkeeper	Neurological examination; EMG	No	None
Todd, 1962	1 weed-sprayer	Neurological examination	No	None
Berkley and Magee, 1963	1 farmer	Neurological examination	No	None
Vietnam				
Decoufle et al., 1992	7,924 veterans	Self-report with neurological examinations in a subset	Self-report	7,364 non-Vietnam veterans
Visintainer et al., 1995	151,377 Michigan veterans who served in Vietnam	No: mortality data only	No	225,651 Non-Vietnam veterans

quantify the concentration of Ah receptors in the central or peripheral nervous systems.

COGNITIVE AND NEUROPSYCHIATRIC EFFECTS

Summary of *VAO*

In *VAO*, the committee concluded that the literature was insufficient to determine whether an association existed between exposure to herbicides and related compounds and chronic cognitive or neuropsychiatric disorders. As suggested by Sharp et al. (1986), the delayed effects of such exposures on human health are difficult to detect, and the health risks may be sufficiently small that they are below the power of present epidemiologic studies to detect.

Although there was no shortage of studies concerning this topic, methodologic problems made it difficult to reach definitive conclusions. Shortcomings in defining exposure included absent or poor exposure assessments; inconsistencies in identifying exposed individuals for study (i.e., some studies relied upon the presence of chloracne for inclusion, while others assumed that all subjects were exposed); and concomitant exposure to different chemicals, mixtures of chemicals, or concentrations of chemicals. Studies of cognitive or neuropsychiatric disorders are also weakened by the small numbers of subjects; poor selection or absence of comparison groups; confounding of the possible effects of herbicides with the effects of stress; and inadequate statistical analyses. Self-reports of exposure and symptoms may not be verified independently.

The committee noted that in order to maximally define the direct effects of dioxin on cognitive and neuropsychiatric function, future studies should focus primarily on occupationally exposed groups for whom levels of exposure were better known and should include neurobehavioral testing in relative proximity to the time of exposure.

VAO also concluded that significantly exposed subjects should be followed for the development of neuropsychological dysfunction in middle and later life. It is possible that minor CNS changes acquired in early adulthood were too subtle to be detected by current neuropsychological testing methods, but they could manifest themselves later when compounded by "normal age-related changes" of the CNS. Theoretically, exposure to neurotoxins could produce "accelerated aging" of the brain due to premature neuronal loss, which could then result in neurobehavioral deficits.

Update of the Scientific Literature

Several papers on this topic have appeared since *VAO*. In the study by Peper et al. (1993) of chronic exposure to environmental polychlorinated dibenzodioxins and dibenzofurans (PCDD/PCDF) at high and low exposures, the group with high- and low-exposure demonstrated multiple neuropsychological changes, including self-reports of memory problems, distractibility, irritability, and fatigue, and objective changes in verbal conceptualization skills, mnestic organization, and psychomotor activity. On the Trail-Making Test, which measures visual exploration speed, deficits correlated with TCDD tissue levels. Combined high- and low-exposure groups, however, deviated only slightly from published norms, with no significant differences. The limitations of this study include the small number of subjects ($N = 19$), the lack of an external control group, and the low estimated amount of exposure. Moreover, there may have been a selection bias in the sample. In consequence, the significance of these findings to the topic of cognitive and neuropsychiatric dysfunction is uncertain.

Decoufle et al. (1992) studied a large sample of Vietnam veterans whose exposure to herbicides was determined by subject reports without confirmation. Reports of psychological dysfunction including posttraumatic stress disorder correlated with self-reports of combat exposure and level of herbicide exposure. The shortcomings of this study are reported in the discussion below on peripheral neuropathy.

Zober et al. (1994) reported the health outcomes in 158 men exposed to TCDD in a factory accident in Germany. Illness episodes handled by hospitalization or outpatient care related to "mental disorders" correlated with severity of chloracne, but not with TCDD blood levels. It is not known whether chloracne documentation close to the time of exposure or TCDD levels many years after exposure represents the better index of actual TCDD exposure. Therefore, it is difficult to draw specific conclusions concerning the relationship between TCDD exposure and mental disorders based on these disparate findings.

In a large mortality study of Vietnam-era veterans in Michigan, proportional mortality ratios were significantly lower for veterans who served in Vietnam than for veterans serving elsewhere for the disease categories of "mental disorders" (not specifically defined) and disorders of "nervous system and sense organs" (Visintainer et al., 1995). The authors did not attempt to separate subjects exposed to herbicides, and they acknowledged that no conclusions could be made in regarding to the specific toxicity of TCDD or Agent Orange. Although some additional publications have appeared on the effect of military service in Vietnam on psychological health outcomes, including PTSD, these reports did not assess the effects of herbicide exposure (Goldberg et al., 1992; Bullman and Kang, 1994).

Conclusions

Strength of Evidence in Epidemiologic Studies

There is inadequate or insufficient evidence of an association between exposure to the herbicides considered in this report and cognitive or neuropsychiatric disorders. The evidence regarding association is drawn from occupational and other studies in which subjects were exposed to a variety of herbicides and herbicide components.

MOTOR/COORDINATION DYSFUNCTION

Summary of *VAO*

In *VAO*, the committee was concluded that there are no definitive studies to determine whether exposure to dioxin or related herbicides is associated with CNS motor/coordination problems. However, follow-up of veterans and, to a lesser extent, environmental observations suggest that motor and coordination difficulties should be assessed further in exposed subjects. It was determined that longitudinal assessments of motor and coordination problems are warranted in exposed subjects, especially those with high exposure, such as the National Institute for Occupational Safety and Health cohort studied by Fingerhut et al. (1991). Vietnam veterans represent the most systematically evaluated group with chronic TCDD exposure, and the findings in this group suggest that CNS disorders may focus on the subtle clinical area of coordination and abnormal involuntary movement disorders. Since this area is a specific subspecialty of neurology, future evaluations should involve specialists in this field. Internationally accepted scales for movement disorders have been developed, and these scales should be used in future studies of such problems.

In addition to assessments that capture the disability related to any objective findings, *VAO* also stressed that in the past decade an increasing concern—unrelated specifically to the question of TCDD and the CNS—has developed scientifically over the possible link between Parkinson's disease and chemicals used as herbicides and pesticides (Semchuk et al., 1992). It was suggested that as Vietnam veterans move into the decades when Parkinson's disease becomes more prevalent, attention to the frequency and character of new cases in exposed versus nonexposed individuals may be highly useful in assessing whether dioxin exposure is a risk factor for eventual Parkinson's disease.

Update of the Scientific Literature

No new data directly addressing this topic have been published since *VAO*. There is, however, a persisting concern about the role of herbicides and pesticides in the pathogenesis of parkinsonism (Semchuk et al., 1993; Butterfield et al., 1993; Golbe, 1993). Using multivariate statistical methods, occupational herbicide use was the third highest predictor of eventual Parkinson's disease risk in the study by Semchuk et al. (1993). Butterfield et al. (1993) examined occupational and environmental factors associated with disease risk in patients with early-onset Parkinson's disease, comparing the findings to a control group. Parkinson's disease was positively associated with herbicide exposure, insecticide exposure, previous residence in a fumigated house, and residence in a rural area at the time of diagnosis. The authors did not specify the type of herbicide or pesticide, so direct extrapolation to the agents used in Vietnam is not possible.

Cases of early-onset parkinsonism are particularly important to testing the hypothesis that the disease relates to a toxic exposure. Patients in this category would presumably have received a heavier dose of toxin than those who developed the disorder at a more typical age in later life. For this reason, the systematic and prospective examination of Vietnam veterans for the development of early-onset parkinsonism assumes particular medical and scientific importance.

Conclusions

Strength of Evidence in Epidemiologic Studies

There is inadequate or insufficient evidence of an association between exposure to the herbicides considered in this report and motor/coordination dysfunction. The evidence regarding association is drawn from occupational and other studies in which subjects were exposed to a variety of herbicides and herbicide components.

CHRONIC PERSISTENT PERIPHERAL NEUROPATHY

Summary of VAO

Although some of the case reports reviewed in VAO suggested that an acute or subacute peripheral neuropathy can develop with exposure to TCDD and related products, other reports with comparison groups did not offer clear evidence that TCDD exposure is associated with chronic peripheral neuropathy. The most rigorously conducted studies argued against a relationship between TCDD or herbicides and chronic persistent neuropathy.

As a group, the studies concerning peripheral neuropathy have been conducted with highly varying methodologies and have lacked uniformity of operational definitions of neuropathy. They have not applied consistent methods to define a comparison population or to determine exposure or clinical deficits. Timing of follow-up may be important, since many, but not all, reports that find neuropathy were based on assessments made only a short time after exposure. It was concluded that careful definition of neuropathy and standardization of protocols will be essential to future evaluations.

Update of the Scientific Literature

Several articles on this topic have appeared since VAO. Decoufle et al.

(1992) compared the self-reported health of 7,924 Vietnam veterans in 1985-86 with their perceived exposure to herbicides and combat in Vietnam. When a subset of subjects was examined neurologically, there was no correlation between the herbicide exposure index used and the occurrence of peripheral neuropathy. The exposure index depended entirely on the subjects' reports and no confirmatory documentation or blood levels of TCDD were obtained. In light of prior studies (CDC, 1988, 1989) that documented no relationship between this self-reported herbicide exposure index and a biological marker of actual dioxin exposure among Vietnam veterans, this study neither confirmed nor refuted a relationship between neuropathy and dioxin exposure among Vietnam veterans. The authors, however, suggested that emotional stress could account for the excessive self-reported symptoms, since complaints were widespread across many body systems, were often vague in quality, and involved many more subjects than were estimated to have been actually exposed to high levels of dioxin.

In the study by Zober et al. (1994), the data were originally thought to suggest an increase in prevalence of disorders of the peripheral nervous system and sense organs. However, reanalysis demonstrated that there was only one case of peripheral neuropathy in the severe chloracne subgroup, and this patient was diabetic, which is a condition also associated with peripheral neuropathy. Their findings are consistent with others who found no evidence of increased occurrence of chronic persistent peripheral neuropathy after TCDD exposure.

Conclusions

Strength of Evidence in Epidemiologic Studies

There is inadequate or insufficient evidence of an association between exposure to the herbicides considered in this report and chronic persistent peripheral neuropathy. The evidence regarding association is drawn from occupational and other studies in which subjects were exposed to a variety of herbicides and herbicide components.

ACUTE AND SUBACUTE TRANSIENT PERIPHERAL NEUROPATHY

The methodology used to establish associations between putative causal agents and persistent chronic neurological deficits relies heavily on epidemiological studies with adequate control or comparison populations. Such methodology can rarely be set in motion with sufficient speed to assess relationships between unexpected chemical exposure and the development of acute or subacute transient neurological disturbance. Because of the very transient nature of the conditions, documenting signs and symptoms in association with documented exposures can be difficult to accomplish in a systematic manner. In such instances, greater reliance must be placed on isolated case histories and less well controlled studies. This section reviews the data from such sources regarding occupational, environmental, and Vietnam herbicide exposure. Because this disorder is of special interest to the DVA, this discussion integrates the studies reviewed in *VAO* with those published more recently.

Review of the Scientific Literature

Occupational Studies A number of reports have suggested that acute or subacute peripheral neuropathies can be associated with occupational exposure to herbicides (Ashe and Suskind, 1950; Baader and Bauer, 1951; Goldstein et al., 1959; Todd, 1962; Berkley and Magee, 1963; Poland et al., 1971; Jirasek et al., 1974). However, only a very limited number of studies on the PNS provide any control or comparison group data. Since peripheral neuropathies can be induced by such common medical and environmental conditions as diabetes and poor nutrition, especially in alcoholics, the presence of neuropathy in an herbicide-exposed population cannot be attributed necessarily to the herbicide without consideration of these other factors. Rigorously defined and examined comparison groups, although especially important in the analysis of peripheral neuropathies, are not available for the topic of acute and subacute neuropathies. The studies cited below provide suggestive but limited evidence of the concept that acute or subacute peripheral neuropathy can develop after exposure to dioxin or related compounds.

Todd (1962) reported a sprayer of 2,4-D weedkiller who developed a gastrointestinal disturbance and, within days, a severe sensory/motor polyneuropathy after contact with the chemical. Recovery occurred gradually over the ensuing months. Berkley and Magee (1963) reported another patient who developed a polyneuropathy four days after exposure to a liquid solution of 2,4-D, which was being sprayed in a cornfield. The neuropathy was purely sensory in type. His symptoms gradually resolved over months. Goldstein et al. (1959) described three patients who had sensory/motor polyneuropathies that developed over several days and progressed over several weeks after exposure to 2,4-D. All had incomplete recovery after several years. Although these patients were not examined neurologically before their exposure, the temporal relationship between the development of their clinical problem and the herbicide exposure was clearly documented. Nonetheless, the possibility that their occurrence was unrelated to the herbicide exposure and represented examples of other disorders, such as idiopathic Guillain-Barre syndrome, cannot be entirely excluded.

Environmental Studies After the Seveso, Italy, chemical explosion, inhabitants from the high-exposure zone were evaluated for signs and symptoms of peripheral nerve disease and compared with inhabitants of a lower-exposure zone. No information is available on acute transient neuropathic effects, since the first reports documented findings in patients evaluated more than six months after the disaster. Boeri et al. (1978) conducted clinical and neurophysiological examination of the peripheral nerves 7 to 11 months after the explosion and reported descriptive differences between 470 volunteer subjects in Zone A (high-exposure group) and 152 volunteer residents of Zone R (low-exposure group). Peripheral nerve problems were frequent in both groups, suggesting to the authors that undefined neuropathic factors predating the explosion may well have been responsible for their findings. Although cranial and peripheral nerve problems were generally more prevalent among the highly exposed group, no statistical analyses were performed on the prevalence data. The electrophysiological studies failed to show any significant abnormalities in either group.

As a complement to the above screening in the first year after exposure, Pocchiari et al. (1979) echoed the observation that neuropathic symptoms were more prevalent in the high-exposure group. No new data were provided. Reporting on symptoms and signs in patients examined eight or more months after the accident, Filippini et al. (1981) compared 308 Seveso residents with 305 nonexposed residents from nearby towns. They examined patients clinically and electrophysiologically, using strict physiological criteria for defining peripheral neuropathy. The authors found no increased risk of "acute" peripheral neuropathy among the exposed residents. However, within the subgroup of exposed subjects who showed clinical signs of significant exposure (chloracne or elevated hepatic enzymes), the risk ratio was 2.8 (CI = 1.2-6.5). Similarly, for Seveso residents with other risk factors for peripheral neuropathy (alcoholism, diabetes, and inflammatory diseases), an elevated risk ratio was also observed (2.6, CI = 1.2-5.6). The authors argued that heavy exposure to dioxin was associated with mild peripheral neuropathy in this two-year follow-up report. Subsequent follow-up studies suggested that there was no increased prevalence of peripheral neuropathy several years after the accident among the high-risk Seveso group (Barbieri et al., 1988; Assennato et al., 1989).

Vietnam Veterans Studies The committee has identified no data on acute or subacute neuropathies related to herbicide exposure in Vietnam. All published data concern chronic effects.

Summary of Acute and Subacute Transient Peripheral Neuropathy

There is some evidence to suggest that neuropathy of acute or subacute onset may be associated with herbicide exposure. This is based primarily on case histories from occupational exposure and the descriptive reports following the Seveso accident. The trend to recovery in the individual cases reported and the negative findings of many long-term follow-up studies of peripheral neuropathy (see section on Chronic Persistent Peripheral Neuropathy) suggest that if a neuropathy indeed develops, it resolves with time.

Conclusions

Strength of Evidence in Epidemiologic Studies

There is limited/suggestive evidence of an association between exposure to the herbicides considered in this report and acute and subacute transient peripheral neuropathy. The evidence regarding association is drawn from occupational and other studies in which subjects were exposed to a variety of herbicides and herbicide components.

CONCLUSIONS FOR NEUROBEHAVIORAL DISORDERS

Strength of Evidence in Epidemiologic Studies

There is inadequate or insufficient evidence to determine whether an association exists between exposure to the herbicides used in Vietnam and disorders involving cognitive and neuropsychiatric dysfunction, motor/coordination deficits, and chronic persistent peripheral neuropathy. The evidence regarding association is drawn from occupational and other studies in which subjects were exposed to a variety of herbicides and herbicide components.

There is limited/suggestive evidence of an association between exposure to the herbicides considered in this report and transient acute or subacute peripheral neuropathy. The evidence regarding association is drawn from occupational and other studies in which subjects were exposed to a variety of herbicides and herbicide components.

Biologic Plausibility

Studies in laboratory animals do not support an association between exposure to TCDD or herbicides and disorders involving cognitive and neuropsychiatric dysfunction, or motor/coordination deficits. New data from animals (Grehl et al., 1993; Grahmann et al., 1993) suggest biological plausibility for an association between TCDD and peripheral neuropathy.

Increased Risk of Disease among Vietnam Veterans

If TCDD is associated with the development of transient acute and subacute peripheral neuropathy, the disorder would become evident shortly after exposure; therefore, there is no evidence that new cases that develop long after service in Vietnam are associated with herbicide exposure that occurred there.

REFERENCES

Ashe W, Suskind R. 1950. Reports on Chloracne Cases. Nitro, WV: Monsanto Chemical Co.

Assennato G, Cervino D, Emmett EA, Longo G, Merlo F. 1989. Follow-up of subjects who developed chloracne following TCDD exposure at Seveso. American Journal of Industrial Medicine 16:119-125.

Baader EW, Bauer H. 1951. Industrial intoxication due to pentachlorophenol. Industrial Medicine and Surgery 20:286-290.

Barbieri S, Pirovano C, Scarlato G, Tarchini P, Zappa A, Maranzana M. 1988. Long-term effects of 2,3,7,8-tetrachlorodibenzo-*p*-dioxin on the peripheral nervous system. Clinical and neurophysiological controlled study on subjects with chloracne from the Seveso area. Neuroepidemiology 7:29-37.

Berkley MC, Magee KR. 1963. Neuropathy following exposure to a dimethylamine salt of 2,4-D. Archives of Internal Medicine 111:133-134.

Boeri R, Bordo B, Crenna P, Filippini G, Massetto M, Zecchini A. 1978. Preliminary results of a neurological investigation of the population exposed to TCDD in the Seveso region. Rivista di Patologia Nervosa e Mentale 99:111-128.

Bullman TA, Kang HK. 1994. The effects of mustard gas, ionizing radiation, herbicides, trauma, and oil smoke on U.S. military personnel: the results of veteran studies. Annual Review of Public Health 15:69-90.

Butterfield PG, Valanis BG, Spencer PS, Lindeman CA, Nutt JG. 1993. Environmental antecedents of young-onset Parkinson's disease. Neurology 43:1150-1158.

Centers for Disease Control. 1988. Health status of Vietnam veterans. II. Physical health. Journal of the American Medical Association 259:2708-2714.

Centers for Disease Control. 1989. Comparison of Serum Levels of 2,3,7,8-tetrachlorodibenzo-*p*-dioxin with Indirect Estimates of Agent Orange Exposure among Vietnam Veterans: Final Report. Atlanta: U.S. Department of Health and Human Services.

Decoufle P, Holmgreen P, Boyle CA, Stroup NE. 1992. Self-reported health status of Vietnam veterans in relation to perceived exposure to herbicides and combat. American Journal of Epidemiology 135:312-323.

Filippini G, Bordo B, Crenna P. 1981. Relationship between clinical and electrophysiological findings and indicators of heavy exposure to 2,3,7,8-tetrachlorodibenzo-*p*-dioxin. Scandinavian Journal of Work, Environment, and Health 7:257-262.

Fingerhut MA, Halperin WE, Marlow DA, Piacitelli LA, Honchar PA, Sweeney MH, Greife AL, Dill PA, Steenland K, Suruda AJ. 1991. Cancer mortality in workers exposed to 2,3,7,8-tetrachlorodibenzo-*p*-dioxin. New England Journal of Medicine 324:212-218.

Golbe LI. 1993. Risk factors in young-onset Parkinson's disease. Neurology 43:1641-1643.

Goldberg J, Eisen SA, True WR, Henderson WG. 1992. Health effects of military service. Lessons learned from the Vietnam experience. Annals of Epidemiology 2:841-853.

Goldstein NP, Jones PH, Brown JR. 1959. Peripheral neuropathy after exposure to an ester of dichlorophenoxyacetic acid. Journal of the American Medical Association 171:1306-1309.

Grahmann F, Claus D, Grehl H, Neundorfer B. 1993. Electrophysiologic evidence for a toxic polyneuropathy in rats after exposure to 2,3,7,8-tetrachlorodibenzo-*p*-dioxin (TCDD). Journal of the Neurological Sciences 115:71-75.

Grehl H, Grahmann F, Claus D, Neundorfer B. 1993. Histologic evidence for a toxic polyneuropathy due to exposure to 2,3,7,8-tetrachlorodibenzo-*p*-dioxin (TCDD) in rats. Acta Neurologica Scandinavica 88:354-357.

Jirasek L, Kalensky K, Kubec K, Pazderova J, Lukas E. 1974. Chronic poisoning by 2,3,7,8-tetrachlorodibenzo-*p*-dioxin. Ceskoslovenska Dermatologie 49:145-157.

Peper M, Klett M, Frentzel-Beyme R, Heller WD. 1993. Neuropsychological effects of chronic exposure to environmental dioxins and furans. Environmental Research 60:124-135.

Pocchiari F, Silano V, Zampieri A. 1979. Human health effects from accidental release of tetrachlorodibenzo-*p*-dioxin (TCDD) at Seveso, Italy. Annals of the New York Academy of Science 320:311-320.

Poland AP, Smith D, Metter G, Possick P. 1971. A health survey of workers in a 2,4,-D and 2,4,5-T plant. Archives of Enivironmental Health 22:316-327.

Semchuk KM, Love EJ, Lee RG. 1992. Parkinson's disease and exposure to agricultural work and pesticide chemicals. Neurology 42:1328-1335.

Semchuk KM, Love EJ, Lee RG. 1993. Parkinson's disease: a test of the multifactorial etiologic hypothesis. Neurology 43:1173-1180.

Sharp DS, Eskenazi B, Harrison R, Callas P, Smith AH. 1986. Delayed health hazards of pesticide exposure. Annual Review of Public Health 7:441-471.

Todd RL. 1962. A case of 2,4-D intoxication. Journal of the Iowa Medical Society 52:663-664.

Visintainer PF, Barone M, McGee H, Peterson EL. 1995. Proportionate mortality study of Vietnam-era veterans of Michigan. Journal of Occupational and Environmental Medicine 37:423-428.

Zober A, Ott MG, Messerer P. 1994. Morbidity follow up study of BASF employees exposed to 2,3,7, 8-tetrachlorodibenzo-*p*-dioxin (TCDD) after a 1953 chemical reactor incident. Occupational and Environmental Medicine 51:469-486.

11

Other Health Effects

INTRODUCTION

A variety of health outcomes are evaluated in this chapter, including chloracne, porphyria cutanea tarda, other metabolic and digestive disorders (diabetes mellitus, alterations in hepatic enzymes, lipid abnormalities, and gastrointestinal ulcers), immune system disorders (immune suppression, autoimmunity), and a number of circulatory and respiratory disorders. Many of them have not been addressed as thoroughly in the epidemiologic literature as the health outcomes described in Chapters 7, 9, and 10.

CHLORACNE

Skin disorders are among the most common health problems encountered in combat, aside from traumatic injuries. Because of the tropical environment and living conditions in Vietnam, veterans developed a variety of skin conditions ranging from bacterial and fungal infections to a condition known as "tropical acne" (Odom, 1993). However, the only dermatologic disorder consistently reported to be associated with Agent Orange and other herbicides, including the contaminant TCDD (2,3,7,8-tetrachlorodibenzo-p-dioxin), is chloracne. Therefore, this discussion will focus on chloracne and its link to TCDD.

Among the numerous industrial chemicals known to cause chloracne, the most potent appears to be TCDD. However, as noted later in this discussion, individual host factors appear to play an important role in determining disease expression. Even at relatively high doses, not all exposed individuals develop chloracne, whereas others with similar or lower exposure demonstrate the condition.

Chloracne has a variable natural history. Longitudinal studies of exposed cohorts suggest that the lesions typically regress and heal over time. However, historical reports indicate that a chronic form of the disease can persist up to 30 years after an exposure (Suskind and Hertzberg, 1984). As with many dermatologic conditions, chloracne can reasonably be suspected on the basis of a careful medical history or appropriate questionnaire information. A key element in diagnosis is the characteristic anatomic distribution. Because acne is such a common dermatologic condition, in any analysis attempting to link acne or chloracne with an environmental or occupational exposure, it is critical that adequate attention be paid to the clinical characteristics, time of onset, and distribution of lesions, and there should be a careful comparison with an appropriate control group. Definitive diagnosis may require histologic confirmation from a biopsy specimen.

Chloracne can be viewed both as a toxic outcome from exposure to TCDD and as a potential clinical marker of TCDD exposure. It is the latter that has generated the most controversy. In this section, the primary focus is on the linkage of chloracne to TCDD exposure. Dose-response relationships between TCDD exposure and chloracne are addressed briefly. The inadequacies of chloracne as a human biomarker of dioxin exposure are discussed in more detail in Chapter 5. A major unresolved issue is whether TCDD exposure below the level required to cause chloracne may cause other adverse health consequences, such as cancer.

Summary of VAO

Chloracne has been linked to TCDD exposure in numerous epidemiologic studies of occupationally and environmentally exposed populations. The data on Vietnam veterans potentially exposed to Agent Orange and other herbicides are less convincing.

Update of the Scientific Literature

Several reports of TCDD exposure in occupational settings have appeared since VAO, some giving updates on previously described populations and others presenting new cohorts. Ott et al. (1993) presented serum TCDD levels on 138 subjects at a BASF plant (79 percent of the cohort still alive) who had been potentially exposed to TCDD and other chemicals in a plant accident in 1953. This was represented as an update of previous reports of this cohort that presented TCDD serum levels correlated with the presence and severity of chloracne. Current TCDD levels ranged from less than 1 to 553 picogram/gram (pg/g) of serum lipid. Using a back extrapolation equation assuming a serum half-life of seven years, the TCDD levels at the time of the accident were calculated to be as high as 12,000 pg/g. Among workers without chloracne, back-extrapolated TCDD (geometric mean) levels were 38 pg/g. Levels among subjects with moderate chlor-acne were 421 pg/g, and among subjects with severe chloracne were 1,701 pg/g.

Zober et al. (1994) reported a retrospective cohort morbidity study using insurance data, comparing 158 men from the BASF plant to 161 nonexposed referents. It is not clear how much this study population overlaps with those in the report by Ott et al. (1993). Back-calculated TCDD levels (geometric mean) ranged from 148 pg/g for a group of exposed men who never developed chloracne to 1,118 pg/g for the severe chloracne group. Back-calculated TCDD levels above an arbitrary cutoff level of 1,000 pg/g were present in 63 percent (33 of 52) of subjects with severe chloracne, 48 percent (29 of 61) of subjects with moderate chloracne, and 24 percent (11 of 45) of subjects with no history of chloracne. The authors noted the very wide range of TCDD levels within each chloracne group and the high degree of overlap in TCDD levels between groups, suggesting either differences in exposure patterns (dermal versus inhaled or ingested) or individual variation in susceptibility.

Schecter et al. (1993) reported seven individuals (three men and four women) from a previously undescribed cohort of 231 workers at a Russian chemical plant who were exposed to dioxins during the manufacture of 2,4,5-T. Five of the seven had been diagnosed with chloracne, and current TCDD levels ranged from 36 to 291 pg/g. This report represented a highly selected group of workers, not a representative cohort, but it did include the first women who demonstrated chloracne and elevated TCDD levels from an occupational exposure.

A cross-sectional investigation of a self-selected group of 153 workers from a BASF plant and from five other chemical plants in Germany also attempted to correlate chloracne with TCDD levels (Von Benner et al., 1994). Its interpretation is limited by the self-referral nature of the study population, leading to uncontrolled selection bias, and the lack of a control population. The prevalence of chloracne by history ranged from 17 percent to 80 percent among the six plant cohorts. The median current TCDD serum level in this population was 60 pg/g serum lipid, compared to a reported background level among the German population of 4.5 pg/g. Lack of data on the dates and levels of exposure precluded back-extrapolation of TCDD levels, and no relationship was observed between current serum TCDD level and a history of chloracne.

Jansing and Korff (1994) described eight employees who developed chloracne after working in a chemical plant in Germany between 1973 and 1976. The plant manufactured trichlorophenol (TCP), and these were apparently newly reported cases. All of the workers were described as having a "long recovery time with a tendency to relapse." Blood TCDD levels were measured, and assuming a half-life of seven years, the extrapolated blood levels at the time of exposure were 545 to 9,894 pg/g. The duration of clinical chloracne was one to ten years, with the duration of disease approximately correlating with extrapolated TCDD level at the time of exposure. Two subjects had extrapolated TCDD levels substantially below the other members of the cohort, which was interpreted by the authors as indicating a particular sensitivity to developing chloracne.

Jung et al. (1994) presented porphyrin and TCDD data on 27 men with present or past chloracne from a study cohort of 170 men who had worked at a German plant manufacturing 2,4-D and 2,4,5-T. There was no correlation between presence of chloracne and TCDD levels or porphyrin levels.

Coenraads et al. (1994) described 118 workers in a Chinese factory making pentachlorophenol (PCP). Forty-four out of 118 (34 percent) showed clinical evidence of chloracne. Most had had the condition for more than 15 years and stated that it began approximately one year after starting work at the plant. Four of the plant's buildings were used in the manufacturing process, and all 40 workers in one of the buildings had clinical chloracne. Interestingly, TCDD levels in the PCP and in the worker's pooled blood samples did not correlate with the prevalence of chloracne among workers in each of the buildings, although polychlorodibenzo-p-dioxin (PCDD) and polychlorodibenzofuran (PCDF) congeners did correlate with chloracne prevalence. Little was known about historical levels of exposure or potential exposures in locations other than the buildings in which the process was carried out.

From these studies, it is apparent that higher levels of exposure to TCDD, as reflected by increased serum levels, are associated in a general way with increased risk of developing chloracne. However, the high degree of variability in TCDD levels among subjects with a history of chloracne and among those with no evidence of the condition suggests a complex dose-response relationship, with highly variable individual susceptibility. In addition, in many subjects, the serum TCDD levels were measured many years after first exposure or onset of chloracne. Based on the current data, it is not possible to ascribe a "threshold" TCDD level associated with chloracne.

Conclusions

Strength of Evidence in Epidemiologic Studies

Evidence is sufficient to conclude that there is a positive association between exposure to the herbicides considered in this report and chloracne. The evidence regarding association is drawn from occupational and other studies in which subjects were exposed to a variety of herbicides and herbicide components.

Biologic Plausibility

The formation of chloracne lesions after administration of TCDD is observed in some species of laboratory animals. Similar observations have not been reported for the herbicides.

Increased Risk of Disease among Vietnam Veterans

Given the large uncertainties concerning the magnitude of potential risk from exposure to herbicides in the occupational, environmental, and veterans studies that have been reviewed, and the lack of information needed to extrapolate from the level of exposure in the studies to that of individual Vietnam veterans, the committee cannot quantify the degree of risk likely to have been experienced by Vietnam veterans because of their exposure to herbicides in Vietnam. Because TCDD-associated chloracne becomes evident shortly after exposure, there is no risk that new cases will occur.

PORPHYRIA CUTANEA TARDA

Porphyria cutanea tarda (PCT) is an uncommon disorder of porphyrin metabolism manifested in patients by thinning and blistering of the skin in sun-exposed areas, as well as by hyperpigmentation (excess pigment in skin) and hypertrichosis (excess hair growth) (Muhlbauer and Pathak, 1979; Grossman and Poh-Fitzpatrick, 1986). The disease is caused by a hereditary or acquired deficiency of uroporphyrinogen decarboxylase (UROD), a cytoplasmic enzyme in the pathway of hemoglobin synthesis (Sweeney, 1986). In the hereditary form, no precipitating exposure is necessary for the appearance of excess uroporphyrin and coproporphyrin in the urine and the development of clinical symptoms.

In cell culture and in rodents (mice and rats), TCDD causes a toxic porphyria resembling PCT in humans (De Verneuil et al., 1983; Cantoni et al., 1984; Smith and De Matteis, 1990).

Summary of *VAO*

The occurrence of clinical PCT is rare and may be influenced by genetic predisposition of individuals with low enzyme levels of uroporphyrinogen decarboxylase. The cases reported have occurred relatively shortly after exposure to specific chemicals, including TCDD, and have improved after removal of the agent. Simultaneous exposure to alcohol and other chemicals, such as hexachlorobenzene, probably increases the risk and severity of PCT. Abnormal porphyrin excretion without clinical illness may occur more commonly than clinical evidence of PCT; this may represent a preclinical stage of PCT.

There is no suggestion of an increase in PCT in studies of Vietnam veterans or the Ranch Hands (the Air Force personnel who handled the herbicides), possibly because of comparatively low dioxin exposure even in Ranch Hand studies, or a fortuitous absence of genetically predisposed individuals who could develop

PCT after TCDD exposure. Further studies of PCT incidence in Vietnam veterans would not be called for, since the biologic and clinical evidence indicate that the rare appearance of PCT occurs soon after heavy TCDD exposure and improves with time. Moreover, the association of PCT with alcoholism makes it difficult to interpret studies of TCDD and PCT that do not simultaneously assess alcohol consumption.

It is possible that a rare individual with asymptomatic hereditary PCT was worsened by exposure to TCDD. Whether such individuals were present in the military cannot be determined, although patients with overt symptomatic disease would likely be excluded from military service. In any individual case, evaluation of potential exposure to chemicals other than TCDD, such as ethanol, estrogens, or hexachlorobenzene, would be necessary to attribute abnormalities to dioxin or herbicide exposure specifically.

The epidemiologic evidence associating PCT and TCDD is sparse because PCT is rare and because of methodological problems. However, case reports and animal studies show that PCT may be associated with TCDD exposure in genetically predisposed individuals.

Update of the Scientific Literature

Jung et al. (1994) presented porphyrin data on former workers in a German pesticide plant that had manufactured 2,4-D and 2,4,5-T. The original cohort working in the plant numbered approximately 300, and possible selection bias among the 170 who completed the examination was not described. Of the 183 men who participated, 170 donated urine and blood samples for analysis of porphyrins. An additional 43 men, including 11 with a current or past history of chloracne and 32 without a history of chloracne, agreed to an adipose tissue biopsy. Among the 170 men tested, 27 had present or past chloracne and 128 had no history of chloracne; for 15 men, the diagnosis was uncertain. The study found no difference in porphyrin levels between subjects with and without chloracne. There was also no relationship between abnormal liver function tests and porphyrin levels and the presence or absence of chloracne, and no relationship between porphyrin levels in urine, RBCs or plasma, and TCDD levels in adipose tissue. Three cases of chronic hepatic porphyria (none with overt PCT and none with chloracne) were identified, a number which did not exceed the expected prevalence in this population.

Calvert et al. (1994) analyzed porphyrin levels and TCDD serum levels in a cross-sectional medical study of the NIOSH cohort of workers who had been previously exposed to TCDD through manufacture of sodium trichlorophenol, 2,4,5-T, or hexachlorophene. The study compared 281 exposed workers with mean serum TCDD level of 220 pg/g lipid to 260 nonexposed referents with mean TCDD level of 7 pg/g lipid (back-extrapolated values assuming a serum half-life of seven years: 1,900 pg/g vs. 6 pg/g). There were no cases of overt

PCT, and three exposed and three unexposed subjects with subclinical PCT. Porphyrin levels did not differ between exposed and unexposed workers, and there was no significant relationship between urinary porphyrin levels and serum TCDD levels.

Von Benner et al. (1994) suggested a possible correlation between TCDD levels and urine coproporphyrin levels in a report of 153 self-referred employees from six chemical plants in Germany. Interpretation of this report is limited by the self-referral nature of the study population, leading to uncontrolled selection bias, and the lack of a control population. There was no indication of clinical PCT among subjects in the cohort.

Taken together, these studies did not support the hypothesis that TCDD caused disturbances in heme metabolism in humans, even at the relatively high exposure levels experienced by these cohorts. In the committee's view, these new data, combined with the studies reviewed in *VAO*, justify moving PCT to the category of limited/suggestive evidence of an association with herbicide exposure. The reports that some persons employed in herbicide production have evidence of increased porphyrins in urine warrant further investigation.

Conclusions

Strength of Evidence in Epidemiologic Studies

There is limited/suggestive evidence of an association between exposure to the herbicides considered in this report and porphyria cutanea tarda. The evidence regarding association is drawn from occupational and other studies in which subjects were exposed to a variety of herbicides and herbicide components.

Biologic Plausibility

There is some evidence that TCDD can be associated with porphyrin abnormalities in laboratory animals, although PCT has not been reported. Porphyria has not been reported in animals exposed to herbicides.

Increased Risk of Disease among Vietnam Veterans

Given the large uncertainties regarding the magnitude of potential risk from exposure to herbicides in the occupational, environmental, and veterans studies that have been reviewed, and the lack of information needed to extrapolate from the level of exposure in the studies reviewed to that of individual Vietnam veterans, the committee cannot quantify the degree of risk likely to have been experienced by Vietnam veterans because of their exposure to herbicides in Vietnam. Because TCDD-associated PCT would become evident shortly after exposure, there is no risk that new cases will occur.

RESPIRATORY DISORDERS

The studies reviewed in this section covered a wide variety of respiratory conditions. In the morbidity studies, a variety of methods were used to assess the respiratory system, including assessing symptoms, performing physical examination of the chest, and assessing lung function tests and chest radiographs. Lung function tests, also called pulmonary function tests, included tests commonly used to detect airflow obstruction (which can occur in conditions such as asthma, chronic bronchitis, and emphysema) and restriction or decrease in lung volumes (which can occur in lung scarring and inflammation). The tests that measure reduced in airflow obstruction include FEV_1 (amount of air that can be forcefully exhaled in one second), FEV_1/FVC ratio (ratio of the amount of air that can be forcefully exhaled in one second to the total amount of air that can be forcefully exhaled), FEF_{25-75} (rate of airflow in the middle range of total volume), and FEF_{max} (rate of airflow at the highest lung volume). The test that measures restriction is the FVC, or forced vital capacity, the total amount of air that can be forcefully exhaled. Chest radiographs, which were used in several studies, can assess whether inhaled agents have damaged the lungs; damage is usually seen as opacities indicating scarring, or inflammation, or both.

Summary of *VAO*

Among the morbidity studies, strong rationales for examining respiratory outcomes were not given. However, in the case of occupational exposures or exposures of military personnel who performed spraying, the respiratory tract could be viewed as a target organ for aerosol or other particulate deposition. Several studies provided spirometry data, including FEV_1, FVC, and FEV_1/FVC ratio (CDC, 1988; Suskind and Hertzberg, 1984; AFHS, 1991; Calvert et al., 1991). Results of chest physical examinations were reported in some studies (AFHS, 1991; Calvert et al., 1991). Although chest radiograph results were provided in several studies, there was no uniform reporting system used, such as the International Labor Organization classification system. For example, in one study (AFHS, 1991), chest films were classified as either normal or abnormal. In another (CDC, 1988), clinical descriptions were provided by radiologists. In another (Pollei et al., 1986), scoring for six specific abnormalities was performed by three radiologists. Questionnaires used to assess smoking histories and various respiratory symptoms, and the resultant symptoms reported from questionnaire data, also varied across studies. The lack of working hypotheses about respiratory disease outcomes associated with herbicides and the nonuniformity in methods and reported results make it difficult to interpret much of the morbidity data, especially reports of symptoms and radiographic data.

Any study examining such respiratory outcomes as chronic bronchitis, decrements in lung function, or radiographic abnormalities must take into account the effects of cigarette smoking. Smoking data were generally not available in the mortality studies, but smoking was taken into account to various degrees in most of the morbidity studies.

Interpretation of many of the mortality studies is limited by the small number of deaths observed. These studies also tend to use the International Classification of Diseases codes for all respiratory diseases, codes 460 to 519, as the mortality outcome. These codes include all diseases of the respiratory tract. Among the diseases covered by these codes are acute respiratory infections, other diseases of the upper respiratory tract, pneumonia, influenza, chronic bronchitis, emphysema, asthma, pleurisy, and pneumoconiosis. This wide range of diverse conditions and the small number of total deaths make it difficult to assess any particular respiratory outcome using mortality studies. In some studies, the ICD codes used were not stated, making comparisons with other studies difficult.

Update of the Scientific Literature

Senthilselvan et al. (1992) investigated the association between self-reported asthma and pesticide use among 1,939 male farmers in Saskatchewan in 1982-83. Pesticide use was categorized as either herbicide or insecticide use. There was no significant association of asthma with herbicide use, although an increase in asthma prevalence was noted among users of carbamate insecticides, which contained a different form of carbamate from that used in herbicides.

Garry et al. (1994) surveyed 1,000 randomly selected state-licensed pesticide appliers in Minnesota. The authors found that the general health of appliers was similar to that of the U.S. population. There was no increase in respiratory disease or other health conditions associated with herbicide use. Interestingly, chronic lung disease and allergy/asthma were significantly increased in fumigant applicators, compared with other pesticide applicators.

Zober et al. (1994) carried out a retrospective cohort morbidity study of 158 men formerly employed at a BASF plant who had been exposed to TCDD in 1953, compared to 161 nonexposed referents. There was no increase in chronic respiratory disease associated with either elevated TCDD levels or with surrogates of exposure, although exposed workers had sought medical attention for respiratory infections significantly more frequently than did referents.

Conclusions

Strength of Evidence in Epidemiologic Studies

There is inadequate or insufficient evidence to determine whether an association exists between exposure to the herbicides and mortality from respiratory diseases; symptoms or history of respiratory illnesses, such as chronic bronchitis, bronchitis, asthma, pleurisy, pneumonia, tuberculosis, and respiratory conditions;

abnormalities on lung or thorax physical examination; pulmonary function test results; and chest radiographs. The evidence regarding association is drawn from occupational and other studies in which subjects were exposed to a variety of herbicides and herbicide components.

IMMUNE SYSTEM DISORDERS

Immunotoxicology is the study of the effects of xenobiotics (chemical compounds that are foreign to the human body) on the immune system. The compounds may produce an impaired immune response (immunosuppression) or an enhanced immune response (immune-mediated disease). Although alterations in the immune system can be related to increases in the incidence of infection and neoplasm (immune suppression) and immune-mediated diseases (allergy and autoimmunity), there has been no observed increase in infectious or immune-mediated disease in the populations examined after exposure to herbicides. However, alterations have been observed in measures of immune function or populations of immune cells. The question of possible increases in neoplastic diseases is dealt with in Chapter 7.

Immune Suppression

The immune system helps defend the host against foreign invaders. It confers resistance to infection by bacteria, viruses, and parasites; it is involved in the rejection of allografts (tissue transplants); and it may eliminate spontaneously occurring tumors (Paul, 1993). Proper function of the immune system is exquisitely sensitive to disruptions in physiologic homeostasis. The immune response is highly redundant, and several different mechanisms may be employed to eliminate an antigen. Therefore, a toxicant can affect one facet of the immune system without altering the ability of the host to survive challenge by an infectious agent.

Suppression of the immune system leads to increased susceptibility to infection and neoplasia. However, the degree of immune suppression necessary to cause disease is unknown and is the subject of intense scientific interest. Immune deficiency may result from genetic abnormalities (e.g., a deficiency in the enzyme adenosine deaminase, leading to severe combined immune deficiency), congenital malformations, surgical accidents, pregnancy, stress, disease (e.g., human immunodeficiency virus [HIV-I] can lead to AIDS), and exposure to immunosuppressive agents (Paul, 1993). Immune suppression can also occur in patients with autoimmune disease (discussed below); for example, in systemic lupus erythematosus, the suppression of complement levels and leukocyte function has been noted. Impaired host defenses can result in severe and recurrent infections with opportunistic microorganisms.   As noted, the immune system may prevent or limit tumor growth, and a high incidence of tumors may follow immune suppression (Paul, 1993).

Allergy and Autoimmunity

A number of diseases involve hyperresponsiveness of the immune system to either foreign allergens (e.g., allergy) or self-antigens (autoimmunity). Allergic responses have been noted to numerous environmental agents, including plant pollens and epithelial products of domestic animals. Allergy is the result of formation of allergen-specific immunoglobulin E (IgE) antibodies, which bind to the surface of mast cells and lead to mast-cell degranulation upon subsequent exposure to antigen. The mediators of allergic reactions, such as histamine, are then released. The alterations discussed below reflect only in vitro immune parameters, not disease incidence. In fact, no increase in allergic disease related to herbicide exposure has been reported in any of the studies reviewed.

In general, the immune response is directed against foreign antigens. However, in some instances, antibodies can be demonstrated that react with endogenous antigens (i.e., autoantibodies). Autoimmune disease is the pathological consequence of an immune response to autologous antigen. Some autoimmune diseases result when autoantibodies activate the complement cascade or interact with "killer" mononuclear cells to induce antibody-dependent cell-mediated cytotoxicity. Others are caused by cytotoxic T cells acting directly on their targets or by injurious cytokines released by activated T cells.

It is important to distinguish the mere presence of an autoimmune response from autoimmune disease. Autoimmunity, as indicated by the presence of autoantibodies, is relatively common, whereas autoimmune disease is relatively rare. Detecting autoantibodies, particularly in high titers and with high affinity, is the first step in diagnosing autoimmune disease in humans. A definite diagnosis of autoimmune disease, however, depends on careful correlation of history and clinical findings with detailed immunologic investigations.

Summary of *VAO*

The effects of herbicide exposure on the level of several immune parameters were presented. The data are divided into two categories: immune suppression and immune enhancement. Some changes in cellular number or function were reported, but no changes in the incidence of disease were noted. Currently, the level of alteration in immune parameters necessary to affect the incidence of disease is unknown.

These data correlate with some of the data observed in animal studies, but much more information is required to determine the mechanism and clinical significance of these alterations in humans. Furthermore, since so many immune parameters have been assessed in these studies, there is a high probability that at least some positive results would be noted based on chance alone, which would undermine the interpretation of the few positive results.

Update of the Scientific Literature

No reports of heightened susceptibility to infectious disease have been identified since *VAO*. In addition, no reports that investigated the association of autoimmune disease or allergy with exposure to herbicides have been identified. Malignant diseases are discussed in Chapter 7. Some new information has appeared, however, on the effects of TCDD on immunological parameters measured in the laboratory.

The study by Jansing and Korff (1994) of eight employees exposed to TCDD in a chemical plant in the Germany between 1973 and 1976 was described previously in this chapter. In addition to assessing chloracne, these investigators determined levels of γ-globulin and lymphocyte subpopulations in the blood. Gamma-globulin was determined by zonal electrophoresis. Four of the eight samples were slightly below the normal range defined by this laboratory. There was also a general correlation between TCDD levels in blood lipids and the decrease in gamma-globulins, although the number of cases was small. The authors also reported that the ratio of the CD4 to CD8 lymphocyte subpopulations was within the normal range.

A long-term follow-up of 138 individuals occupationally exposed to TCDD in a trichlorophenol production facility in 1953 was described by Ott et al. (1994). In addition to measuring TCDD concentration in the blood, the authors were able to perform a number of clinical laboratory tests. The immune system parameters investigated included IgA, IgG, and IgM levels, complement components C3 and C4, and the following lymphocyte markers: CD3 for mature T cells, CD4 for T-helper cells, CD8 for T cytotoxic cells, CD4CDW29 for T-helper/inducer cells, CD11 for natural killer cells and monocytes, and CD19 for B cells. However, the tests for complement components C3 and C4 and for T-helper/inducer cells were added late in the study and data were available for only half of the participants. The results were compared with a reference population comprising men between 50 and 69 years of age who participated in routine occupational medical examinations during the years 1989-91. None of the immune system parameters measured was significantly different from those in the reference group. The total lymphocyte count, however, was 13 percent lower in the study population than in the reference group. In regression analyses, slight increases in the IgA and IgG levels and marginal increases of complement components C3 and C4 were seen with higher TCDD concentrations. A marginal decline in T cells and in the total lymphocyte count was seen and appeared to be positively correlated with TCDD concentration. Chloracne was associated with marginal decreases in the percentages of natural killer cells, T cells, and T-suppressor cells.

A cross-sectional study of 153 occupationally exposed employees of six chemical plants in West Germany was reported by Von Benner et al. (1994). They found no significant correlation of cell-mediated immunity, as measured by multiple skin tests, with TCDD concentration. There was, however, a slight decrease in total protein concentration and IgM in serum as TCDD increased. A minimal decrease in the white-blood-cell count was also recorded as TCDD levels increased.

Svensson et al. (1994) measured the levels of several organochloride compounds—polychlorinated dioxins (PCDD), dibenzofurans (PCDF), and biphenyls (PCB)—in the blood of Baltic Sea fishermen. The subjects were divided into "high" consumers and "low" consumers of fish. The high consumers, who had higher levels of the organochloride compounds, had a lower proportion of natural killer cells, identified by the CD56 marker. There were no changes in other lymphocyte populations or immunoglobulin levels.

Using monoclonal antibodies in flow cytometry, Neubert et al. (1993) studied a variety of surface markers on lymphocyte subpopulations of workers exposed to TCDD and other polychlorinated dibenzofurans (TCDF) at the Dekonta Company, in Hamburg, Germany. Sixty-two volunteers were studied with various body burdens of TCDD or TCDF. Since there was no control group, comparisons were made between volunteers with low or medium levels and with higher levels. No differences were observed in the number of total leukocytes or in absolute or relative numbers of granulocytes and total lymphocytes, nor were there clear-cut changes in the percentages of the main lymphocyte subpopulations in individuals with different body burdens. There was, however, a trend toward an increase in the percentage or absolute number of cells carrying the CD4 and CD45RO biomarkers, representing helper/inducer and memory subpopulations of T cells. Similarly, there was no decrease in the percentage or absolute number of total B cells bearing the markers CD20 or CD19. However, a minor subpopulation of CD19+CD20+CD21+ mature B cells was decreased in 40 percent of the volunteers, in both the higher- and lower-level exposure groups. In a follow-up study, Neubert et al. (1994) measured in vitro proliferation of lymphocytes from workers exposed to PCDD and/or PCDF. The investigators performed regression analyses of the data evaluating the proliferative responses against the body burdens. There was no indication of a dose-dependent decrease in proliferative capacity. There was, in fact, a slight trend toward enhanced proliferation in response to phytohemagglutinin at higher body burdens.

Conclusions

Strength of Evidence in Epidemiologic Studies

There is inadequate or insufficient evidence to determine whether an association exists between exposure to the herbicides considered in this report and immune suppression or autoimmunity. The evidence regarding association is drawn from occupational and other studies in which subjects were exposed to a variety of herbicides and herbicide components.

OTHER METABOLIC AND DIGESTIVE DISORDERS

Diabetes, hepatic enzymes, lipid abnormalities, and ulcers have been reported in the scientific literature as possibly associated with TCDD or herbicide exposure. Assessment of these metabolic and digestive disorders in association with exposure to herbicides and TCDD involves the medical evaluation of a wide array of clinical signs and symptoms, laboratory parameters, and other diagnostic tools. These diagnostic criteria and their use in the clinical evaluation of these four health parameters are described below.

Diabetes Mellitus

Diabetes mellitus is a syndrome of disordered metabolism and hyperglycemia due to an absolute or relative deficiency of insulin secretion, a reduction in its biologic effectiveness, or both. There are two major types of diabetes: type I (insulin-dependent) and type II (non-insulin-dependent). Type I diabetes occurs most commonly among juveniles but occasionally among adults, whereas type II diabetes occurs predominantly in adults and only occasionally in juveniles. More than 90 percent of the estimated 7 million diabetics in the United States are classified as type II diabetics (Karam, 1992). Many of these patients initially exhibit few or no symptoms, although polyuria (increased urination) and polydipsia (excessive thirst) may be present.

Diabetes is associated with high levels of serum glucose. Plasma glucose levels in excess of 140 mg/dl after an overnight fast are generally suggestive of an abnormal glucose tolerance, which is a prerequisite for the diagnosis of diabetes. The presence of obesity or a strongly positive family history for mild diabetes suggests a high risk for the development of type II diabetes.

Summary of VAO

Limited information suggests the possibility of increased glucose intolerance and diabetes in chemical workers and Ranch Hand veterans exposed to TCDD, but the data are inconclusive. Additional information on the pharmacokinetics of dioxin metabolism, particularly with regard to total body fat, is necessary in order to interpret epidemiologic studies indicating an association between TCDD exposure and serum glucose levels.

Update of the Scientific Literature

Ott et al. (1994) reported on 138 workers at a BASF plant who had been potentially exposed to TCDD and other chemicals in a plant accident in 1953. Evaluation of this cohort took place in 1989 and 1990, when the median age of employees was 61 years. The relationship between fasting serum glucose and

TCDD level was studied, adjusting for age, body-mass index, and smoking. There were no remarkable differences between the exposed and referent groups. A marginal increase in the log of the fasting serum glucose level was observed with current TCDD level, but not with back-calculated TCDD level. Because TCDD level may be a function of lipid content of the body, it is possible that the weak positive association between current TCDD and glucose levels is secondary to the link between diabetes and obesity.

Zober et al. (1994) followed 158 workers at the BASF plant through 1989. There is considerable overlap between the subjects in this study and the study by Ott et al. (1994). The authors compared the coded diagnoses and conditions reported in the medical insurance claims for these employees with 161 age-matched control employees without TCDD exposure. Exposed employees were stratified in three groups based on history of chloracne—severe, moderate, and none; they were also stratified with low and high back-calculated TCDD level groups (<1,000 vs. ≥1,000 ppt). There was no adjustment for obesity in this study. Diabetes was diagnosed significantly less frequently in the exposed groups than the controls. The rate of diabetes did not increase with chloracne severity, and the high TCDD subgroup had no increase compared to the controls.

In 1991 and 1993, 153 employees of six chemical factories in Germany were studied (Von Benner et al., 1994). The workers had been involved in the production of trichlorophenol from 1953 to 1983, during which time they were they were exposed to TCDD. The median TCDD level was 60 ppt (range + 1.0-2,252 ppt). An unknown number of these employees were also included in the BASF cohort reported by Ott et al. (1994) and Zober et al. (1994). The authors stated that only limited conclusions could be drawn about causality, because of the selection bias, lack of a control group, and the cross-sectional design of the study. There was no correlation between serum TCDD levels and blood glucose level; 2.6 percent of the 158 employees were diabetics. There was a positive correlation between increasing body-mass index and increasing blood sugar.

Liver Toxicity

Increases in the serum activity of certain hepatic enzymes—including aspartate aminotransferase (AST or SGOT), and alanine aminotransferase (ALT or SGPT), as well as gamma-glutamyltransferase (GGT), d-glucaric acid, and others are commonly noted in many kinds of liver disorders. The relative sensitivity and specificity of these enzymes for liver disease vary, and several different tests may be required for a diagnosis. The only regularly reported abnormality in liver function associated with TCDD exposure in humans is elevation in GGT. Estimates of the serum activity of this enzyme provide a sensitive indicator of alcohol and drug hepatotoxicity, infiltrative lesions of the liver, parenchymal liver disease, and biliary tract obstruction (Berkow and Fletcher, 1987). Elevations are noted with many chemical and drug exposures without evidence of liver injury.

The confounding effects of alcohol ingestion (frequently associated with increased GGT) make interpretation of changes in GGT in exposed individuals difficult (Calvert et al., 1992). Moreover, elevation in GGT may be considered a normal biologic adaptation to chemical, drug, or hormone exposure.

In animal species that exhibit sensitivity to TCDD, the liver represents one of the primary metabolic organs; studies show that TCDD is transported to the liver, where it is stored and metabolized (Lakshman et al., 1986; Piper et al., 1973). TCDD is metabolized by enzymes in the liver to form derivatives that can dissolve in water and therefore be more easily eliminated from the body than TCDD itself, which is water-insoluble. Changes in hepatic enzyme levels after TCDD exposure in animals have been observed, although there is considerable variation among species (see Chapter 3).

Summary of VAO

Changes in liver function in humans exposed to TCDD are limited to an increase in GGT; results are inconsistent regarding ALT and d-glucaric acid excretion. These metabolic "adaptations" to chemical exposure have been seen in industrial workers as well as Ranch Hand veterans. Any study suggesting an association between TCDD exposure and changes in hepatic enzymes or occurrence of liver disease must consider known associations with alcohol, hepatitis, or other toxic chemical exposures. Given the long observation period since TCDD exposure occurred in most studies and consideration of other known risk factors, it seems very unlikely that there is any association between TCDD or herbicide exposure (at levels seen to date in humans) and liver dysfunction.

Update of the Scientific Literature

Ott et al. (1994) reported on 138 workers at a BASF plant who had been potentially exposed to TCDD and other chemicals in a plant accident in 1953. The relationships between severe liver function indicators and TCDD level were studied, adjusting for age, body-mass index, and smoking. Alcohol consumption was not controlled for in the analysis. Based on regression analyses, none of the tests was significantly correlated with current TCDD level. Only one test, for alkaline phosphatase, was significantly correlated in a positive direction, with back-calculated TCDD level. This was also the only test that was significantly associated with chloracne status, showing higher values with increasing chloracne.

Zober et al. (1994) followed 158 of the BASF workers through 1989. There is considerable overlap between the subjects in this study and the study by Ott et al. (1994). There was no control for alcohol use in this study. There were nonsignificant increases in the frequency of chronic liver disease, among the total exposed group versus the controls, as well as among the moderate and severe chloracne subgroups versus the controls. The frequency was also marginally higher in the high TCDD group (31.5 percent) versus the low TCDD group (21.2 percent), or versus the controls (23.0 percent).

Von Benner et al. (1994) studied 153 employees of six chemical factories in Germany in 1991 and 1993. An unknown number of these employees were also included in the BASF cohort reported by Ott et al. (1994) and Zober et al. (1994). There was no correlation between serum TCDD levels and abnormalities in liver function tests. The authors interpreted this to mean that "there was no persistent and/or clinically significant isolated effect of TCDD on the parameters of liver functioning." In contrast, there were "plausible" correlations between self-reported alcohol consumption and increases in SGOT and GGT levels.

Lipid Abnormalities

Hyperlipidemia, or elevation in cholesterol, triglycerides, or the lipoprotein carriers of these lipids [very low density lipoprotein (VLDL), low-density lipoprotein (LDL), and high-density lipoprotein (HDLP)] has been described in relation to hereditary and dietary factors. The clinical manifestations of these changes relate primarily to the incidence of ischemic cardiovascular disease and other forms of atherosclerosis. Measurement of lipid and lipoprotein levels is essential to the diagnostic evaluation of hyperlipidemia. However, the measurements should be adjusted for diet and sex, because the concentration of lipids varies with nutritional, endocrine, and gender differences. There is frequently a substantial time delay between onset of lipid changes and clinical manifestations of disease, often 20 to 40 years (Stanbury et al., 1978).

Summary of VAO

The variable results in the reviewed literature do not allow clear-cut attribution of lipid abnormalities to TCDD exposure. It is possible that levels of TCDD were increased in those subjects with hypercholesterolemia (elevated levels of serum cholesterol) because of the concentration of the chemical in lipids or because of obesity. In industrial exposures, increases have been modest and variable. A positive association was noted between serum TCDD levels and triglycerides among Ranch Hands. Further research on the pharmacokinetics of TCDD and its relation to the percentage of fat in the body will be important in understanding the significance of these associations.

The problem of interpreting the observed association in epidemiologic studies between serum TCDD and lipid levels is complicated by the role of obesity as both a risk factor for lipid abnormalities and a major determinant of the storage and metabolism of TCDD in the body (see Chapter 5). Body fat must be taken into account in analyses of this kind to ensure the validity of the results.

Update of the Scientific Literature

Ott et al. (1994) reported on 138 workers at a BASF plant who had been potentially exposed to TCDD and other chemicals in a plant accident in 1953. The relationships between four lipids (cholesterol, triglycerides, HDL, and LDL) and TCDD level were studied, adjusting for age, body-mass index, and smoking. There were no remarkable differences between the exposed and reference groups.

Gastrointestinal Ulcers

There are usually no specific physical signs in patients with gastrointestinal ulcers, and the symptoms of gastric ulcer are often nonspecific. The typical pattern of epigastric pain is variable, and many patients with this symptom may not have an ulcer when examined endoscopically, whereas patients with ulcers demonstrated by endoscopy may report no pain. Endoscopy is generally recommended only in patients whose symptoms persist despite treatment. Acid secretory values are of relatively little clinical value in diagnosis of ulcer disease (Samiy et al., 1987). In many patients, the disease is associated with the presence of *Helicobacter pylori* (*H. pylori*).

Summary of VAO

The risk of ulcers in populations exposed to TCDD or herbicides has not been sufficiently studied to determine an association. However, detection of a specific association is unlikely, given the frequency of ulcer disease and the many factors that are known to be related to the onset of symptomatic ulcer disease. Furthermore, given the length of time that has elapsed since veterans' last exposure to TCDD in Vietnam, it is unlikely that new cases of ulcer disease will occur.

Update of the Scientific Literature

Zober et al. (1994) followed 158 workers at a BASF plant who were potentially exposed to TCDD during a 1953 plant accident. The workers were followed through 1989. There is considerable overlap between the subjects in this study and the study by Ott et al. (1994). There were no increases in the frequency of ulcers in the exposed group versus the controls (even in the highest TCDD subgroup), and no increases with increasing severity of chloracne.

Conclusions

Strength of Evidence in Epidemiologic Studies

There is inadequate or insufficient evidence to determine whether an association exists between exposure to the herbicides considered in this study and diabetes, liver toxicity, lipid abnormalities, or gastrointestinal ulcers. The evidence regarding association is drawn from occupational and other studies in which subjects were exposed to a variety of herbicides and herbicide components.

Biologic Plausibility

The liver is the site of TCDD storage and metabolism in laboratory animals. Some of the herbicides have also induced liver toxicity in laboratory animals. There have been no reports of an association between TCDD or herbicide exposure and diabetes in laboratory animals. Hyperlipidemia has been reported in laboratory animals following exposure to TCDD, but not following exposure to the herbicides. Specific digestive disorders have not been reported.

CIRCULATORY DISORDERS

The circulatory diseases reviewed in this section cover a wide variety of conditions. The studies reviewed are divided into two categories: morbidity studies and mortality studies. In the morbidity studies, a variety of methods were used to assess the circulatory system, including analysis of symptoms or history, physical examination of the heart and peripheral arteries, Doppler measurement of peripheral pulses, electrocardiograms, and chest radiographs. Doppler measurements and physical examination of the pulses in the arms and legs are used to detect decreased strength of the pulses, which can be caused by thickening and hardening of the arteries. Electrocardiograms can be used to detect heart conditions and abnormalities such as arrhythmias (abnormal heart rhythms), heart enlargement, and previous heart attacks. Chest radiographs can be used to assess whether the heart is enlarged, which can result from heart failure and other heart conditions.

Summary of VAO

The circulatory outcomes addressed in these studies include: mortality from circulatory diseases (including overall circulatory disease mortality and various subgroups of cardiovascular disease); symptoms or history of circulatory illnesses, such as heart disease, hypertension, coronary artery disease, angina, or myocardial infarction; abnormalities detected during physical examinations; electrocardiogram results; and chest radiographs.

The usefulness of the mortality studies was limited, because in most studies there were no a priori hypotheses provided regarding herbicide exposure and particular circulatory outcomes. Their usefulness is also limited by assessment of independent risk factors for circulatory disease.

Among the morbidity studies, strong rationales for examining circulatory outcomes were not given. However, the Air Force Health Study (1991) has reported associations between serum TCDD and both diabetes and blood lipids. This suggests a rationale for examining, in future studies, coronary artery disease in subjects exposed to dioxins, because of the possible association between risk factors for coronary artery disease and serum TCDD level. In the morbidity studies, a wide range of outcomes was assessed, and the presentation of results varied across studies. Symptoms or history of heart disease were difficult to assess across studies, because each study gathered unique noncomparable data. Data derived from physical examination differed among the studies.

Update of the Scientific Literature

The majority of human studies have not found a significant relationship between herbicide or TCDD exposures and the development of circulatory and renal disorders. Three reports were identified in which cardiovascular and/or renal effects were identified. Only one of these studies (Air Force Health Study) found significant associations between dioxin levels and several lipid-related variables (Wolfe et al., 1992). These data are potentially significant, since they were derived from the first large-scale study of dose-response relationships in humans. The cardiovascular and renal effects observed may be related to diabetes mellitus, since no consistent evidence of an adverse effect of dioxin was seen in nondiabetics. There was a significant increased risk of essential hypertension for Ranch Hand workers in the high-current-dioxin category (> 33.3 ppt) relative to background (< 10 ppt), when the effect of body fat was not considered. The adjusted mean level for systolic and diastolic pressures was increased for Ranch Hands in the high-current-dioxin category. However, the reverse analysis of participants suffering from hypertension did not show an association with dioxin, suggesting lack of dose-response relationships. The assessment of peripheral vascular function found a significant association between dioxin and decreased peripheral pulses. Because these effects of dioxin were related to body fat content, causal relationships could not be established, because it is unknown whether dioxin increases fat or whether fat decreases dioxin elimination (see Chapter 5).

Von Benner et al. (1994) reported on the dose-effect relationship between serum TCDD level (median = 60 ppt) and disease in 153 occupationally exposed employees. Possible correlations were found for elevated systolic blood pressure, but not for diastolic blood pressure. However, this relationship was difficult to evaluate, because age and body-mass index also had a significant effect.

Zober et al. (1994) followed 158 workers at a BASF plant who were potentially exposed to TCDD during a 1953 plant accident. The workers were followed through 1989. There is considerable overlap between the subjects in this study and the study by Ott et al. (1994). There were no increases in the frequency of ischemic heart disease in the exposed group versus the controls (even in the highest TCDD subgroup); and no increases with increasing severity of chloracne.

Conclusions

Strength of Evidence in Epidemiologic Studies

There is inadequate or insufficient evidence to determine whether an association exists between exposure to the herbicides considered in this report and the following circulatory outcomes: circulatory disease mortality and various subgroups of cardiovascular disease; symptoms or history of circulatory illnesses, such as heart disease, hypertension, coronary artery disease, angina, or myocardial infarction; or abnormalities detected from physical examination, electrocardiogram results, and chest radiographs. The evidence regarding association is drawn from occupational and other studies in which subjects were exposed to a variety of herbicides and herbicide components.

REFERENCES

Air Force Health Study. 1991. An Epidemiologic Investigation of Health Effects in Air Force Personnel Following Exposure to Herbicides. Serum Dioxin Analysis of 1987 Examination Results. 9 vols. Brooks AFB, TX: USAF School of Aerospace Medicine.

Berkow R, Fletcher A, eds. 1987. The Merck Manual of Diagnosis and Therapy. 15th ed. Rahway, N.J.: Merck.

Calvert GM, Sweeney MH, Morris JA, Fingerhut MA, Hornung RW, Halperin WE. 1991. Evaluation of chronic bronchitis, chronic obstructive pulmonary disease, and ventilatory function among workers exposed to 2,3,7,8-tetrachlorodibenzo-*p*-dioxin. American Review of Respiratory Disease 144:1302-1306.

Calvert GM, Hornung RV, Sweeney MH, Fingerhut MA, Halperin WE. 1992. Hepatic and gastrointestinal effects in an occupational cohort exposed to 2,3,7,8-tetrachlorodibenzo-*para*-dioxin. Journal of the American Medical Association 267:2209-2214.

Calvert GM, Sweeney MH, Fingerhut MA, Hornung RW, Halperin WE. 1994. Evaluation of porphyria cutanea tarda in U.S. workers exposed to 2,3,7,8-tetrachlorodibenzo-*p*-dioxin. American Journal of Industrial Medicine 25:559-571.

Cantoni L, Dal Fiume D, Ruggieri R. 1984. Decarboxylation of uroporphyrinogen I and III in 2,3,7,8-tetrachlorodibenzo-*p*-dioxin induced porphyria in mice. International Journal of Biochemistry 16:561-565.

Centers for Disease Control. 1988. Health status of Vietnam veterans. II. Physical health. Journal of the American Medical Association 259:2708-2714.

Coenraads PJ, Brouwer A, Olie K, Tang N. 1994. Chloracne. Some recent issues. Dermatologic Clinics 12:569-576.

De Verneuil H, Sassa S, Kappas A. 1983. Effects of polychlorinated biphenyl compounds, 2,3,7,8-tetrachlorodibenzo-*p*-dioxin, phenobarbital and iron on hepatic uroporphyrinogen decarboxylase. Implications for the pathogenesis of porphyria. Biochemical Journal 214:145-151.

Garry VF, Kelly JT, Sprafka JM, Edwards S, Griffith J. 1994. Survey of health and use characterization of pesticide appliers in Minnesota. Archives of Environmental Health 49:337-343.

Grossman ME, Poh-Fitzpatrick MB. 1986. Porphyria cutanea tarda: diagnosis, management, and differentiation from other hepatic porphyrias. Dermatologic Clinics 4:297-309.

Jansing PJ, Korff R. 1994. Blood levels of 2,3,7,8-tetrachlorodibenzo-*p*-dioxin and gamma-globulins in a follow-up investigation of employees with chloracne. Journal of Dermatological Science 8:91-95.

Jung D, Konietzko J, Reill-Konietzko G, Muttray A, Zimmermann-Holz HJ, Doss M, Beck H, Edler L, Kopp-Schneider A. 1994. Porphyrin studies in TCDD-exposed workers. Archives of Toxicology 68:595-598.

Karam J. 1992. Diabetes mellitus, hypoglycemia, and lipoprotein disorders. In: Schroeder SA, Tierney LM, McPhee SJ, Papadakis MA, Krupp, MA, eds. Current Medical Diagnosis and Treatment. Norwalk, CT: Appleton and Lange.

Lakshman MR, Campbell BS, Chirtel SJ, Ekarohita N, Ezekiel M. 1986. Studies on the mechanism of absorption and distribution of 2,3,7,8-tetrachlorodibenzo-*p*-dioxin in the rat. Journal of Pharmacology and Experimental Therapeutics 239:673-677.

Muhlbauer JE, Pathak MA. 1979. Porphyria cutanea tarda. International Journal of Dermatology 18:767-780.

Neubert R, Maskow L, Webb J, Jacob-Muller U, Nogueira AC, Delgado I, Helge H, Neubert D. 1993. Chlorinated dibenzo-*p*-dioxins and dibenzofurans and the human immune system. 1. Blood cell receptors in volunteers with moderately increased body burdens. Life Sciences 53:1995-2006.

Neubert R, Maskow L, Delgado I, Helge H, Neubert D. 1994. Chlorinated dibenzo-*p*-dioxins and dibenzofurans and the human immune system. 2. In vitro proliferation of lymphocytes from workers with quantified moderately increased body burdens. Life Sciences 56:421-436.

Odom R. 1993. Dermatological Disorders in Vietnam Veterans. Presentation to the Institute of Medicine Committee to Review the Health Effects in Vietnam Veterans of Exposure to Herbicides. February 8, 1993.

Ott MG, Messerer P, Zober A. 1993. Assessment of past occupational exposure to 2,3,7,8-tetrachlorodibenzo-*p*-dioxin using blood lipid analyses. International Archives of Occupational and Environmental Health 65:1-8.

Ott MG,Zober A, Germann C. 1994. Laboratory results for selected target organs in 138 individuals occupationally exposed to TCDD. Chemosphere 29:2423-2437.

Paul W, ed. 1993. Fundamental Immunology. 3rd ed. Raven Press, New York.

Piper WN, Rose JQ, Gehring PJ. 1973. Excretion and tissue distribution of 2,3,7,8-tetrachlorodibenzo-*p*-dioxin in the rat. Environmental Health Perspectives 5:241-244.

Pollei S, Mettler FA Jr, Kelsey CA, Walters MR, White RE. 1986. Follow-up chest radiographs in Vietnam veterans: are they useful? Radiology 161:101-102.

Samiy A, Douglas R, Barondess JA, (eds). 1987. Textbook of Diagnostic Medicine. Philadelphia: Lea and Febiger.

Schecter A, Ryan JJ, Papke O, Ball M, Lis A. 1993. Elevated dioxin levels in the blood of male and female Russian workers with and without chloracne 25 years after phenoxy herbicide exposure: the UFA 'Khimprom' incident. Chemosphere 27:253-258.

Senthilselvan A, McDuffie HH, Dosman JA. 1992. Association of asthma with use of pesticides: results of a cross-sectional survey of farmers. American Review of Respiratory Diseases 146:884-887.

Smith AG, De Matteis F. 1990. Oxidative injury mediated by the hepatic cytochrome P-450 system in conjunction with cellular iron. Effects on the pathway of haem biosynthesis. Xenobiotica 20:865-877.

Stanbury J, Frederickson D, Wyngaardern J. 1978. The Metabolic Basis of Inherited Disease. 4th ed. New York: McGraw-Hill.

Suskind RR, Hertzberg VS. 1984. Human health effects of 2,4,5-T and its toxic contaminants. Journal of the American Medical Association 251:2372-2380.

Svensson BG, Hallberg T, Nilsson A, Schutz A, Hagmar L. 1994. Parameters of immunological competence in subjects with high consumption of fish contaminated with persistent organochlorine compounds. International Archives of Occupational and Environmental Health 65:351-358.

Sweeney GD. 1986. Porphyria cutanea tarda, or the uroporphyrinogen decarboxylase deficiency diseases. Clinical Biochemistry 19:3-15.

Von Benner A, Edler L, Mayer K, Zober A. 1994. 'Dioxin' investigation program of the chemical industry professional association. Arbeitsmedizin Sozialmedizin Praventivmedizin 29:11-16.

Wolfe WH, Michalek JE, Miner JC, Roegner RH, Grubbs WD, Lustik MB, Brockman AS, Henderson SC, Williams DE. 1992. The Air Force Health Study: An epidemiologic investigation of health effects in Air Force personnel following exposure to herbicides, serum dioxin analysis of 1987 examination results. Chemosphere 25:213-216.

Zober A, Ott MG, Messerer P. 1994. Morbidity follow up study of BASF employees exposed to 2,3,7, 8-tetrachlorodibenzo-*p*-dioxin (TCDD) after a 1953 chemical reactor incident. Occupational and Environmental Medicine 51:479-486.

APPENDIXES

APPENDIX
A

Information Gathering

LITERATURE SEARCHES

The primary charge to this committee was to analyze the scientific and medical literature published on the health effects of herbicides used in Vietnam. Appendix A of *VAO* contains a complete description of the methods used to perform the literature searches and dissemination. Since we were to focus on reviewing literature published since the completion of *VAO*, databases were searched for articles published between 1993 and 1995. Also, outside consultants were not utilized in the analysis of the new epidemiological studies, as they were for *VAO*, since there were far fewer studies to review for the present report. Indexing and critiquing of all epidemiological studies was performed by the committee and Institute of Medicine staff.

ORAL AND WRITTEN TESTIMONY
PRESENTED TO THE COMMITTEE

A public meeting was held on April 21, 1995, in Washington, D.C., to solicit scientific information on the health effects of exposure to dioxin and other chemical compounds in herbicides used in Vietnam during the Vietnam era. In order to reach a broad range of interested individuals, more than 1,000 notices of the meeting were sent to more than 1,000 members of veterans organizations, Congress, government agencies, academic institutions, environmental groups, chemical companies, pulp and paper industry, medical research associations, and other groups, as well as to those who attended the first committee's public meeting in

September 1992. At the 1995 public meeting (see list), which was attended by approximately 100 people, 15 individuals presented oral testimony. Written testimony was also received and was accorded the same weight as the oral testimony.

Oral Testimony Presented at the Public Meeting
April 21, 1994

Session I

Betty Mekdeci, Executive Director, Association of Birth Defect Children, Orlando, FL
William Lewis, New Jersey Agent Orange Commission, Trenton, NJ
Steven Stellman, Ph.D., M.P.H., American Health Foundation, New York City, NY

Session II

Linda Schwartz, R.N., M.S.N., Yale School of Medicine, New Haven, CT
Karen Webb, Wife of Vietnam Veteran, Hampton, GA
John Gullo, Vietnam Veteran, Clinton, MT
Jenny LeFevre, Widow of Vietnam Veteran, Shady Side, MD
Hope Tinoco, Wife of Vietnam Veteran, Olathe, KS (written testimony presented by Jenny LeFevre)
Turner Camp, M.D., Veterans of Foreign Wars of the United States, Washington, DC
Robert Golden, Ph.D., Environmental Risk Sciences, Washington, DC
J. B. Harris, J.D., Private Attorney, Washington, DC
Charles Stone, Stone and Associates, Silver Spring, MD

Session III

E. R. Zumwalt, Admiral, U.S. Navy (Ret.), Arlington, VA

Open Session

Jeffrey Land, Legislative Assistant, U.S. Congress
Karen Webb, Wife of Vietnam Veteran, Hampton, GA

Written Testimony Presented to the Committee

Thomas Allen, Vietnam Veteran, Canvas, WV
Topic: Personal account of being diagnosed with lupus, which he believes to be related to Agent Orange exposure.

William Barber, Vietnam Veterans Agent Orange March, Mt. Pleasant, PA

Topic: Results of personal research, including scientific articles, on the link between Agent Orange exposure and peripheral neuropathy.

Noel Benefield, Waiuku, New Zealand

Topic: Questions the use of chloracne as a suitable marker of exposure to herbicides by non-Ranch Hand servicemen in Vietnam. Also, he believes that rashes that occurred among soldiers in Vietnam may have been due to Agent White rather than Agent Orange.

June Borton, Mother of Vietnam Veteran, Swanton, OH

Topic: Personal account of son's health problems, including death from amyotrophic lateral sclerosis, which she believes to be related to exposure to motor oil and Agent Orange.

Richard Cain, Vietnam Veteran, Jasper, AL

Topic: Personal account of health problems that he believes are related to exposure to Agent Orange.

Turner Camp, M.D., Veterans of Foreign Wars Medical Consultant, Washington, DC

Topic: Relationship between the findings and recommendations of the first IOM report and DVA compensation policies. He expressed concern about the lack of compensation for metabolic disorders, especially diabetes, in Vietnam veterans exposed to Agent Orange and pointed out that the results of the Ranch Hand study suggest an association between disorders of lipid metabolism and diabetes and herbicide exposure. Dr. Camp requested clarification of the findings of the first IOM study on peripheral neuropathy and proposed a future reevaluation of Agent Orange.

John Casanos, Vietnam Veteran, Otter Rock, OR

Topic: Personal account of Mr. Casanos's health problems, which he believes to be related to his exposure to Agent Orange.

Richard Christian, American Legion, Washington, DC

Topic: Provided copies of testimony by Dr. Ruth Shearer, consultant in genetic toxicology, to Congress in 1984 and 1985 regarding Agent Orange and provided a copy of a GAO report concerning the efforts of DHHS and CDC to study the health effects of Agent Orange in Vietnam veterans. Request for the committee to review the connection between chondrosarcoma and Agent Orange exposure. He also provided a letter from Philip Landrigan, M.D., who reviewed the case of Roger Solberg, a Vietnam veteran who died of chondrosarcoma. Dr. Landrigan concluded that "Mr. Solberg's death from chondrosarcoma could have been caused by his military exposure to dioxin."

Billy Churchill, Vietnam Veteran, Searcy, AR

Topic: Personal account of health problems, including emphysema and dermatological problems, which he believes to be related to Agent Orange exposure.

George Claxton, Vietnam Veterans of America, Washington, DC
Topic: Results of personal research on the health effects of TCDD.
Joe Cole, Vietnam Veteran, Olympia, WA
Topic: Welfare reform and how it might affect benefits to Vietnam veterans.
William W. Dean, Vietnam Veteran, Apple Valley, MN
Topic: Personal account of health problems, including multiple bilateral
    fibromatosis tumors (MBF), which he believes to be related to his exposure
    to Agent Orange.   Mr. Dean also provided the results of his research on
    exposures that may be related to MBF and requested that the DVA compen-
    sate Vietnam veterans for benign soft-tissue tumors, including Dupuytrevis
    contractures.
Michael Eckstein, Vietnam Veterans of America, Bayonne, NJ
Topic: Service-connected benefits for Vietnam veterans and reasons why pe-
    ripheral neuropathy should be considered service-connected.
Manual Gonzales, Vietnam Veteran, Address Unknown
Topic: Personal account of health problems, especially diabetes, which he feels
    are related to his exposure to Agent Orange.
Keith Horsley, M.D., Australian Department of Veterans' Affairs, Woden, Aus-
    tralia
Topic: Update on Australian regulations covering compensation for diseases
    related to herbicide exposure.
Industry Task Force on 2,4-D Research Data, Belhaven, NC
Topic: Results of recent research on 2,4-D, including a report from the EPA and
    other publications.
Harold Jackson, Vietnam Veteran, Houston, TX
Topic: Personal account of health problems, including peripheral neuropathy
    and autoimmune disease, which he believes to be related to Agent Orange
    exposure.
Thomas Joyce, Vietnam Veteran, Waitsfield, VT
Topic: Results of personal research into health effects of exposure to Agent
    Orange.   He also provided information on herbicide formulations used in
    Vietnam.
Renate Kimbrough, M.D., Institute for Evaluating Health Risks, Washington,
    DC
Topic: Results of the Ranch Hand studies, specifically metabolic disorders,
    including altered lipid metabolism and diabetes.
Robert Ku, Ph.D., DABT, CIH, Syntex USA Inc., Palo Alto, CA
Topic: Results of research on dioxin conducted by Syntex and others.
George Losoncy, Vietnam Veteran, Temple, PA
Topic: Personal account of health problems, including alopecia, which he feels
    are related to exposure to Agent Orange.   Mr. Losoncy is also requesting that
    the committee look closely at the relationship between exposure to Agent
    Orange and dermatological effects.

John Martignetti, Vietnam Veteran, Bethlehem, NH

Topic: Personal account of health problems, including chloracne and multiple sclerosis, which he believes to be related to Agent Orange exposure.

Carol Mathews, Widow of Vietnam Veteran, Mendota, IL

Topic: Personal account of husband's health problems and death from multiple myeloma at age 43, which she believes were related to his exposure to Agent Orange. She also believes that their daughter's asthma and allergies are related to her father's exposure to Agent Orange.

Cheryl Mertens, Widow of Vietnam Veteran, Niantic, CT

Topic: Personal account of husband's health problems, which she believes to be related to his exposure to Agent Orange.

Terry Miller, Vietnam Veteran, Mendota, IL

Topic: Personal account of health problems, including chloracne, migraines, and ulcers, and of daughter's health problems, including hernia, thyroid disease, and asthma, which he believes are related to his exposure to Agent Orange.

William Morgan, Vietnam Veteran, Caldwell, WV

Topic: Personal account of health problems, including macular degeneration and dermatological problems, which he believes to be related to exposure to Agent Orange.

Rocky Notnes, Hinton, AB, Canada

Topic: Mr. Notnes has several friends in the United States who are Vietnam veterans. He wrote to express frustration with the difficulties his friends face in lobbying the DVA for compensation for health problems that they believe are related to Agent Orange exposure.

James Pirkle, M.D., M.P.H., Centers for Disease Control and Prevention, Atlanta, GA

Topic: Comments and articles from the CDC concerning the health effects of exposure to dioxin and other chemical compounds in herbicides used in Vietnam.

Ronald Rick, Lino Lakes, MN

Topic: Results of personal research on reproductive effects of Agent Orange.

Brenda Sanders, Widow of Vietnam Veteran, Plano, TX

Topic: Personal account of family's health problems, which she believes are related to her husband's exposure to Agent Orange.

Arnold Schecter, M.D., M.P.H, SUNY-Health Science Center, Binghamton, NY

Topic: Information on his research, including books and scientific articles, on health effects resulting from exposure to dioxin and on the research on the health effects of Agent Orange being conducted in Vietnam.

John Sherlock, Vietnam Veteran, Levittown, PA

Topic: Personal account of battle with testicular cancer, which he believes to be related to Agent Orange exposure.

Micheal Sovick, Oklahoma Agent Orange Foundation, Lexington, OK

Topic: Chemical composition and use of defoliants other than Agent Orange, including Red, Red/White, and Green. Critiqued the section on immune system disorders from the 1993 IOM report and provided a copy of Dr. Ellen Silbergeld's testimony before the Senate Committee on Veterans' Affairs on November 2, 1993, where she criticized the first IOM report.

Jack Spey, Ranch Hand Vietnam Society, Fort Walton Beach, FL

Topic: The Ranch Hand cohort study and the findings from the study indicating that morbidity and mortality rates are not higher among the Ranch Hand cohort.   Mr. Spey also believes that the IOM "has allowed itself to mix science with the politics surrounding Agent Orange" in the past and should stick to a more scientific focus for the current report.

Charles Stone, Stone and Associates, Silver Spring, MD

Topic: Summary of oral testimony regarding health effects of Agent Orange in Vietnam veterans presented at the April 21, 1995, public meeting.

John Thomas, Vietnam Veteran, Miami, FL

Topic: Personal account of psychological and behavioral problems, which he believes to be a result of his exposure to Agent Orange, and a description of how he believes Agent Orange could cause aggressive, violent behavior.

Ed La Venture, Vietnam Veteran, Menomonie, WI

Topic: Health effects of Agent Orange in the children of Vietnam veterans. He also listed the symptoms that his own children are experiencing, such as epilepsy and asthma, which he believes to be related to his exposure to Agent Orange.

Shelia Winsett, Friend of Vietnam Veteran, Jasper, AL

Topic: Personal account of Vietnam veteran Gary Jack's health problems and eventual death from cardiac failure.

Richard Zalucky, Vietnam Veteran, Troy, NY

Topic: Personal account of health problems, including diagnosis of prostate cancer at age 46, which he believes to be related to exposure to Agent Orange.

APPENDIX
B

Risk of Disease in Vietnam Veterans
Bryan Langholz and Malcolm Pike

ESTIMATION OF MEAN MAXIMUM SERUM TCDD LEVEL

The current best estimate of the average half-life of TCDD body-burden concentration (per unit of fat serum lipids) in people is 8.4 years (weighted average of values from studies reported in Table 5 of Michalek et al., 1996). Since the dropoff in TCDD body-burden concentration is approximately exponential (Johnson et al., 1992; Wolfe et al., 1994), this half-life figure can be expressed as:

$$\exp(-\lambda t_{1/2}) = 1/2$$

where $t_{1/2}$ = 8.4 years and λ is the TCDD body-burden concentration decay rate. Thus

$$\lambda = \ln(1/2)/(-8.4) = 0.0825 \text{ per year.}$$

If the body-burden concentration decay rate, λ, is known, one may estimate the TCDD body-burden concentration at the time of last exposure (t = 0) from a measurement made t years later. The measured concentration t years after last exposure, c_t, is related to the concentration at last exposure, c_0, by the equation

$$c_t = c_0 \exp(-\lambda t). \tag{1}$$

Equation (1) has been used by some authors to estimate c_0 from measurements made at varying times after last exposure, and we have made equivalent calculations for a number of studies, as indicated in Table B-1.

For persons with brief exposure, c_0 is directly related to the dose of TCDD received (per unit body fat) at time $t = 0$. The appropriate dose to apply to the person for purposes of risk assessment is not immediately clear. The effective exposure between time 0 and time t would appear likely to be the sum of the immediate effect of the TCDD exposure at time 0 plus the integrated effect of the TCDD as it is "released" into the serum and reabsorbed or excreted from the body, i.e.,

$$\text{effective cumulative dose by time t} = \alpha c_0 + \beta c_0[(1 - \exp(-\lambda t)]/\lambda \qquad (2)$$

where α and β are unknown constants.

For persons with longer exposure, c_0 will generally represent their highest body-burden due to the relatively long half-life of TCDD. If exposure began at time t_b, then equation (2) will require an additional term to allow for the exposure between t_b and t_0; this term could be large if exposure took place over an extended period of time. This issue is discussed at some length by Johnson et al. (1992).

The true value of λ will vary between studies to a limited but unknown extent, since it is known that λ varies between persons and is inversely related to weight—i.e., the rate decreases with increasing weight (Wolfe et al., 1994). In addition to the uncertainty in the value of λ, in many of these studies precise data are not available on the time between the last exposure and the sample collection for TCDD measurement, and most importantly, precise data are not available on the time during which the dose was accumulated.

Despite these known inaccuracies, the values in the table are most valuable in giving some estimate of relative exposures, and thus to direct attention to the studies in which exposure was the greatest. Under any of the risk models that are generally considered in relating exposure to risk, the risk will be greatest at the highest dose. Under additive models the excess risk increases proportional to dose, while under other models the risk at higher doses is generally even greater (relative to the risk at lower doses). Thus, a risk that is not observed at a high dose casts serious doubt on the results of studies that see a risk at a much lower dose. It should be noted that the c_0 values calculated for the industrial cohorts in the table are relatively too low, since these exposures will have been accumulated over a lengthy period.

APPLICATION OF ESTIMATED MEAN MAXIMUM TCDD LEVELS TO ESTIMATION OF RISK OF DISEASE IN VIETNAM VETERANS

An initial quantitative risk estimate of the degree of risk likely to have been experienced by Vietnam veterans from their exposure to herbicides in Vietnam can be made based on the results from the NIOSH study (Fingerhut et al., 1991) and the estimated mean maximum TCDD levels from the NIOSH study and from various Vietnam veterans groups shown in Appendix B, Table 1 if certain simplifying assumptions are made. One can extrapolate the risks observed in the NIOSH cohort of production workers to Vietnam veterans if one assumes that: a) TCDD was the agent responsible for any association between exposure to herbicides and particular cancers; b) the evidence of elevated relative risks for these cancers reflects a causal relationship; c) the time patterns of exposure were unimportant to risk, so that the long-term exposures of workers and the short-term exposures of veterans carry comparable risk; and d) there is a linear relationship between serum TCDD and the excess relative risk in both groups.

The NIOSH workers with ≥ 1 year of exposure and ≥ 20 years latency had an estimated mean maximum serum TCDD level of 2,620 ppt. This compares with an estimated mean maximum serum TCDD level of 199 ppt in Ranch Hand veterans. If the increase (above 1.0) in relative risk for the NIOSH workers is 'x', then the increase (above 1.0) in relative risk for the Ranch Hand veterans is estimated as $(x/2620) \times 199 = 0.076x$. Non-Ranch Hand veterans had an average measured level of TCDD no different from controls, so that no additional disease risk can be attributed overall for such veterans.

The estimated relative risks for the Ranch Hand veterans are:

Cancer Site	Relative Risk in NIOSH study (≥ 1 year exposure, ≥ 20 years latency)	Estimated Mean Relative Risk for Ranch Hand Veterans
Respiratory	1.42	1.03
STS	9.22	1.62
Prostate	1.52	1.04
Multiple Myeloma	2.62	1.12

In addition to the 4 cancers given in this table, the committee also found sufficient evidence of an association between herbicides and/or TCDD exposure and Hodgkin's disease (HD) and non-Hodgkin's lymphoma (NHL).

The relative risk (RR) for HD in the NIOSH study (≥ 1 year exposure, ≥ 20 years latency) was 2.8 based on a single case of HD. This suggests that the mean relative risk for Ranch Hand veterans is about 1.1 (with a wide confidence interval). The other studies of HD discussed in Chapter 7 do not provide any further information to check on the appropriateness of this estimate.

The RR for NHL in the NIOSH study (≥ 1 year exposure, ≥ 20 years latency) was 0.9 based on 2 cases of NHL. The nested case-control study of production and spraying workers reported by Kogevinas et al. (1995) found a relative risk of 3.6 for "medium" and "high" exposure based on 7 cases. Assuming that these

TABLE B-1   Estimated mean maximum serum TCDD levels
(ppt in serum lipids)

Reference	Exposed Group	Date of Serum Sampling	Details of Exposed Group
Gross et al., 1984	Vietnam veterans	~1983 ~15 years since exposure	"Heavily exposed" "Lightly exposed" Controls
Kahn et al., 1988	Vietnam veterans	~1986 ~18 years since exposure	"Heavily exposed" Controls
CDC, 1988	Vietnam veterans	~1985 ~17 years since exposure	Exposed: Low Medium High Controls
Kang et al., 1991	Vietnam veterans		Vietnam veterans Non-Vietnam veterans Controls
Wolfe et al., 1988 Wolfe et al., 1990	Ranch Hand personnel	~1985 ~17 years since exposure	Exposed Controls
Fingerhut et al., 1990 Salvan et al., 1994	Herbicide manufacturing workers (NIOSH study)	~22 years since exposure	All exposed < 1 yr. exposed ≥ 1 yr. exposed < 1 yr. exposed; ≥ 20 yrs. since first exposure ≥ 1 yr. exposed; ≥ 20 yrs. since first exposure
Manz et al., 1991	Occupationally exposed (Germany)	~1985 exposed up to 1984 in some cases	"High" exposure "Medium" & "Low" exposure

N	Observed Mean	Estimated Mean Level at Maximum	Remarks
3	37	127[a]	[a]Estimated from information
5	5		given in the reference.
10	6		
9	46	203[a]	[a]Estimated from information given in
10	7		the reference. "Heavily exposed" are
			Ranch Hand or Chemical Corp veterans.
	4[a]		[a]No relation with exposure
298			level. No Ranch Hand or
157			Chemical Corp personnel.
191			
97			
36	13*		
79	13*		
80	16*		
147	49	199[a]	[a]Estimated from information given in the
49	5		reference. These results are from MMWR
			(1988): larger JAMA (1990) report only
			gives medians—it appears from
			a comparison of medians in the two papers
			that the figures quoted here may be
			too high by a factor of approximately
			$26/12.4 = 2.1$
253	233	1,434[a]	[a]Estimated from information
134	69	425[a,b]	given in the reference
119	418	2,573[a]	
81	78	462[a,b]	[b]Estimated by assuming the
			same ratio to measured mean
			as in "All exposed"
95	462	2,620[a]	
37	296	?	Supersedes Beck et al. (1989).
11	73	?	

TABLE B-1   Continued

Reference	Exposed Group	Date of Serum Sampling	Details of Exposed Group
Patterson et al., 1989	Missouri chemical plant workers	1985 ~13 yrs. since exposure	Exposed Not exposed
Smith et al., 1992	Pesticide applicators (New Zealand)		
Ott et al., 1993	BASF 1953 accident clean-up workers	~35 yrs. since accident	Exposed Controls
Littorin et al., 1994	Herbicide manufacturing workers (Sweden, part of IARC study)	~1993 ~16 yrs. since exposure	Exposed Controls
Mocarelli et al., 1991	Seveso residents	"Immediately" after accident	Zone A; age ≤16; severe chloracne
Mocarelli et al., 1988			Zone A: adults; no chloracne
Cerlesi et al., 1989			Zone B
			Zone R

*Adipose tissue value.

N	Observed Mean	Estimated Mean Level at Maximum	Remarks
8	363	1,023[a]	[a]Estimated from information
5	15*		given in the reference.
9	53	229[a]	[a]Estimated from information
			given in the reference.
138	15[a]	520[b]	[a]Geometric means.
102	3[a]		[b]Weighted average from information
			given in Fig. 1 of reference.
5	17	61[a]	[a]Estimated from information
5	2		given in the reference.
10	19,144	19,144	Zone B and Zone R means estimated from the 5,240 mean figure for Zone A residents without chloracne, and the relative amount
9	5,240	5,240	of TCDD found in the soil.
	68	68	
	20	20	

workers had exposures comparable to the NIOSH cohort we estimate the relative risk of Ranch Hand veterans at 1.20.

Use of Further Information on Exposure

The above estimates for Ranch Hand veterans is indicative of individual risk insofar as the individual is a Ranch Hand veteran. With added validated information on individual exposure (such as serum TCDD level) a more accurate estimate of risk may be calculated using the same method that was used here for the Ranch Hand veterans as a group.

Serum TCDD levels measured in non-Ranch Hand Vietnam veterans many years after Vietnam service have been found to be no different from levels in controls. This suggests that, as a group, such Vietnam veterans had no excess exposure to TCDD. There may well have been some groups of non-Ranch Hand Vietnam veterans who were exposed to higher levels of TCDD, but for reason of their small size or other reason not currently discernible, this exposure is not demonstrated in the distribution of serum TCDD as measured in non-Ranch Hand Vietnam veterans. If such groups or individuals can be identified with validated information on exposure (such as current serum TCDD level) then their risks may be calculated using the same method that was used here for the Ranch Hand veterans as a group.

Linear Extrapolation from the High Dose (Long Exposure), Long Latency NIOSH Results

The NIOSH study is the only study with risk estimates and serum TCDD measurement on a large enough sample to make reasonable inferences about exposure and risk. The sample of workers with TCDD measurements was not a random sample of the group but Salvan et al. (1994) make a convincing argument that they are representative of the NIOSH cohort as a whole.

The statistical model we have chosen specifies that the relative risk of a specific cancer given a maximum, i.e., back-extrapolated, serum TCDD of c is $(1+\beta c)$. This linear model has the property that the mean predicted relative risk is the predicted relative risk at the mean exposure. There are few data with which to validate the choice of this linear form of the relative risk. The relative risks observed for the low dose, long latency NIOSH subgroup are certainly consistent with this model, but there is little power to detect deviations. This model is generally considered conservative.

TCDD Concentrations with Time after Exposure

As discussed in Chapter 5, there has been new research on the Ranch Hand cohort validating the use of the one-compartment model in back-extrapolating serum TCDD levels to the level at the time of last exposure. We note that prior to *VAO*, the only extensive data on the change in serum TCDD with time was from blood samples at two time points from Ranch Hand volunteers. Since then a third sample has been collected and improved statistical methods have been developed that account for the 'censoring' at low levels (Michalek et al., 1996). A mean half-life of 8.7 years (95% CI = 8.0-9.5) was computed. This estimate is based on measurements made on blood where the first sample was collected a median of 15 years after last exposure. Results of half-life investigation of 27 individuals exposed in the Seveso accident yielded a similar mean half-life of 8.2 years (95% CI = 7.2-9.7; Needham et al., 1994). In this study, the first samples were taken shortly after exposure so that the similarity of results to the Ranch Hand volunteer study strengthens the use of a one-compartment model. The other half-life study was based on samples at two time points on 48 production workers (Flesch-Janys et al., 1994). This study was reported as showing a *median* half-life of 6.9 years. Since half-life estimates tend to be skewed to the right, the mean half-life is likely to be somewhat larger than this. It appears therefore that the mean half-life of production workers with long exposure is likely to be close to that observed in the other two studies. This indicates that the use of the same mean half-life for NIOSH workers and the Veterans is reasonable.

Use of Back-extrapolated Serum TCDD as a Measure of Dose

The back-extrapolated serum TCDD is essentially estimating the serum level at the time last exposed. For short-term exposures, this will be highly correlated with cumulative dose. This should apply reasonably well to the Vietnam veterans who were exposed for a maximum period of their tour of duty. For long-term exposures, back-extrapolated serum TCDD will underestimate cumulative dose because some (possibly a significant amount) of TCDD has left the body by the time of last exposure. For example, suppose that during the first year of exposure an individual's exposure results in a 100 ppt serum concentration. If the individual is exposed for another 8 years, only about 50 ppt from that first years' exposure will be left in the blood at that time. This pattern of exposure was common for workers in the NIOSH cohort. This implies that the mean-maximum serum TCDD levels from the NIOSH workers are an *underestimate* of their mean cumulative exposure. Since the risk estimates generated by the methodology presented in this Appendix are based on a low-dose extrapolation from the mean-maximum serum TCDD concentration in the NIOSH workers, this methodology over-estimates the risk in veterans, if cumulative exposure is the appropriate measure.

REFERENCES

Beck H, Eckart K, Mathar W, Wittkowski R. 1989. Levels of PCDDs and PCDFs in adipose tissue of occupationally exposed workers. Chemosphere 18:507-516.

Centers for Disease Control. 1988. Serum 2,3,7,8-tetrachlorodibenzo-*p*-dioxin levels in U.S. Army Vietnam-era veterans. The Centers for Disease Control Veterans Health Studies [see comments]. Journal of the American Medical Association 260:1249-1254.

Cerlesi S, di Domenico A, Ratti S. 1989. Recovery yields of early analytical procedures to detect 2,3,7,8-tetrachloro-dibenzo-*p*-dioxin (TCDD) in soil samples at Seveso, Italy. Chemosphere 18:989-1003.

Fingerhut M, Halperin W, Marlow DA, Piacitelli L, Honchar P, Sweeney M, Greife A, Dill P, Steenland K, Suruda A. 1990. Mortality Among U.S. Workers Employed in the Production of Chemicals Contaminated with 2,3,7,8-tetrachlorodibenzo-*p*-dioxin (TCDD). Final Report. PB 91-12591, Industrywide Studies Branch, Division of Surveillance, NIOSH, Cincinnati, OH.

Fingerhut MA, Halperin WE, Marlow DA, Piacitelli LA, Honchar PA, Sweeney MH, Greife AL, Dill PA, Steenland K, Suruda AJ. 1991. Cancer mortality in workers exposed to 2,3,7,8-tetrachlorodibenzo-*p*-dioxin. New England Journal of Medicine 324:212-218.

Flesch-Janys D, Gurn P, Konietzko J, Manz A, Päpke O. 1994. First results of an investigation of the elimination of polychlorinated dibenzo-p-dioxins and dibenzofurans (PCDD/F) in occupationally exposed persons. Organohalogen Compounds 21: 93-99.

Gross ML, Lay JO, Lippstreu D, Lyon PA, Kangas N, Harless RL, Taylor SE. 1984. 2,3,7,8-tetrachlorodibenzo-*p*-dioxin levels in adipose tissue of Vietnam veterans. Environmental Research 33:261.

Johnson ES, Parsons W, Weinberg CR, Shore DL, Mathews J, Patterson DG Jr, Needham LL. 1992. Current serum levels of 2,3,7,8-tetrachlorodibenzo-*p*-dioxin in phenoxy acid herbicide applicators and characterization of historical levels. Journal of the National Cancer Institute 84:1648-1653.

Kahn PC, Gochfeld M, Nygren M, Hansson M, Rappe C, Velez H, Ghent-Guenther T, Wilson WP. 1988. Dioxins and dibenzofurans in blood and adipose tissue of Agent Orange-exposed Vietnam veterans and matched controls. Journal of the American Medical Association 259:1661-1667.

Kang HK, Watanabe KK, Breen J, Remmers J, Conomos MG, Stanley J, Flicker M. 1991. Dioxins and dibenzofurans in adipose tissue of U.S. Vietnam veterans and controls. American Journal of Public Health 81:344-349.

Kogevinas M, Kauppinen T, Winkelmann R, Becher H, Bertazzi PA, Bueno de Mesquita HB, Coggon D, Green L, Johnson E, Littorin M, Lynge E, Marlow DA, Mathews JD, Neuberger M, Benn T, Pannett B, Pearce N, Saracci R. 1995. Soft tissue sarcoma and non-Hodgkin's lymphoma in workers exposed to phenoxy herbicides, chlorophenols, and dioxins: two nested case-control studies. Epidemiology 6:396-402.

Littorin M, Hansson M, Rappe C, Kogevinas M. 1994. Dioxins in blood from Swedish phenoxy herbicide workers (4). Lancet 344:611-612.

Manz A, Berger J, Dwyer JH, Flesch-Janys D, Nagel S, Waltsgott H. 1991. Cancer mortality among workers in chemical plant contaminated with dioxin. Lancet 338:959-964.

Michalek JE, Pirkle JL, Caudill SP, Tripathi RC, Patterson DG, Needham LL. 1996. Pharmacokinetics of TCDD in veterans of Operation Ranch Hand: 10 year follow-up. Journal of Exposure Analysis and Environmental Epidemiology 47:102-112.

Mocarelli P, Pocchiari F, Nelson N. 1988. Preliminary report: 2,3,7,8-tetrachlorodibenzo-*p*-dioxin exposure to humans - Seveso, Italy. Morbidity and Mortality Weekly Report 37:733-736.

Mocarelli P, Needham LL, Marocchi A, Patterson DG Jr, Brambilla P, Gerthoux PM, Meazza L, Carreri V. 1991. Serum concentrations of 2,3,7,8-tetrachlorobdibenzo-*p*-dioxin and test results from selected residents of Seveso, Italy. Journal of Toxicology and Environmental Health 32:357-366.

Needham L, Gerthoux P, Patterson D, Brambilla P, Pirkle J, Tramacere P, Turner W, Beretta C, Sampson E, Mocarelli P. 1994. Half-life of 2,3,7,8-tetrachlorodibenzo-*p*-dioxins in serum of Seveso adults: interim report. Organohalogen Compounds 21:81-85.

Ott MG, Messerer P, Zober A. 1993. Assessment of past occupational exposure to 2,3,7,8-tetrachlorodibenzo-*p*-dioxin using blood lipid analyses. International Archives of Occupational and Environmental Health 65:1-8.

Patterson DG Jr, Fingerhut MA, Roberts DW, Needham LL, Haring L, Sweeney M, Marlow DA, Andrews JS Jr, Halperin WE. 1989. Levels of polychlorinated dibenzo-*p*-dioxins and dibenzofurans in workers exposed to 2,3,7,8-tetrachlorodibenzo-*p*-dioxin. American Journal of Industrial Medicine 16:135-146.

Salvan A, Dankovic D, Stayner L, Gilbert S, Steenland K, Fingerhut M. 1994. An approach to the quantitative assessment of cancer risk in relation to occupational exposure to dioxin: limitations and variability TCDD dose-rate estimates. Imformatik, Biometrie und Epidemiologie in Medizin und Biologie 25: 292-300.

Smith AH, Patterson DG Jr, Warner ML, Mackenzie R, Needham LL. 1992. Serum 2,3,7,8-tetrachlorodibenzo-*p*-dioxin levels of New Zealand pesticide applicators and their implication for cancer hypotheses. Journal of the National Cancer Institute 84:104-108.

Wolfe W, Michalek J, Miner JC, Petersen M. 1988. Serum 2,3,7,8-tetrachlorodibenzo-*p*-dioxin levels in Air Force Health Study participants: preliminary report. Morbidity and Mortality Weekly Report 37:309-311.

Wolfe WH, Michalek JE, Miner JC, Rahe A, Silva J, Thomas WF, Grubbs WD, Lustik MB, Karrison TG, Roegner RH, Williams DE. 1990. Health status of Air Force veterans occupationally exposed to herbicides in Vietnam. I. Physical health. Journal of the American Medical Association 264:1824-1831.

Wolfe WH, Michalek JE, Miner JC, Pirkle JL, Caudill SP, Patterson DG Jr, Needham LL. 1994. Determinants of TCDD half-life in veterans of Operation Ranch Hand. Journal of Toxicology and Environmental Health 41:481-488.

APPENDIX
C

Committee and Staff Biographies

COMMITTEE BIOGRAPHIES

David Tollerud, M.D., M.P.H. (Chairman) is Associate Professor and Chief of the Division of Occupational and Environmental Medicine, Department of Environmental and Occupational Health, at the University of Pittsburgh. He received his M.D. from Mayo Medical School and his M.P.H. from the Harvard School of Public Health. He served as a Medical Staff Fellow in the Environmental Epidemiology Branch, National Cancer Institute; Pulmonary Fellow at Brigham and Women's and Beth Israel Hospitals in Boston; Assistant Professor of Medicine at the University of Cincinnati; and Associate Professor of Environmental and Occupational Health at the University of Pittsburgh Graduate School of Public Health. He is a Fellow of the American College of Occupational Environmental Medicine and the American College of Chest Physicians, a member of numerous professional societies, including the American Thoracic Society, the American Association of Immunologists, the Clinical Immunology Society, the American Public Health Association, and the American Association for the Advancement of Science, and a member of the editorial board of the *Journal of the American Industrial Hygiene Association.*

Michael Aminoff, M.D., is Professor of Neurology, Director of the Clinical Neurophysiology Laboratories, and Director of the Movement Disorders Clinic and the Epilepsy Program at the University of California Medical Center, San Francisco. He has published extensively on topics related to clinical neurology and neurophysiology, has authored or edited 13 textbooks, and is on the editorial board of several medical and scientific journals.

Jesse Berlin, Sc.D., is Research Associate Professor of Biostatistics in Medicine at the University of Pennsylvania School of Medicine, where he has been since 1989. He received his doctorate in Biostatistics from the Harvard School of Public Health in 1988. He has participated in both the design and analysis of a wide variety of clinical and epidemiologic investigations. Dr. Berlin's principal research interest lies in the application of meta-analysis to epidemiologic studies. Dr. Berlin also serves as an Associate Editor for the *Journal of General Internal Medicine* and as a Deputy Editor for the *Online Journal of Clinical Trials.*

Karen Bolla, Ph.D., is Associate Professor of Neurology, Psychiatry and Behavioral Sciences at the Johns Hopkins School of Medicine, and Environmental Health Sciences - Division of Occupational Medicine, Johns Hopkins School of Public Health. She is currently the director of Neuropsychology at the Johns Hopkins Bayview Medical Center. She has been appointed a guest investigator at the National Institutes on Drug Abuse, Intramural Research Program. Dr. Bolla's primary clinical and research interests concern the neurobehavioral effects of occupational and environmental neurotoxins and drugs of abuse.

Graham A. Colditz, M.D., Dr. P.H., is Associate Professor of Medicine at the Harvard Medical School, Associate Professor of Epidemiology at the Harvard School of Public Health and an Epidemiologist in the Department of Medicine, Channing Laboratory, Brigham and Women's Hospital. He has extensive experience in lifestyle and health, having worked as Co-investigator on the Nurses' Health Study since 1982. This wide range of studies includes screening and mortality; benign breast disease and risk of breast cancer; diet and activity, and risk of fractures in women. He has published numerous studies on chronic conditions that affect women including heart disease, breast and other cancers, fractures, gall stones, and obesity. In addition to his work with the Nurses' Health Study, Dr. Colditz is responsible for the design and implementation of several Epidemiologic courses at the Harvard School of Public Health and the Harvard Medical School.

Seymour Grufferman, M.D., Dr. P.H., is Professor and Chairman of the Department of Family Medicine and Clinical Epidemiology at the University of Pittsburgh School of Medicine. He is a pediatrician and cancer epidemiologist with a longstanding research interest in the epidemiology of Hodgkin's disease. He is Principal Investigator for a large N.I.H. grant to do an international case-control study of Hodgkin's disease in children. He was recently elected to a Fellowship in the American Association for the Advancement of Sciences for his contributions to the epidemiology of the leukemias and lymphomas. Dr.

Grufferman is Director of the Family Medicine Division of the Children's Hospital of Pittsburgh, PA and he also holds an appointment as Senior Research Associate in Epidemiology and Biostatistics at the European Institute of Oncology in Milan, Italy. He is on the editorial board of the *Journal of Epidemiology and Biostatistics.*

S. Katharine Hammond, Ph.D., is Associate Professor of Environmental Health Sciences at the University of California, Berkeley, School of Public Health. She received her BA from Oberlin College, her Ph.D. in chemistry from Brandeis University, and her MS in environmental health sciences from Harvard School of Public Health, where she holds an appointment as Visiting Lecturer in Industrial Hygiene. Her research has focused on assessing exposure for epidemiological studies; among the exposures she has evaluated are those associated with work in the semiconductor industry, diesel exhaust, and environmental tobacco smoke. She served as a consultant to the U.S. Environmental Protection Agency Scientific Advisory Board in its review of the environmental tobacco smoke documents that culminated in the publication of *Respiratory Health Effects of Passive Smoking: Lung Cancer and Other Disorders,* and she is currently on the Acrylonitrile Advisory Panel for the National Cancer Institute.

David Kriebel, Sc.D., received his doctorate in occupational epidemiology from the Harvard School of Public Health in 1986. After postdoctoral work at Harvard, the University of Massachusetts Medical Center, and the Center for the Study and Prevention of Cancer in Florence, Italy, he joined the Department of Work Environment at the University of Massachusetts, Lowell, where he is now Associate Professor. In addition to teaching graduate courses in epidemiology, Dr. Kriebel also conducts research in two broad areas. The first is the early detection of the nonmalignant respiratory effects of occupational exposures to dusts and gases, and the second is the development of improved methods for the utilization of quantitative exposure data in epidemiologic models.

Peter C. Nowell, M.D., is Professor of Pathology and Laboratory Medicine at the University of Pennsylvania School of Medicine, where he received his M.D., and is also Deputy Director of the University's Cancer Center. His early work, demonstrating that bone marrow could be successfully transplanted to ameliorate radiation injury, ultimately helped lead to marrow transplantation procedures for treating hematopoietic malignancies. His co-discovery, with Dr. David Hungerford, of the Philadelphia chromosome was the first observation of a consistent cytogenetic alteration in human cancer. Some of his current research on lymphocyte growth regulation focuses on chronic lymphoid tumors that do not have consistent genetic alterations. He has served on the Advisory Committee to the Director of the National Institutes of Health, and has received numerous honors, including election to the National Academy of Sciences and the American Philosophical Society.

Andrew Olshan, Ph.D., is Assistant Professor in the Department of Epidemiology, School of Public Health, at the University of North Carolina, Chapel Hill. He received his Ph.D. in epidemiology from the University of Washington. He was a postdoctoral fellow in medical genetics at the University of British Columbia from 1987 to 1989 and Assistant Professor in the Department of Clinical Epidemiology and Family Medicine, University of Pittsburgh, from 1989 to 1991. He is a member of several professional societies, including the Society for Epidemiologic Research, the American Society of Human Genetics, the International Genetic Epidemiology Society, and the Teratology Society. His major areas of interest include cancer and perinatal epidemiology, particularly male-mediated effects on abnormal reproduction and development.

Malcolm C. Pike, Ph.D., is Professor of Epidemiology and Flora L. Thornton Chair of the Department of Preventive Medicine at the University of Southern California School of Medicine. He received his Ph.D. in Mathematical Statistics from the University of Aberdeen in Scotland. He was formerly Director of the Imperial Cancer Research Fund's Cancer Epidemiology Unit and the University of Oxford. He is a member of the Institute of Medicine of the National Academy of Sciences. Dr. Pike's main areas of research is the prevention of female cancers.

Kenneth S. Ramos, Ph.D., is Professor in the Department of Physiology and Pharmacology, College of Veterinary Medicine and Chairman of the Faculty of Toxicology at Texan A&M University. Dr. Ramos received his Ph.D. degree from the University of Texas at Austin. He is a member of several professional societies, including the Society of Toxicology, Society for In Vitro Biology, American Society for Cell Biology, and American Society for Pharmacology and Experimental Therapeutics. He serves in the editorial boards of the *Journal of Biochemical Toxicology, Journal of Toxicology and Environmental Health, Annual Review of Pharmacology and Toxicology, Toxicology In Vitro,* and *American Journal of Physiology.* His primary research interests are in the area of cellular and molecular toxicology with emphasis on the study of chemically-induced deregulation of cell growth and differentiation.

Noel R. Rose, M.D., Ph.D., is Professor of Pathology and of Molecular Microbiology and Immunology at the Johns Hopkins University and holds joint appointments in the Departments of Medicine and of Environmental Health Sciences. He is also Director of the World Health Organization Collaborating Center for Autoimmune Diseases and of the Johns Hopkins Reference Laboratory. Dr. Rose directs the University's training program in immunotoxicology and is active as a consultant in immunotoxicology. He has also served on panels of the National Institutes of Health, the Food and Drug Administration, the National Center for Toxicological Research, the National Research Council, and other governmental agencies.

STAFF BIOGRAPHIES

Michael Stoto, Ph.D., the director of the Division of Health Promotion and Disease Prevention, oversaw the conduct of the study. He received an A.B. in statistics from Princeton University and a Ph.D. in statistics and demography from Harvard University, and was formerly Associate Professor of public policy at Harvard's John F. Kennedy School of Government. A member of the professional staff since 1987, Dr. Stoto directed the IOM's effort in support of the Public Health Service's *Healthy People 2000* project and has worked on IOM projects addressing a number of issues in public health, health statistics, health promotion and disease prevention, vaccine safety and policy, and AIDS. Dr. Stoto served as study director for the IOM committee that produced *Veterans and Agent Orange: Health Effects of Herbicides Used in Vietnam*, and recently led the staff responsible for *HIV and the Blood Supply: An Analysis of Crisis Decisionmaking*. Dr. Stoto is co-author of *Data for Decisions: Information Strategies for Policy Makers* and numerous articles in statistics, demography, health policy, and other fields. He is a member of the American Public Health Association, the American Statistical Association, the International Union for the Scientific Study of Population, the Population Association of America, and other organizations.

David A. Butler, Ph.D., is a Senior Project Officer in the Division of Health Promotion and Disease Prevention of the Institute of Medicine. He received B.S. and M.S. degrees in engineering from the University of Rochester, and a Ph.D. in public policy analysis from Carnegie-Mellon University. He worked as a researcher in the Energy and Environmental Policy Center at Harvard University's John F. Kennedy School of Government, and was Research Associate in the Department of Environmental Health at the Harvard School of Public Health. Prior to joining the IOM, he served as an analyst for the Environment Division of the United States Congress Office of Technology Assessment. Dr. Butler's research interests include exposure assessment and risk analysis.

Cynthia Abel is a Program Officer in the Division of Health Promotion and Disease Prevention of the Institute of Medicine. She received a B.A. in government and political science and expects to receive a M.P.P. (public policy) this year from the University of Maryland. Most recently, she worked with the Institute of Medicine (IOM) committee that produced *Veterans and Agent Orange: Health Effects of Herbicides Used in Vietnam* and the IOM committee that issued the report *HIV and the Blood Supply: An Analysis of Crisis Decisionmaking.* She has also worked with several other IOM committees in the area of health promotion and disease prevention and the National Research Council's committee that produced the report *Safety Issues at the Defense Production Reactors: A Report to the U.S. Department of Energy.*

Deborah Katz, M.P.H., is a Research Assistant in the Division of Health Promotion and Disease Prevention of the Institute of Medicine. She received a B.S. in zoology from the University of Massachusetts and a Master of Public Health from George Washington University. Ms. Katz previously worked at several health consulting firms in Washington, D.C. which specialized in occupational and environmental health issues. She was also the research assistant on an IOM study which evaluated the clinical program set up by the Department of Defense to provide medical examinations to veterans of the Persian Gulf war.